CLASSICS OF CARDIOLOGY

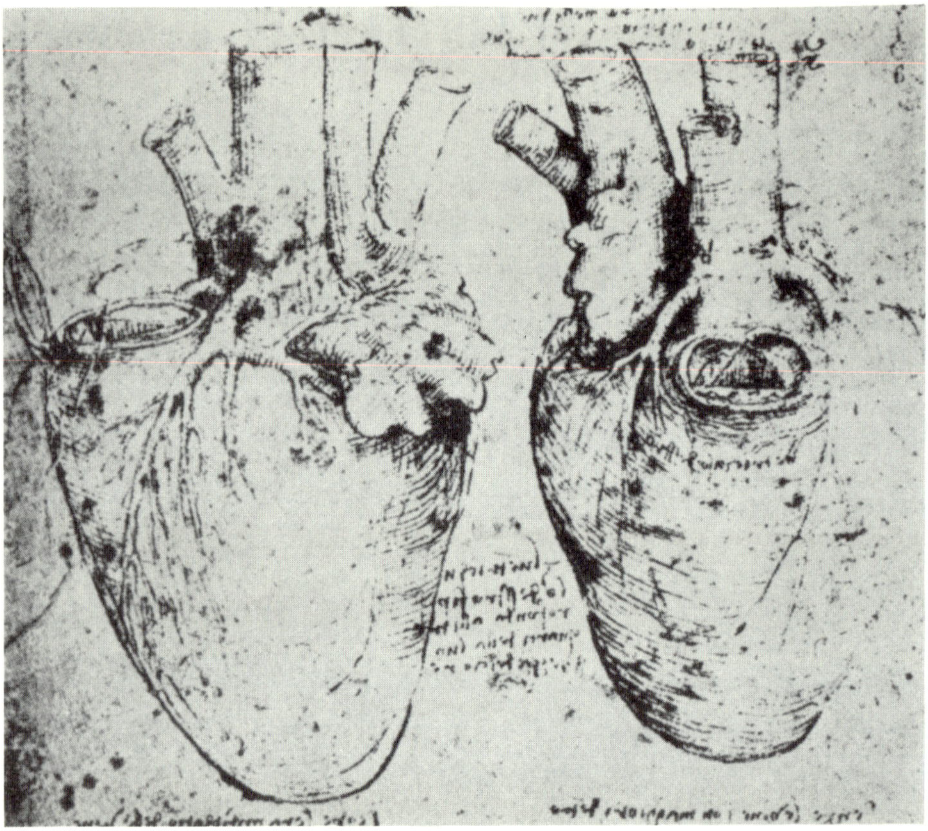

Anatomic drawings of the heart by Leonardo da Vinci (1512)

(Courtesy Carnegie Institution of Washington.)

CLASSICS OF CARDIOLOGY

former title: *Cardiac Classics*

A Collection of Classic Works on the
Heart and Circulation with Comprehensive
Biographic Accounts of the Authors

Fifty-Two Contributions by Fifty-One Authors

BY

FREDRICK A. WILLIUS, M.D., M.S. in Med.

Former Chief, Section of Cardiology, Professor Emeritus of Medicine,
The Mayo Foundation for Medical Education and Research,
The Graduate School, The University of Minnesota

AND

THOMAS E. KEYS, A.B., M.A.

Librarian, The Mayo Clinic; Assistant Professor of the History
of Medicine, Mayo Foundation for Medical Education and Research,
The Graduate School, The University of Minnesota

VOLUME ONE

ROBERT E. KRIEGER PUBLISHING COMPANY
MALABAR, FLORIDA
1983

Reprint of the 1961 edition published in two volumes by Dover as an unabridged and unaltered republication of the work first published by the C.V. Mosby Company in 1941 under the former title: CARDIAC CLASSICS

Printed and Published by
ROBERT E. KRIEGER PUBLISHING COMPANY, INC.
KRIEGER DRIVE
MALABAR, FL 32950

Printed in the United States of America

Library of Congress Cataloging in Publication Data

Main entry under title:
Classics of cardiology.

Vol. 3 edited by John A. Callahan, Thomas E. Keys, and Jack D. Key.
Vols. 1-2 are a reprint of the 1961 ed. published by Dover; v. 3 is original ed.
Bibliography: p.
Includes index.
1. Heart—Diseases—Addresses, essays, lectures. 2. Cardiology—Addresses, essays, lectures. 3. Cardiologists—Biography. 4. Cardiology—History—Sources.
I. Willius, Frederick Arthur, 1888- II. Keys, Thomas Edward, 1908-
[DNLM: 1. Cardiovascular system—Collected works. WG 5 C614]
RC682.C56 1982 616.1 82-7830
ISBN 0-89874-514-4 (v.1) AACR2
ISBN 0-89874-515-2 (v.2)
ISBN 0-89874-516-0 (v.3)

FOREWORD

The era of specialization which has characterized medical education and practice in the past few years has greatly extended our knowledge of all fields of medicine. The advances represented in changing conceptions of disease, new methods of treatment, and radical revision of practice have introduced into medical education an important problem, that of correlation of accumulated facts and theories. An understanding of this correlation is difficult to attain but is equally essential to the medical student, the general practitioner, the specialist, and particularly the teacher. While it is usually true that advances in any field of endeavor have been accomplished through specialization, it is also true that the principles upon which practice should be based have been, and probably will continue to be, set up by those who possess an adequate knowledge of general medicine and can, therefore, correlate this with that acquired through intensive investigation of any special field. In the further development of specialization it is essential that education should focus on the fact that the broader the knowledge of general medicine, the more likely will investigations in any special field prove to be of permanent value.

Medical literature today represents these advances, and voluminous as the literature is, it has the virtue of reiteration, which is essential in education. In the appraisal of medical literature, students and practitioners are likely to overlook the writings of those who established the fundamentals upon which subsequent progress has been made. These epoch-making contributions are also evidence of the fact that in the study of disease thorough and accurate observation is the first requirement and supersedes other methods. In the diseases of the heart and circulation this fact is particularly true and in no field of medicine is sound clinical sense so important. The morbidity and mortality of heart disease is a challenge to the medical profession which is already being met, for recent statistics in this country show a decrease in this mortality rate. It is of particular importance, therefore, that any information which will aid the profession to understand better these diseases should be widely disseminated.

It is, therefore, appropriate that Dr. Willius and Mr. Keys have selected a representative group of classics pertaining to the heart and circulation and have added to the interest of these by accounts of the lives of the authors whose works are included and by a comprehensive correlation of the influence of these classics on the development of cardiology.

DONALD C. BALFOUR.

Rochester, Minn.

. . . . If you do remember,
I send it through the rivers of your blood,
Even to the court, the heart, to the seat o' the brain:
And through the cranks and offices of man,
The strongest nerves and small inferior veins
From me receive that natural competency
Whereby they live.

—William Shakespeare: Act 1, Scene 1, *Coriolanus*

PREFACE

The preparation of this volume of classics on the heart and circulation was occasioned by several motivating influences. Our personal appreciation of the older medical writings was the first influence to encourage us to undertake this project. After the expenditure of considerable time and effort, we came to the realization that the inaccessibility of numerous rare works undoubtedly deterred many physicians, as well as medical students, from availing themselves of these treasures of the past. Furthermore, the accelerated tempo of modern times and the voluminous current medical literature allow many but little time for the culture of yesteryear. However, the importance of these older writings remains unchallenged and many of them contain such accurate descriptions based on masterful observation that they endure as integral parts of the modern concepts of our day.

One cannot read and contemplate the classics without being aroused by a desire to express apologies to the old masters, for there are many moderns who have written certain lines, believed to be original, only to find that the same observations and thoughts were expressed many years before. It is reasonable to conclude that the classics of medical antiquity form the basis of modern medicine and that the physician of today relinquishes many cultural advantages when he avoids acquaintance with his distinguished predecessors. It is our hope that this volume will reward the reader with the same measure of profit and pleasure that we have derived from the wisdom of these great masters.

Dr. Robert Watt of Glasgow more than 125 years ago wrote: "The reading of the student is too often confined to systems and to compilations which are generally the work of men of no experience or of men writing under the influence of preconceived opinions. To obtain correct views of medicine, it is necessary to have recourse to original authors, to such as write from actual observation, who have seen and treated the diseases they describe."

We do not presume that we have incorporated all the cardiac classics in the present volume, but we have selected from them those which have been of special interest to us and which, we believe, have contributed in a large measure to the development and progress of present-day cardiology. We have selected contributions that deal with the anatomy and physiology of the heart and circulation, descriptions of disease, pathologic and therapeutic contributions, methods of diagnosis, and the like.

We have attempted faithfully to reproduce the original writings, and where translations from other languages have been undertaken, it is our sincere hope that we have accurately expressed the author's meaning. With few exceptions we have reproduced the writings in their entirety, remembering our own feeling of keen disappointment in other years in reading a medical masterpiece that had been radically abridged solely by the personal discretion of the compiler. There are, however, instances in which the unusual length of a classic or tedious repetition made certain deletions advisable. It is our belief that the rather complete reproduction of these works is of much greater value and permits the reader more fully to appreciate and understand the personality and the philosophy of the author, than might be true had deletion been practiced.

We have presented the various classics in their chronologic order and have prefaced each with a biographic account of the author. Chronologic sequence has been carried out with the purpose of permitting the progress of cardiology to be recorded and compared with contemporary historic events. Whenever possible, note is made of discrepancies between the date of discovery and the date of publication of the contributions included. The order of their inclusion in this volume has been formulated according to date of publication; discrepancies are discussed either in the biographic accounts or in footnotes. Certain disagreement concerning dates occurs among various historians, and in so far as possible we have been guided by the date given by Garrison.

The first classic included in this volume is the epoch-making contribution of William Harvey, published in 1628. We have deliberately avoided earlier writings, being convinced that Harvey's work is in reality the fundamental contribution on which the modern concepts of the anatomy and physiology of the heart and circulation are based. Genuine progress in the field of cardiology first became evident when the views of Harvey became generally accepted. Our final classic is Dr. J. B. Herrick's account of coronary thrombosis which appeared in 1912.

We wish to acknowledge with gratitude the splendid resources of the Library of The Mayo Clinic and to express our appreciation for the splendid cooperation of its staff of librarians. We are deeply appreciative of the assistance rendered us by Dr. Maurice Walsh of the Mayo Clinic and Dr. Erich Hausner, formerly of the Mayo Foundation, in translations of works from the French and Latin. Our appreciation also is extended to Mr. James Eckman, our editor, of the Division of Publications of The Mayo Clinic, whose encouragement and suggestions have been of great help to us, and also many others whose technical assistance has been indispensable.

FREDRICK A. WILLIUS
THOMAS E. KEYS

Rochester, Minn.

CONTENTS

VOLUME ONE

ILLUSTRATIONS

VOLUME ONE

VOLUME TWO

Page

CLASSICS OF CARDIOLOGY

CLASSICS OF CARDIOLOGY

THE INFLUENCE OF CERTAIN CARDIAC CLASSICS ON THE DEVELOPMENT OF MODERN CARDIOLOGY

IN THE history of medicine are recorded the heroic efforts of man over the unknown, the conflicts against ignorance, superstition, and prejudice; relentless self-sacrifice in the search for truth, indomitable courage in the face of failure and disappointment, all a part of the marvelous yet uncompleted pageant of present-day medicine. In the chronologic presentation of these classics on the heart and circulation it is possible to trace the development of cardiology to its present position. It is probable that the advancement of knowledge in the century to follow the present one will be greater and more dramatic than that of the three preceding centuries comprising the scope of this volume, but if this prediction materializes, it will be only because our illustrious predecessors have built their structure well and wisely.

There is no doubt that William Harvey's epoch-making contribution, published in 1628, on the anatomy and the physiology of the heart and circulation laid the foundation for subsequent discoveries and advancements in this field. Earlier observations are uncertain, isolated, and lack co-ordinated continuity; some are erroneous and speculative, products of the ages of scientific ignorance, religous prejudice, and superstition. We do not mean to deny the fact that certain earlier observations were noteworthy; but their sporadic occurrence in the space of time hardly permits their inclusion in this consideration. Even Harvey's views were bitterly contested by many of his contemporaries, who found it simpler to disagree on the premise of erroneous doctrines accepted as fact, rather than to open their minds to the comprehension of new data demonstrated by dissection and experiment. Harvey proved the circulation of the blood and the manner in which it was accomplished; he also predicted the existence of the capillary circulation, which he referred to as "pores." He preceded the era of the microscope, and the use of his magnifying glass was of course inadequate for the demonstration of this minute anastomosis. However, through remarkably clear reasoning he realized that some manner of communication between the terminal arterial and venous tributaries must exist in order to correlate the various observations which were evident from his thorough and painstaking investigations.

In 1640, Pierre Gassendi recorded the demonstration of the existence of the foramen ovale in the adult heart. Gassendi witnessed this demonstration, which was made by a surgeon named Payanus in Aix during the dissection of a human body. This early settlement of a controversial issue of that era is of unusual interest and reveals the meticulous care exercised by some of the older anatomists in carrying out their dissections.

With the advent of and improvement in the microscope, the opportunity of demonstrating the capillary circulation, and thereby verifying Harvey's prediction, was accorded Marcello Malpighi, who vividly described these minute vascular structures in the lung and mesentery of the frog. These observations were recorded in 1661, in his classic letters to Borelli, professor of science at Pisa, his friend and erstwhile idol.

Three years later, in 1664, Niels Stensen revealed the true muscular nature of the heart. This was a most important observation, because subsequent studies on the activity of the heart found confirmation in this fundamental demonstration.

Thus, the teaching of correct basic anatomic and physiologic principles, though limited in scope, was the pioneer influence for the better understanding and recognition of departures from normal in the fields of physiology, pathology, and clinical medicine.

In 1705, William Cowper clearly described disease of the aortic valve with aortic insufficiency. This was accomplished through keen observation by correlating the symptoms of the patient and alterations detected in the pulse with the abnormal findings in the heart as revealed by postmortem examination. It must be recalled that this observation antedated the discovery of auscultation by more than a century.

Antony van Leeuwenhoek, in 1708, published his conception of "that motion which we call the pulse." Although his observations in this study were inaccurate and his conclusions erroneous, his noteworthy contributions in microscopy place him deservedly among science's immortals, for his mechanical ingenuity and inordinate patience enabled many brilliant successors to contribute generously to the advancement of cardiology.

A quarter of a century later (1733) Stephen Hales, a scientifically minded clergyman, published the results of his rather unique experiments on blood pressure and blood velocity. This was the first outstanding contribution on the physiology of the cardiovascular system following the exposition of Harvey. These observations were made possible by the correct teaching of basic anatomic principles and yet little or nothing was known regarding hemodynamics. These experiments, conducted on living animals, were the first in which an attempt at actual measurement of blood pressure and blood velocity in various parts of the circulatory system was undertaken. They revealed certain fundamental facts upon which the modern concepts of today are largely dependent.

In 1749, Jean Baptiste De Sénac made a most extraordinary observation which without a doubt is the very beginning of the relatively modern quinidine therapy of cardiac arrhythmia. Although more than a century and a half elapsed before the medical world became cognizant of the value of quinidine, De Sénac clearly described the beneficial effects of quinine in "rebellious palpitation."

Albrecht von Haller, in 1755, described calcification of the heart and pericardium in a very clear and vivid manner. This observation was based on a study of post-mortem material.

In 1761, the interesting and important observations of John Baptist Morgagni were published. They appeared in the form of letters collected in five books under the title of *The Seats and Causes of Diseases, etc.* (trans.). This work comprises the descriptions of a wide variety of diseases, with post-mortem observations. The remarkably accurate and interesting manner of presentation of Morgagni prompted us to reprint his observations on mitral stenosis, heart block, calcareous stenosis of the aortic valve with insufficiency, coronary sclerosis, and aneurysm of the aorta. Studies of this character were of great importance in the development of medicine because they represented the correlation of clinical symptoms and signs with dissection after death. Although the concepts of pathology were still ill-defined, observations of changes in tissue were recorded even though their nature and significance were not always understood. Such records served to stimulate others to pursue similar investigations with a determined curiosity.

Also in 1761, Leopold Auenbrugger published the results of his investigations dealing with a new diagnostic method, percussion of the thorax. This work preceded the introduction of auscultation by fifty-eight years. He introduced the Preface of his work with the following words, "I here present the Reader with a new sign which I have discovered for detecting diseases of the chest. This consists in the Percussion of the human thorax, whereby, according to the character of the peculiar sound thence elicited, an opinion is formed of the internal states of that cavity" (trans.). The tremendous influence of this discovery on the science and art of physical diagnosis requires no special comment. It enabled the physician to use an additional method of clinical investigation, since his methods were still limited to his own senses of perception.

In 1772, William Heberden's classic description of angina pectoris was first published, and again it appeared in 1802 in his *Commentaries on the History and Cure of Diseases.* Heberden, an outstanding scholar of his day, was possessed of the art of clear and accurate description, so that his vivid portrayal of the symptoms of angina pectoris, recorded in remarkable clarity, stands unchallenged today and is without a doubt one of the most cherished and brilliant masterpieces of the past.

William Withering, in 1785, published the results of years of study and observation and gave to the world a drug of inestimable and enduring value, digitalis. He was a botanist of wide experience, in addition to being a much respected physician. His concise comments on the use and actions of the foxglove *(Digitalis purpurea)* in cardiac dropsy, his remarkable understanding of the indications and contraindications of the drug, his admonitions regarding its indiscriminate employment, and his warnings relative to overdosage endure today as the very basis of digitalis therapy. Withering was one of science's most humble servants, as the introductory sentence of his Preface testifies: "After being frequently urged to write upon this subject, and as often declining to do it, from apprehension of my own inability, I am at length compelled to take up the pen, however unqualified I may still feel myself for the task." His dissertation becomes more interesting and remarkable when it is recalled that the era in which he lived saw therapeutics in the zenith of empiricism. Drugs of unknown and uncertain action were administered by the method of trial and error, standardization of preparations was unknown or uncertain, and therapeutics to a large extent became a tradition perpetuated by word of mouth.

In 1788, Matthew Baillie picturesquely described the findings after death in a case of congenital dextrocardia with complete situs transversus. In this publication he philosophized in a very interesting and understanding manner on the origin of the condition. Baillie is particularly noted for his interest in pathology, and he was probably the first physician to emphasize morbid anatomy as a definitive branch of medical science. He investigated the morbid changes in various organs and attempted to correlate them in the individual case. His studies unquestionably wrought an important influence in the field of pathology and in no small measure contributed to the groundwork of that science.

John Hunter, the celebrated English surgeon, rather unwittingly contributed to the progress of cardiology through the personal records of his own illness. He suffered severe, recurrent attacks of angina pectoris, and his observations and descriptions of the symptoms and signs of the disorder were the first recorded by a physician suffering from this disease. The intimate aspects of his illness are extremely interesting, as are also his various and sundry therapeutic attempts at relief in an era in which therapeutic effort was, to say the least, extremely discouraging. This account was published by his brother-in-law, Everard Home, in 1794, three years after Hunter's death. Post-mortem examination of Hunter revealed marked sclerosis of the coronary arteries which was vividly described in the following words: "The coronary arteries had their branches which ramify through the substance of the heart in the state of bony tubes, which were with difficulty divided by the knife, and their transverse sections did not collapse, but remained open." This is one of the early accounts demonstrating the coexistence of angina pectoris and coronary sclerosis.

In 1806, Jean Nicolas Corvisart published his treatise on diseases of the heart. This was a comprehensive consideration of the diseases of the heart and great vessels according to the knowledge of that era. He emphasized percussion as an important diagnostic method, and his influence undoubtedly had great influence in its survival, for Auenbrugger's teachings had not been enthusiastically received by his contemporaries. Laënnec, one of Corvisart's illustrious students, was greatly stimulated by his able teacher, as evidenced by the frequent citation of Corvisart in Laënnec's treatise on auscultation.

William Charles Wells, in 1812, published one of the earliest clinical accounts of the cardiac participation in rheumatic fever, which he designated as rheumatism of the heart. His observations preceded the discovery of auscultation and his observations comprised the record of symptoms referable to the heart and alterations occurring in the pulse, notably tachycardia and irregularity. In several instances post-mortem examination confirmed Wells's clinical suspicions. The recognition of rheumatic fever as a causative factor in heart disease was to become an important contribution in the field of etiology.

Clinical observations were recorded with greater frequency as the nineteenth century progressed, and one of the striking developments was the evident desire to correlate symptoms and signs of disease with post-mortem observations. A typical instance of keen observation was that of John Cheyne, who, in 1818, described an unusual form of periodic breathing in an instance of fatty heart, which was again described in 1846 by William Stokes, and ultimately became known as "Cheyne-Stokes respiration." In both of these accounts of the disorder, the descriptions are vividly clear and impressive, and testify to the art of careful observation and expression.

In 1819 a new and very fruitful method of clinical examination was introduced in René T. H. Laënnec's epoch-making contribution of auscultation. With the acceptance and refinement of this method, progress in the diagnosis of diseases of the heart advanced in great strides. This discovery was, in a large measure, directly responsible for the great advances in cardiology that were destined to occur in Laënnec's century. In fairly rapid succession, many important observations and discoveries ensued, of which we are able to reproduce only certain outstanding classics.

Caleb Hillier Parry, in 1768, was the first to recognize exophthalmic goiter and its cardiovascular phenomena. This work, however, was not published until 1825.*

Two years later (1827) Robert Adams presented his classic description of heart block, which was again described by William Stokes in 1854, and the cerebral phenomena at times present in this disorder later became known as the "Adams-Stokes syndrome."

In 1831, James Hope published a remarkably complete treatise on diseases of the heart and great vessels. Numerous interesting and graphic descriptions are contained in this work. Of unusual interest are his dis-

*We again wish to remind the reader that the chronologic sequence of presentation in this volume is governed by the year of publication, and not necessarily by the year in which the observation or work was carried out.—F. A. W., 1940.

cussions of cardiac asthma, stenosis of the pulmonary valves, and cardiac neurosis. Of particular importance is Hope's discussion of cardiac asthma, because this syndrome was then only rarely identified as being of cardiac origin.

Sir Dominic John Corrigan, in 1832, published his classic description of the pulse in aortic insufficiency. This observation was important from more than the standpoint of diagnosis, for it stimulated interest and thought on the vascular mechanics of this valvular lesion. Here again is portrayed accurate and masterful description of keen observation.

In 1835, Jean-Baptiste Bouillaud, an eminent physician of his era, among other important contributions described the pathologic aspects of endocarditis according to the knowledge of his time and undoubtedly stimulated others to inquire further into the endocarditides.

Six years later, William Senhouse Kirkes described and discussed emboli resulting from intracardiac coagula and corrected the existing tenets ascribing the remote lesions to local disease (so-called capillary phlebitis). This work was especially important in supporting the theory of emboli. Minute and gross visceral infarction is described in a clear and understanding manner.

Additional observations regarding the signs of already recognized diseases began to appear, and in 1861 Paul Louis Duroziez described the auscultatory findings audible in certain peripheral arteries, notably the femoral arteries, in the presence of aortic insufficiency. He referred to this phenomenon as the "double intermittent murmur over the femoral (crural) arteries" (trans.), which later was to be known as "Duroziez' sign."

In this era of medicine, the teaching of clinical cardiology largely centered around murmurs, and much emphasis was placed on the description of their character, slight variations in timbre and intensity, timing and transmission. This period of the history of cardiology witnessed many significant advances and stimulated physicians to search for new and additional diagnostic methods to penetrate still further the secrets of the normal, as well as of the diseased, heart. It was in 1862 that Austin Flint, an American physician, published his important contribution, "On Cardiac Murmurs," which appeared in the *American Journal of the Medical Sciences.* This paper deals comprehensively with murmurs in general and contains the description of the murmur, later to be known as the "Austin Flint murmur."

In 1867, Pierre Carl E. Potain called attention to the importance and significance of another peripheral phenomenon of heart disease in his observations on the pulsations of the jugular veins. Evidence more or less remote from the heart was gradually being accumulated and correlated, helping to lay the foundation for the innumerable signs that now constitute the diagnostic armamentarium of the present-day physician.

In the same year, Sir Thomas Lauder Brunton enriched the world with the important contribution relative to the ameliorating effects of amyl nitrite in the anginal syndrome. Preceding this discovery, sufferers from angina pectoris had received little or no relief from the therapeutic agents available to them. In this study the vasodilating action of amyl nitrite, first suspected by Dr. B. W. Richardson, was confirmed. The drug was discovered by Balard, but Brunton was the first to suggest its use on a practical therapeutic basis. Studies of this character were extremely important in the attack on the existing therapeutic empiricism of that era.

A year later (1868) Heinrich Irenaeus Quincke clearly described the capillary and venous pulse. Quincke was another keen observer who called attention to more remote signs of the impaired heart. These observations were significant and continue to be of great practical importance today.

In 1870, Sir Samuel Wilks very clearly described the disease later to be known as "bacterial endocarditis," under the title "capillary embolism or arterial pyaemia." This contribution was important in that it called attention to the necessity for separating old valvular defects (healed endocarditis) from associated or superimposed vegetative lesions resulting in the dissemination of emboli.

Ludwig Traube, two years later (1872), described a significant disturbance in the pulse which he termed "pulsus alternans." He clearly distinguished it from the simulating condition, pulsus bigeminus. Traube's contribution has endured as a very valuable sign and today continues to guide the clinician in his appraisal of the course of the failing heart.

In 1876, Sir William Richard Gowers graphically described certain changes found in the retinal vessels in the presence of arterial hypertension. This demonstration was destined to be of great importance, as testified to by the extensive development of retinoscopy in recent years. He fully appreciated the fact that the retinal arteries, visible by special means, afforded the physician an opportunity of actually observing vessels during the life of the patient and of comparing the retinas of normal individuals with those of patients afflicted with cardiovascular-renal disease. At the time that Gowers conducted these studies, the concept of primary renal damage occupied a very prominent position, and the concept of generalized vascular disease in relationship to hypertension had not yet been clearly conceived.

A year later (1877), Julius Friedrich Cohnheim in his chapter on thrombosis and embolism of his work on the *Pathology of the Circulation* (trans.) described paradoxical embolism. This work called attention to a new significance attending otherwise innocuous imperfections of the septa of the heart and demonstrated the manner in which, in the presence of these imperfections, thrombi arising in the venous system can be transported to the periphery of the arterial system.

In 1879, Henri Roger described the uncomplicated congenital defect of the interventricular septum and masterfully described the prolonged murmur, extending through both systole and diastole, pathognomonic of this defect. The murmur is still frequently known as the "Roger murmur."

In the same year, William Murrell, undoubtedly influenced by the work of his worthy predecessor, Sir Thomas Lauder Brunton, published his studies on the effects of nitroglycerin in angina pectoris. In this investigation, conducted during a controversial period because of a lack of standardization of drugs, he pursued his studies in a determined manner and compared the effects of nitroglycerin with those of amyl nitrite. This contribution made available another valuable drug for the mitigation of the anginal seizure. It also stressed the importance of standardization of drugs.

Six years later (1885) Pierre Carl Potain made another important contribution to cardiology. He published his studies on gallop rhythm and presented his views on the genesis and significance of this condition.

Augustus D. Waller, in 1887, after extensive physiologic studies on the action currents of the heart by means of the capillary electrometer, published his work on a method of leading the currents from the surface of the body by means of paired electrodes. Previous work in this field had necessitated direct contact with the heart. His studies clearly paved the way for clinical electrocardiography, an almost indispensable method of modern cardiology.

In the same year, John Alexander MacWilliam recorded the results of his experiments dealing with direct faradization of the heart, and produced profound alterations in rate and rhythm. He clearly described the abnormal rhythms now known as "auricular fibrillation," "auricular flutter," "ventricular tachycardia" and "ventricular fibrillation." His work, moreover, was a steppingstone to clinical electrocardiography, particularly from the standpoint of the ultimate correlation of graphs revealing abnormal waves with actual visualization of induced disturbances in the hearts of animals.

A year later (1888), Graham Steell described the pulmonary diastolic murmur, under the title of "The Murmur of High Pressure in the Pulmonary Artery." This was destined to be known as the "Graham Steell murmur," and is so designated today.

In the same year, A. Fallot described the interesting and unusual combination of congenital cardiac defects consisting of pulmonary stenosis, interventricular septal defect, dextroposition of the aorta, and hypertrophy of the right ventricle. This became known as the *tetralogy of Fallot* and is frequently referred to as the *maladie bleue.*

At this time, very little was known regarding the intrinsic physiology of the cardiac impulse and its dissemination through the substance of the heart. It was in 1893 that Wilhelm His, Jr., accurately described the minute fasciculus that conducts the impulse from the auricles to the ventricles: the auriculoventricular bundle. This structure is still frequently designated as the "bundle of His." This contribution was of paramount importance in the clearer understanding of the intricate mechanism of cardiac conduction and inevitably led to further discoveries in this field.

In 1896, Francis Henry Williams of Boston reported his observations on the fluoroscopic examination of the heart and aorta. Although his studies were not the first recorded, they are extremely noteworthy and we have chosen to include them in this volume. Williams' observations were published a year following Roentgen's original observations and surely represent pioneer efforts in this remarkable branch of science.

The following year (1897), Sir William Henry Broadbent presented his classic description of adherent pericarditis and described the recession of the intercostal spaces as a sign of this disease, a sign which was to become known as "Broadbent's sign." Simulating findings have since been frequently misinterpreted, yet Broadbent emphatically discussed the limitations of interpretation.

In 1903, Willem Einthoven devised the string galvanometer, the original modern electrocardiograph. During his extensive experience with the capillary electrometer in the study of the action currents of the heart, he was aware of the inherent error existing in this method and sought to devise a method of registration wherein this error would be obviated. The world owes this humble scientist a tremendous debt of gratitude for his brilliant gift, for with the advent of electrocardiography, remarkable progress has been made, and many of the secrets of the heart have gradually become bared. Electrocardiography is today virtually an indispensable method in the thorough appraisal of the heart.

A year later (1904), during the time that the issue between the myogenic and neurogenic theories of heart contraction was controversial, Ludwig Aschoff presented his epoch-making work on rheumatic myocarditis. He described the characteristic lesion of rheumatic fever, which has come to be known as the "Aschoff nodule." This was a monumental work and did much to crystallize the present-day concepts of the pathology of this yet unsolved disease, and it established a histopathologic picture that was destined to exert a great influence in classifying examples of true myocarditis. Other myocardial abnormalities, later to be proved noninflammatory in nature, were before this universally shuffled into the rather vague category of "myocarditis."

It was not until 1907 that the sino-auricular node was demonstrated by the painstaking microscopic studies of Arthur Keith and Martin Flack. They also predicted the function of this node to be the "pacemaker" of the heart, that is, the point of origin of the cardiac impulse. This discovery proved to be of great importance in bridging certain gaps in the more comprehensive understanding of the intrinsic anatomy and physiology of the heart.

Sir James Mackenzie contributed generously to the modern concepts of cardiology, but the identification and clarification of auricular fibrillation was probably one of his greatest achievements. The conclusive publication of this work appeared in 1908, although he described this form of arrhythmia in 1902, believing then that it represented "nodal rhythm." His clinical observations on the pulse and the differentiation and segregation of the various irregularities of the pulse were made possible by his adoption of the simultaneous recording of arterial and venous pulse waves by means of the polygraph. This mechanical method of registration was eventually supplanted by the electrocardiograph, in a great measure through the comprehensive studies of Mackenzie's brilliant student, Sir Thomas Lewis.

At this time another outstanding physician was molding the form of modern medicine, and his varied contributions are still the byword of present-day medical students. Sir William Osler's influence on modern medicine was profound. We have chosen to reproduce his article on chronic infectious endocarditis, published in 1909, wherein the description of the cutaneous nodules of subacute bacterial endocarditis is found. These pathognomonic lesions are widely known today as "Osler's nodes."

Our final contributor, one of the few masters still living, is our beloved American, Dr. James Bryan Herrick. His classic description of coronary thrombosis, appearing in 1912 in the *Journal of the American Medical Association,* clearly opened a new era in which the clinical recognition of this disease was to become the rule rather than the exception. Although this report was preceded by that of Dr. Adam Hammer of St. Louis and Vienna in 1878, Herrick's paper attracted much wider attention and therefore appears to have had a more profound influence on the modern concepts of the disease than that of Hammer.

It has been impossible to include all noteworthy contributions of the past in this volume of CARDIAC CLASSICS, and there will be some critics who will disapprove of certain inclusions while others will question certain exclusions. In the anticipation of such criticisms we can but state, simply, that we have conscientiously attempted to make this collection of classics comprehensive, and have selected from the great literature of the three centuries preceding our own those contributions which have particularly appealed to us and which, we believe, have profoundly influenced the progress of this branch of medical science. We have, as far as possible, avoided the inclusion of the works of living physicians, well realizing the possibilities for controversy which would have arisen if such a plan had been extensively adopted. There are, of course, many notable contributions by our living contemporaries, who, however, must remain patient until some future compilers honor them in a manner similar to that adumbrated by the present collection.

1628

WILLIAM HARVEY

ON THE MOTION OF THE HEART AND BLOOD IN ANIMALS

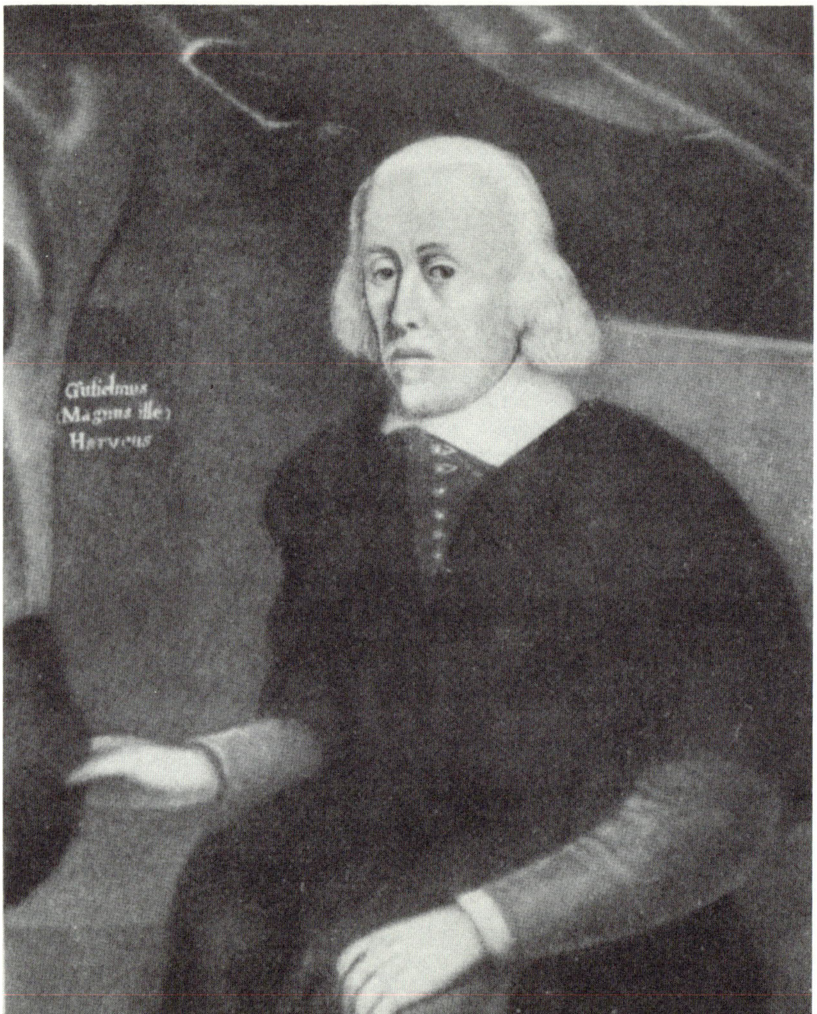

WILLIAM HARVEY

Painting by unknown contemporary

(Courtesy Ciba Symposia.)

WILLIAM HARVEY

(1578-1657)

"Cor, Imperator, Rex"

"I was almost tempted to think with Fracastorius that the motion of the heart was only to be comprehended by God."

—William Harvey, Chapter I, *De motu cordis.*

WILLIAM HARVEY, born in 1578 as the eldest son of Thomas Harvey of Folkestone, Kent, had his preliminary education at the Canterbury Grammar School and was admitted as a student of Caius' College, Cambridge, in 1593. Dr. Caius, the founder and long the master according to Power (p. 13), in addition to his knowledge of Greek, introduced the study of practical anatomy into England. Through his influence, his college was allowed to use the bodies of two criminals annually for the purposes of dissection. It is not definitely known whether or not Harvey was permitted to watch or to participate in dissections, but it is known that he was graduated from this school, Bachelor of Arts, in 1597. His collegiate education probably was a general one and included a sound knowledge of Greek and Latin plus an acquaintanceship with dialectics and with physics.

In choosing Padua for the study of medicine, Harvey was no doubt drawn by the renown of its medical school, made famous by the great Vesalius and by the work of the successor of Vesalius, Hieronymus Fabricius. Harvey supposedly entered Padua in 1598, but there is no record of his being there before the year 1600.

The theater in which Fabricius lectured still exists. It is now an ancient structure containing seats which rise perpendicularly, one above the other. But when Harvey was at Padua the theater was new, and the government had placed an inscription over the entrance to commemorate the genius of Fabricius. Fabricius must have been a source of great inspiration to Harvey and it was under him that the young student became an expert in anatomy. Harvey makes reference in "De motu cordis" to his former teacher as "the celebrated Hieronymus Fabricius of Aquapendente, a most skilful anatomist, and venerable old man." While Harvey was receiving his medical training at Padua, Fabricius was perfecting his knowledge concerning the valves of the veins. Sylvius of Louvilly (Jacques DuBois, 1478-1555), the teacher of Vesalius at Paris, had known and described the valves at an early date. But Fabricius rediscovered them in 1574 (Power, p. 25). Fabricius, as Harvey so skillfully points out, did not rightly understand the function of the valves. Fabricius thought their purpose was to prevent overdistention of the vessels when blood flowed from the larger into the smaller veins, but that they were not needed in the arteries because the blood was always in a state of ebb and flow! Harvey pointed out that the true function of the valves was to prevent venous reflux and, therefore, this prevention of contrary motion was a great factor in the circulation of the blood.

After a five-year stay at Padua, Harvey received his diploma as Doctor of Physics (1602), with the right to practice and teach arts and medicine in every land and seat of learning. Apparently, Harvey had made a great impression on his superiors, for his diploma further stated, "He had conducted himself so wonderfully well in the

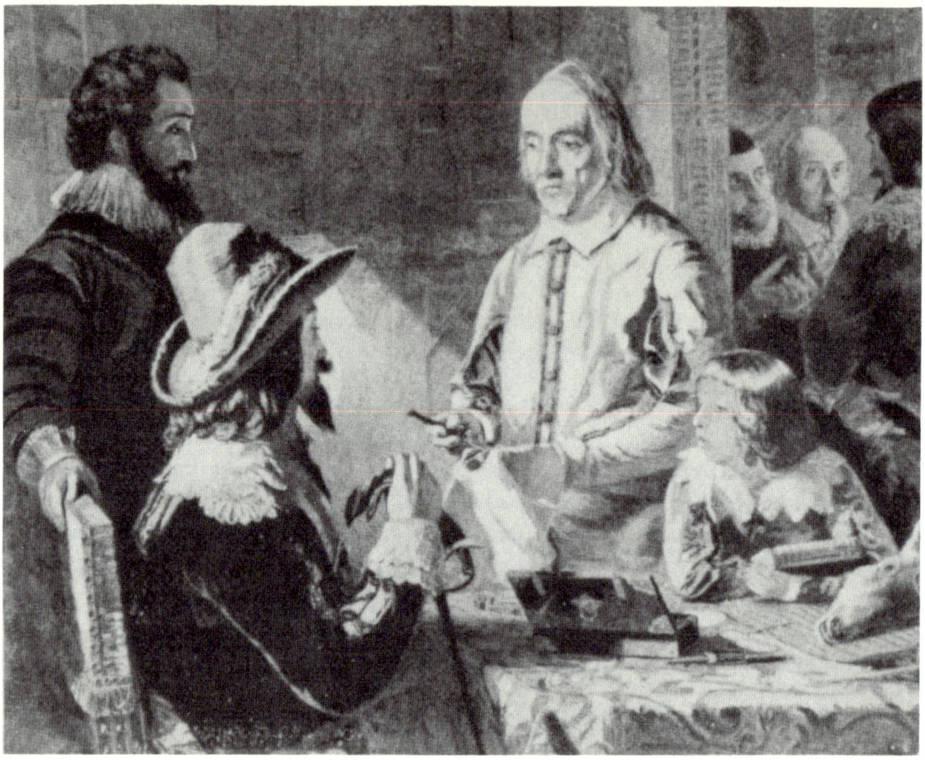

WILLIAM HARVEY EXPOUNDING HIS CONCEPTION OF THE CIRCULATION OF THE BLOOD TO KING CHARLES I OF ENGLAND

Painting by Robert Hannah

(Courtesy Ciba Symposia.)

examination, and had shown such skill, memory, and learning that he had far surpassed even the great hopes which his examiners had formed of him.'' (Quoted by Power, pp. 26-27.)

On his return to England in the same year, Harvey also received the degree of Doctor of Medicine from the University of Cambridge. Two years later (1604), Harvey settled in London, married the daughter of a physician (Lancelot Browne, physician to Queen Elizabeth and to King James I) by whom, it is to be regretted, he had no children. He then entered the practice of his profession and was elected a fellow of the College of Physicians in 1607. In 1609 he was duly appointed physician to St. Bartholomew's Hospital.

In 1615 Harvey was appointed to the office of Lumleian lecturer, a highly esteemed position under the sponsorship of the College of Physicians. He continued in this capacity until 1656, when he resigned his post. Harvey's lectures (on anatomy and surgery as qualified by the Lumleian Trust) were first delivered from April 16 to 18, 1616. On April 23 of that same year, Shakespeare died at Stratford-on-Avon. Garrison (p. 249) and others have pointed out the resemblance of Harvey's finely formed head to that of the world's greatest dramatist. And it may be possible that Harvey was influenced somewhat by his great contemporary.

The manuscript notes of his first course of lectures are now the sacred property of the British Museum. The second portion of his notes (as described by Power, pp. 64-66) contains an account of the thorax and its contents. After a full discussion of the situation and functions of the various abdominal viscera, Harvey next considered the thorax, and his remarkable words contain his first written description of his memorable discovery. These words are initialed to show that Harvey believed the idea was original.

''It is plain from the structure of the heart that the blood is passed continuously through the lungs to the aorta as by the two clacks of a water bellows to raise water.

''It is shown by the application of a ligature that the passage of the blood is from the arteries into the veins.

''Whence it follows that the movement of the blood is constantly in a circle, and is brought about by the beat of the heart. It is a question, therefore, whether this is for the sake of nourishment or rather for the preservation of the blood and the limbs by the communication of the heat, the blood cooled by warming the limbs being in turn warmed by the heart.''

Therefore, it is apparent that Harvey knew of the circulation, at least, by the year 1616, at the age of thirty-seven, and twelve years before the publication of ''De motu cordis.''

In 1618 Harvey was appointed Physician Extraordinary to James I and, on the death of that monarch, his son, Charles I, appointed Harvey a physician-in-ordinary. Besides being physician to the King's household, Harvey was physician to several distinguished noble families. Included among his patients was Francis Bacon (1561-1626), whose great genius did not impress the mind of Harvey, who said of one of Bacon's works, ''He writes philosophy like a Lord Chancellor.''

The year 1628 marks the highest point in the career of William Harvey. From Frankfort-on-the-Main came his matured account in Latin of the circulation of the blood. The Italians claimed Andrea Cesalpino[1] (1524-1603), professor of medicine

[1]Erasistratus (circa 310-250 B.C.) of Keos, the first experimental physiologist, described the aortic and pulmonary valves, the chordae tendineae of the heart and had the idea of the capillary system. He also conceived that the heart was a pump and expressed the first theory of the circulation. (See Finlayson, J.: Hierophilus and Erasistratus. Glasgow M. J. 39: 321-352, 1893.) Others in addition to Cesalpino who contributed more or less meritorious theoretical accounts of the circulatory system included Ibn an- Nafis, of Egypt and Syria (c. 1288-1289), Servetus (1509-1553), the Spaniard, and Realdo Colombo (1516-1559), the successor of Vesalius at Padua.

at Pisa, as having discovered the circulation during the period from 1571-1593 prior to Harvey (1616). Cesalpino described the lesser circulation, but his observations did not lead him to a clear recognition of the greater circulation. Cesalpino is deserving of credit, however, and it is possible that Harvey knew of his work while he was a student at Padua. In his first chapter of ''De motu cordis,'' Harvey suggests that he sought to discover the motions and uses of the heart ''from actual inspection and not from the writings of others.'' For this purpose he resorted to vivisection, ligation and perfusion. He experimented on several living animals whose hearts were observable with the naked eye, and also on some smaller animals whose hearts he could observe with the aid of a magnifying glass. As an anatomist, and an outstanding one, he was further able to confirm much of his proof of the circulation on the basis of his many dissections of human bodies.

The mainstay of Harvey's argument—that the actual quantity of blood as measured made it physically impossible for the blood to do other than return to the heart by the venous route—not only gave him definite proof of the circulation but also, as Garrison (p. 247) has so well stated, insured that his computation was the first idea of measurement in any biologic investigation. This quantitative demonstration gave impetus to the rise of physiology.

After the publication of ''De motu cordis,'' there can be no doubt that Harvey's prestige as a physician suffered somewhat. He was severely attacked by the pedantic thinkers of the time. But this disturbance was more than counterbalanced by the acceptance during his lifetime of his most important contribution.

Harvey, at an early date (1613), had been elected to the office of censor in the College of Physicians. He was reappointed to this office in 1625 and again in 1629. In 1628 he was appointed Treasurer of the ''College,'' to which office he was reappointed in 1629. In the same year he received the commands of the King to accompany the Duke of Lennox, who was sent to travel abroad. He continued to travel with the Duke until the winter of 1631-1632, at which time he returned to England. In 1632 he drew up a set of rules for the new library of the College of Physicians. Early in 1633, Harvey again received the commands of the King, this time to attend Charles I on his journey to Scotland. During this trip he wrote his treatise on the ''Bass Rock.''

In 1634, the story of the Lancashire witches ran rampant through England. As was the case in the Salem witchcraft episode in New England in 1692, the accusations were the result of a child's perjury. Dr. Harvey was called upon to examine the bodies of some of the arrested ''witches'' and some of those permitted to live. Owing to his testimony and that of others, four of the seven convicted ''witches'' were pardoned. Harvey's attitude is all the more remarkable, considering that his contemporary in medicine, Sir Thomas Browne (1605-1682), supposedly a model of tolerance, affirmed that he believed in witchcraft (Smith, vol. 1, p. 445), and the great Carl Linnaeus (1707-1778), born 129 years later than Harvey, displayed in his ''Nemesis Divina,'' written for his son, that he believed in supernatural punishments (Smith, vol. 2, pp. 540, 541).

Another interesting experience occurred to Harvey in 1635. In this year he was ordered by the King to perform necropsy on the body of Thomas Parr, who is said to have died at the ripe age of one hundred and fifty-two years and nine months. The notes of this necropsy were not printed until 1669, when they were published in Bett's ''On the Source and Quality of Blood.'' From these notes it appears that Harvey believed ''Old Tom Parr'' would have lived even longer had he remained in his native home, Shropshire, and not transported himself to London and altered his diet by living with a nobleman!

Harvey's friendship with the King resulted in his being suspected, and rightly, of being an enthusiastic Loyalist. In the early part of the Civil War (1642), a mob of citizen-soldiers entered Harvey's lodgings, stole his goods, and scattered his papers. These papers included the records of a large number of dissections, his observations on the development of insects, and a series of notes on comparative anatomy.

In 1645 Harvey was elected to the honorable position of warden of Merton College at the University of Oxford. This was the school of which the famous John of Gaddesden (circa 1350), one of the earliest Englishmen to write a complete treatise on medicine,[2] had been a fellow. Because of the tumult of the Cromwellian Civil War, Harvey held this position for only one year.

The surrender of Oxford in 1645 marks the period of Harvey's severance from the Court and his gradual retirement from public life, occasioned in part by his being affected with gout, from which he suffered recurrent attacks. During this time he was preparing his essay "De generatione animalium," which was published in 1651. In his investigation of the embryo, handicapped as he was by not having a microscope, he formed a wrong idea of fecundation. He believed the fertilization of the ovum to be something "incorporeal—as iron touched by the magnet is endowed with its own powers." Garrison (p. 248) suggests that the true importance of "De generatione" was "that it subverted the ancient concept that life is engendered out of corruption (or putrefaction)."

The College of Physicians was promised, by an anonymous donor, a library of books, a museum of numerous objects of curiosity, and a variety of surgical instruments. Before the building was completed the name of the generous benefactor became known, and the College responded in 1652 by creating a statue of Harvey.

But the College still felt indebted to Harvey and chose him as its president in 1654. He, however, did not accept this honor, recognizing the influences of the infirmities in his health. The attacks of gout continued, and he died on June 3, 1657, from a cerebral hemorrhage. He was buried in the family vault at Hempstead in Essex.

Abraham Cowley (1618-1667) wrote of Harvey:

> "Harvey sought for Truth, in Truth's own book,
> The creatures, which by God himself was writ;
> And wisely thought 'twas fit,
> Not to read comments only upon it,
> But on th' original itself to look."

[2]*Rosa Anglica,* printed in 1492.

EXERCITATIO

ANATOMICA DE MOTV CORDIS ET SAN-GVINIS IN ANIMALI-BVS,

GVILIELMI HARVEI ANGLI,

Medici Regii, & Professoris Anatomiæ in Collegio Medicorum Londinensi.

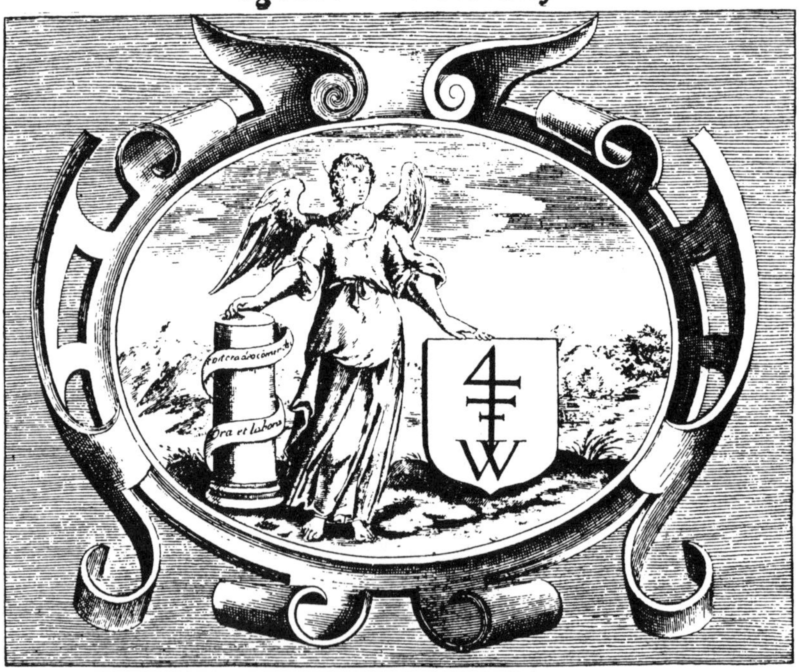

FRANCOFVRTI,

Sumptibus GVILIELMI FITZERI.

ANNO M. DC. XXVIII.

AN ANATOMICAL DISQUISITION ON THE MOTION OF THE HEART AND BLOOD IN ANIMALS*

By

WILLIAM HARVEY, M.D.

INTRODUCTION

AS WE are about to discuss the motion, action, and use of the heart and arteries, it is imperative on us first to state what has been thought of these things by others in their writings, and what has been held by the vulgar and by tradition, in order that what is true may be confirmed, and what is false set right by dissection, multiplied experience, and accurate observation.

Almost all anatomists, physicians, and philosophers, up to the present time, have supposed with Galen, that the object of the pulse was the same as that of respiration, and only differed in one particular, this being conceived to depend on the animal, the respiration on the vital faculty; the two, in all other respects, whether with reference to purpose or to motion, comporting themselves alike. Whence it is affirmed, as by Hieronymus Fabricius of Aquapendente, in his book on "Respiration," which has lately appeared, that as the pulsation of the heart and arteries does not suffice for the ventilation and refrigeration of the blood, therefore were the lungs fashioned to surround the heart. From this it appears, that whatever has hitherto been said upon the systole and diastole, on the motion of the heart and arteries, has been said with especial reference to the lungs.

But as the structure and movements of the heart differ from those of the lungs, and the motions of the arteries from those of the chest, so seems it likely that the other ends and offices will thence arise, and that the pulsations and uses of the heart, likewise of the arteries, will differ in many respects from the heavings and uses of the chest and lungs. For did the arterial pulse and the respiration serve the same ends; did the arteries in their diastole take air into their cavities, as commonly stated, and in their systole emit fuliginous vapours by the same pores of the flesh and skin; and further, did they, in the time intermediate between the diastole and the systole, contain air, and at all times either air, or spirits, or fuliginous vapours, what should then be said to Galen, who wrote a book on purpose to show that by nature the arteries contained blood, and nothing

**Exercitatio anatomica de motu cordis et sanguinis in animalibus,* London, 1628. Translated by Robert Willis, Barnes, Surrey, England, 1847.

but blood; neither spirits nor air, consequently, as may be readily gathered from the experiments and reasonings contained in the same book? Now if the arteries are filled in the diastole with air then taken into them (a larger quantity of air penetrating when the pulse is large and full), it must come to pass, that if you plunge into a bath of water or of oil when the pulse is strong and full, it ought forthwith to become either smaller or much slower, since the circumambient bath will render it either difficult or impossible for the air to penetrate. In like manner, as all the arteries, those that are deep-seated as well as those that are superficial, are dilated at the same instant, and with the same rapidity, how were it possible that air should penetrate to the deeper parts as freely and quickly through the skin, flesh, and other structures, as through the mere cuticle? And how should the arteries of the foetus draw air into their cavities through the abdomen of the mother and the body of the womb? And how should seals, whales, dolphins and other cetaceans, and fishes of every description, living in the depths of the sea, take in and emit air by the diastole and systole of their arteries through the infinite mass of waters? For to say that they absorb the air that is infixed in the water, and emit their fumes into this medium, were to utter something very like a mere figment. And if the arteries in their systole expel fuliginous vapours from their cavities through the pores of the flesh and skin, why not the spirits, which are said to be contained in these vessels, at the same time, since spirits are much more subtile than fuliginous vapours or smoke? And further, if the arteries take in and cast out air in the systole and diastole, like the lungs in the process of respiration, wherefore do they not do the same thing when a wound is made in one of them, as is done in the operation of arteriotomy? When the windpipe is divided, it is sufficiently obvious that the air enters and returns through the wound by two opposite movements; but when an artery is divided, it is equally manifest that blood escapes in one continuous stream, and that no air either enters or issues. If the pulsations of the arteries fan and refrigerate the several parts of the body as the lungs do the heart, how comes it, as is commonly said, that the arteries carry the vital blood into the different parts, abundantly charged with vital spirits, which cherish the heat of these parts, sustain them when asleep, and recruit them when exhausted? And how should it happen that, if you tie the arteries, immediately the parts not only become torpid, and frigid, and look pale, but at length cease even to be nourished? This, according to Galen, is because they are deprived of the heat which flowed through all parts from the heart, as its source; whence it would appear that the arteries rather carry warmth to the parts than serve for any fanning or refrigeration. Besides, how can the diastole (of the arteries) draw spirits from the heart to warm the body and its parts, and, from without, means of cooling or tempering them? Still further, although some affirm that the lungs, arteries, and heart have all the same offices, they yet maintain that the heart is the workshop of the spirits, and that the arteries contain and transmit them; denying, however, in opposition to the opinion of Columbus, that the lungs can either make or contain spirits; and then they assert, with Galen, against Erasistratus, that it is blood, not spirits, which is contained in the arteries.

These various opinions are seen to be so incongruous and mutually subversive, that every one of them is not unjustly brought under suspicion. That it is blood and blood alone which is contained in the arteries is made manifest by the experiment of Galen, by arteriotomy, and by wounds; for from a single artery divided, as Galen himself affirms in more than one place, the whole of the blood may be withdrawn in the course of half an hour, or less. The experiment of Galen alluded to is this: "If you include a portion of an artery between two ligatures, and slit it open lengthways, you will find nothing but blood"; and thus he proves that the arteries contain blood only. And we too may be permitted to proceed by a like train of reasoning: if we find the same blood in the arteries that we find in the veins, which we have tied in the same way, as I have myself repeatedly ascertained, both in the dead body and in living animals, we may fairly conclude that the arteries contain the same blood as the veins, and nothing but the same blood. Some, whilst they attempt to lessen the difficulty here, affirming that the blood is spiritous and arterious, virtually concede that the office of the arteries is to carry blood from the heart into the whole of the body, and that they are therefore filled with blood; for spiritous blood is not the less blood on that account. And then no one denies that the blood as such, even the portion of it which flows in the veins, is imbued with spirits. But if that portion which is contained in the arteries be richer in spirits, it is still to be believed that these spirits are inseparable from the blood, like those in the veins; that the blood and spirits constitute one body (like whey and butter in milk, or heat [and water] in hot water), with which the arteries are charged, and for the distribution of which from the heart they are provided, and that this body is nothing else than blood. But if this blood be said to be drawn from the heart into the arteries by the diastole of these vessels, it is then assumed that the arteries by their distension are filled with blood, and not with the ambient air, as heretofore; for if they be said also to become filled with air from the ambient atmosphere, how and when, I ask, can they receive blood from the heart? If it be answered: during the systole; I say, that seems impossible; the arteries would then have to fill whilst they contracted; in other words, to fill, and yet not become distended. But if it be said: during the diastole, they would then, and for two opposite purposes, be receiving both blood and air, and heat and cold; which is improbable. Further, when it is affirmed that the diastole of the heart and arteries is simultaneous, and the systole of the two is also concurrent, there is another incongruity. For how can two bodies mutually connected, which are simultaneously distended, attract or draw anything from one another; or, being simultaneously contracted, receive anything from each other? And then it seems impossible that one body can thus attract another body into itself, so as to become distended, seeing that to be distended is to be passive, unless, in the manner of a sponge, previously compressed by an external force, whilst it is returning to its natural state. But it is difficult to conceive that there can be anything of this kind in the arteries. The arteries dilate, because they are filled like bladders or leathern bottles; they are not filled because they expand like bellows. This I think easy of demonstration; and indeed conceive that I have already proved it. Nevertheless, in that book of Galen headed 'Quod Sanguis continetur in Arteriis,' he quotes an experiment to prove the contrary: An artery having been exposed, is opened longitudinally, and a reed or other pervious tube, by which the blood is prevented from being lost, and the wound is closed, is inserted into the vessel through the opening. "So long," he says, "as things are thus arranged, the whole artery will pulsate; but if you now throw a ligature about the vessel and tightly compress its tunics over the tube, you will no longer see the artery beating beyond the ligature." I have never performed this experiment of Galen's, nor do I think that it could very well be performed in the living body, on account of the profuse flow of blood that would take place from the vessel which was operated on; neither would the tube effectually close the wound in the vessel without a ligature; and I cannot doubt but that the blood would be found to flow out between the tube and the vessel. Still Galen appears by this experiment to prove both that the pulsative faculty extends from the heart by the walls of the arteries, and that the arteries, whilst they dilate, are filled by that pulsific force, because they expand like bellows, and do not dilate because they are filled like skins. But the contrary is obvious in arteriotomy and in wounds; for the blood spurting from the arteries escapes with force, now farther, now not so far, alternately, or in jets; and the jet always takes place with the diastole of the artery, never with the systole. By which it clearly appears that the artery is dilated by the impulse of the blood; for of itself it would not throw the blood to such a distance, and whilst it was dilating; it ought rather to draw air into its cavity through the wound, were those things true that are commonly stated concerning the uses of the arteries. Nor let the thickness of the arterial tunics impose upon us, and lead us to conclude that the pulsative property proceeds along them from the heart. For in several animals the arteries do not apparently differ from the veins; and in extreme parts of the body, where the arteries are minutely subdivided, as in the brain, the hand, etc., no one could distinguish the arteries from the veins by the dissimilar characters of their coats; the tunics of both are identical. And then, in an aneurism proceeding from a wounded or eroded artery, the pulsation is precisely the same as in the other arteries, and yet it has no proper arterial tunic. This the learned Riolanus testifies to, along with me, in his Seventh Book.

Nor let any one imagine that the uses of the pulse and the respiration are the same, because under the influence of the same causes, such as running, anger, the warm bath, or any other heating thing, as Galen says, they become more frequent and forcible together. For, not only is experience in opposition to this idea, though Galen endeavors to explain it away, when we see that with excessive repletion the pulse beats more forcibly, whilst the respiration is diminished in amount; but in young persons the pulse is quick, while respiration is slow. So also is it in alarm, and amidst care, and under anxiety of mind; sometimes, too, in fevers, the pulse is rapid, but the respiration is slower than usual.

These and other objections of the same kind may be urged against the opinions mentioned. Nor are the views that are entertained of the offices and pulse of the heart, perhaps, less bound up with great and most inextricable difficulties. The heart, it is vulgarly said, is the fountain and workshop of the vital spirits, the centre from whence life is dispensed to the several parts of the body; and yet it is denied that the right ventricle makes spirits; it is rather held to supply nourishment to the lungs; whence it is maintained that fishes are without any right ventricle (and indeed every animal wants a right ventricle which is unfurnished with lungs), and that the right ventricle is present solely for the sake of the lungs.

1. Why, I ask, when we see that the structure of both ventricles is almost identical, there being the same apparatus of fibres, and braces, and valves, and vessels, and auricles, and in both the same infarction of blood, in the subjects of our dissections, of the like black colour, and coagulated—why, I say, should their uses be imagined to be different, when the action, motion, and pulse of both are the same? If the three tricuspid valves placed at the entrance into the right ventricle prove obstacles to the reflux of blood into the vena cava, and if the three semilunar valves, which are situated at the commencement of the pulmonary artery be there, that they may prevent the return of blood into the ventricle; wherefore, when we find similar structures in connexion with the left ventricle, should we deny that they are there for the same end, of preventing here the egress, there the regurgitation of the blood?

2. And again, when we see that these structures, in point of size, form, and situation, are almost in every respect the same in the left as in the right ventricle, wherefore should it be maintained that things are here arranged in connexion with the egress and regress of spirits, there, i.e., in the right, of blood. The same arrangement cannot be held fitted to favor or impede the motion of blood and of spirits indifferently.

3. And when we observe that the passages and vessels are severally in relation to one another in point of size, viz., the pulmonary artery to the pulmonary veins; wherefore should the one be imagined destined to a private or particular purpose, that to wit, of nourishing the lungs, the other to a public and general function?

4. And, as Realdus Columbus says, how can it be conceived that such a quantity of blood should be required for the nutrition of the lungs; the vessel that leads to them, the vena arteriosa or pulmonary artery being of greater capacity than both the iliac veins?

5. And I ask further; as the lungs are so close at hand, and in continual motion, and the vessel that supplies them is of such dimensions, what is the use or meaning of the pulse of the right ventricle? And why was nature reduced to the necessity of adding another ventricle for the sole purpose of nourishing the lungs?

When it is said that the left ventricle obtains materials for the formation of spirits, air to wit, and blood, from the lungs and right sinuses of the heart, and in like manner sends spiritous blood into the aorta, drawing fuliginous vapours from thence, and sending them by the arteria venosa into the lungs, whence spirits are at the same time obtained for transmission into the aorta, I ask how, and by what means, is the separation effected? And how comes it that spirits and fuliginous vapours can pass hither and thither without admixture or confusion? If the mitral cuspidate valves do not prevent the egress of fuliginous vapours to the lungs, how should they oppose the escape of air? And how should the semilunars hinder the regress of spirits from the aorta upon each supervening diastole of the heart? And, above all, how can they say that the spiritous blood is sent from the arteria venalis (pulmonary veins) by the left ventricle into the lungs without any obstacle to its passage from the mitral valves, when they have previously asserted that the air entered by the same vessel from the lungs into the left ventricle, and have brought forward these same mitral valves as obstacles to its retrogression? Good God! how should the mitral valves prevent regurgitation of air and not of blood?

Further, when they dedicate the vena arteriosa (or pulmonary artery), a vessel of great size, and having the tunics of an artery, to none but a kind of private or single purpose, that, namely, of nourishing the lungs, why should the arteria venalis (or pulmonary veins), which is scarcely of similar size, which has the coats of a vein, and is soft and lax, be presumed to be made for many—three or four, different uses? For they will have it that air passes through this vessel from the lungs into the left ventricle; that fuliginous vapours escape by it from the heart into the lungs; and that a portion of the spiritous or spiritualized blood is distributed by it to the lungs for their refreshment.

If they will have it that fumes and air—fumes flowing from, air proceeding towards the heart—are transmitted by the same conduit, I reply, that nature is not wont to institute but one vessel, to contrive but one way for such contrary motions and purposes, nor is anything of the kind seen elsewhere.

If fumes or fuliginous vapours and air permeate this vessel, as they do the pulmonary bronchia, wherefore do we find neither air nor fuliginous vapours when we divide the arteria venosa? Why do we always find this vessel full of sluggish blood, never of air? Whilst in the lungs we find abundance of air remaining.

If any one will perform Galen's experiment of dividing the trachea of a living dog, forcibly distending the lungs with a pair of bellows, and then tying the trachea securely, he will find, when he has laid open the thorax, abundance of air in the lungs, even to their extreme investing tunic, but none in either pulmonary veins, or left ventricle of the heart. But did the heart either attract air from the lungs, or did the lungs transmit any air to the heart, in the living dog, by so much the more ought this to be the case in the experiment just referred to. Who, indeed, doubts that, did he inflate the lungs of a subject in the dissecting-room, he would instantly see the air making its way by this route, were there actually any such passage for it? But this office of the pulmonary veins, namely, the transference of air from the lungs to the heart, is held of such importance, that Hieronymus Fabricius, of Aquapendente, maintains the lungs were made for the sake of this vessel, and that it constitutes the principal element in their structure.

But I should like to be informed wherefore, if the pulmonary vein were destined for the conveyance of air, it has the structure of a blood-vessel here. Nature had rather need of annular tubes, such as those of the bronchia, in order that they might always remain open, not have been liable to collapse; and that they might continue entirely free from blood, lest the liquid should interfere with the passage of the air, as it so obviously does when the lungs labour from being either greatly oppressed or loaded in a less degree with phlegm, as they are when the breathing is performed with a sibilous or rattling noise.

Still less is that opinion to be tolerated which (as a two-fold matter, one aëreal, one sanguineous, is required for the composition of vital spirits) supposes the blood to ooze through the septum of the heart from the right to the left ventricle by certain secret pores, and the air to be attracted from the lungs through the great vessel, the pulmonary vein; and which will have it consequently, that there are numerous pores in the septum cordis adapted for the transmission of the blood. But, in faith, no such pores can be demonstrated, neither in fact do any such exist. For the septum of the heart is of a denser and more compact structure than any portion of the body, except the bones and sinews. But even supposing that there were foramina or pores in this situation, how could one of the ventricles extract anything from the other—the left, e.g., obtain blood from the right, when we see that both ventricles contract and dilate simultaneously? Wherefore should we not rather believe that the right took spirits from the left, than that the left obtained blood from the right ventricle, through these foramina? But it is certainly mysterious and incongruous that blood should be supposed to be most commodiously drawn through a set of obscure or invisible pores, and air through perfectly open passages, at one and the same moment. And why, I ask, is recourse had to secret and invisible porosities, to uncertain and obscure channels, to explain the passage of the blood into the left ventricle, when there is so open a way through the pulmonary veins? I own it has always appeared extraordinary to me that they should have chosen to make, or rather to imagine, a way through the thick, hard, and extremely compact substance of the septum cordis, rather than to take that by the open vas venosum or pulmonary vein, or even through the lax, soft and spongy substance of the lungs at large. Besides, if the blood could permeate the substance of the septum, or could be imbibed from the ventricles, what use were there for the coronary artery and vein, branches of which proceed to the septum itself, to supply it with nourishment? And what is especially worthy of notice is this: if in the foetus, where everything is more lax and soft, nature saw herself reduced to the necessity of bringing the blood from the right into the left side of the heart by the foramen ovale, from the vena cava through the arteria venosa, how should it be likely that in the adult she should pass it so commodiously, and without an effort, through the septum ventriculorum, which has now become denser by age?

Andreas Laurentius,[1] resting on the authority of Galen[2] and the experience of Hollerius, asserts and proves that the serum and pus in empyema, absorbed from the cavities of the chest into the pulmonary vein, may be expelled and got rid of with the urine and faeces through the left ventricle of the heart and arteries. He quotes the case of a certain person affected with melancholia, and who suffered from repeated fainting fits, who was relieved from the paroxysms on passing a quantity of turbid, fetid, and acrid urine; but he died at last, worn out by the disease; and when the body came to be opened after death, no fluid like that he had micturated was discovered either in the bladder or in the kidneys; but in the left ventricle of the heart and cavity of the thorax plenty of it was met with; and then Laurentius boasts that he had predicted the cause of the symptoms. For my own part, however, I cannot but wonder, since he had divined and predicted that heterogenous matter could be discharged by the course he indicates, why he could not or would not perceive, and inform us that, in the natural state of things, the blood might be commodiously transferred from the lungs to the left ventricle of the heart by the very same route.

Since, therefore, from the foregoing considerations and many others to the same effect, it is plain that what has heretofore been said concerning the motion and function of the heart and arteries must appear obscure, or inconsistent or even impossible to him who carefully considers the entire subject; it will be proper to look more narrowly into the matter; to contemplate the motion of the heart and arteries, not only in man, but

[1]Lib. ix, cap. xi quest. 12.
[2]De Locis Affectis., lib. vi, cap. 7.

in all animals that have hearts; and further, by frequent appeals to vivisection, and constant ocular inspection, to investigate and endeavor to find the truth.

CHAPTER I

THE AUTHOR'S MOTIVES FOR WRITING

When I first gave my mind to vivisections, as a means of discovering the motions and uses of the heart, and sought to discover these from actual inspection, and not from the writings of others, I found the task so truly arduous, so full of difficulties, that I was almost tempted to think, with Fracastorius, that the motion of the heart was only to be comprehended by God. For I could neither rightly perceive at first when the systole and when the diastole took place, nor when and where dilatation and contraction occurred, by reason of the rapidity of the motion, which in many animals is accomplished in the twinkling of an eye, coming and going like a flash of lightning; so that the systole presented itself to me now from this point, now from that; the diastole the same; and then everything was reversed, the motions occurring, as it seemed, variously and confusedly together. My mind was therefore greatly unsettled, nor did I know what I should myself conclude, nor what believe from others; I was not surprised that Andreas Laurentius should have said that the motion of the heart was as perplexing as the flux and reflux of Euripus had appeared to Aristotle.

At length, and by using greater and daily diligence, having frequent recourse to vivisections, employing a variety of animals for the purpose, and collating numerous observations, I thought that I had attained to the truth, that I should extricate myself and escape from this labyrinth, and that I had discovered what I so much desired, both the motion and the use of the heart and arteries; since which time I have not hesitated to expose my views upon these subjects, not only in private to my friends, but also in public, in my anatomical lectures, after the manner of the Academy of old.

These views, as usual, pleased some more, others less; some chid and calumniated me, and laid it to me as a crime that I had dared to depart from the precepts and opinion of all anatomists; others desired further explanations of the novelties, which they said were both worthy of consideration, and might perchance be found of signal use. At length, yielding to the requests of my friends, that all might be made participators in my labours, and partly moved by the envy of others, who, receiving my views with uncandid minds and understanding them indifferently, have essayed to traduce me publicly, I have been moved to commit these things to the press, in order that all may be enabled to form an opinion both of me and my labours. This step I take all the more willingly, seeing that Hieronymus Fabricius of Aquapendente, although he has accurately and learnedly delineated almost every one of the several parts of animals in a special work, has left the heart alone untouched. Finally, if any use or benefit to this department of the republic of letters should accrue from my labours, it will, perhaps, be allowed that I have not lived idly, and, as the old man in the comedy says:

> For never yet hath any one attained
> To such perfection, but that time, and place,
> And use, have brought addition to his knowledge;
> Or made correction, or admonished him,
> That he was ignorant of much which he
> Had thought he knew; or led him to reject
> What he had once esteemed of highest price.

So will it, perchance, be found with reference to the heart at this time; or others, at least, starting from hence, the way pointed out to them, advancing under the guidance of a happier genius, may make occasion to proceed more fortunately, and to inquire more accurately.

CHAPTER II

OF THE MOTIONS OF THE HEART, AS SEEN IN THE DISSECTION OF LIVING ANIMALS

In the first place, then, when the chest of a living animal is laid open and the capsule that immediately surrounds the heart is slit up or removed, the organ is seen now to move, now to be at rest;—there is a time when it moves, and a time when it is motionless.

These things are more obvious in the colder animals, such as toads, frogs, serpents, small fishes, crabs, shrimps, snails and shell-fish. They also become more distinct in warm-blooded animals, such as the dog and the hog, if they be attentively noted when the heart begins to flag, to move more slowly, and, as it were, to die: the movements then become slower and rarer, the pauses longer, by which it is made much more easy to perceive and unravel what the motions really are, and how they are performed. In the pause, as in death, the heart is soft, flaccid, exhausted, lying, as it were, at rest.

In the motion, and interval in which this is accomplished, three principal circumstances are to be noted:

1. That the heart is erected, and rises upward to a point, so that at this time it strikes against the breast and the pulse is felt externally.

2. That it is everywhere contracted, but more especially towards the sides, so that it looks narrower, relatively longer, more drawn together. The heart of an eel taken out of the body of the animal and placed upon the table or the hand, shows these particulars; but the same things are manifest in the heart of small fishes and of those colder animals where the organ is more conical or elongated.

3. The heart being grasped in the hand, is felt to become harder during its action. Now this hardness proceeds from tension, precisely as when the forearm is grasped, its tendons are perceived to become tense and resilient when the fingers are moved.

4. It may further be observed in fishes, and the colder blooded animals, such as frogs, serpents, etc., that the heart, when it moves, becomes of a paler colour, when quiescent of a deeper blood-red colour.

From these particulars it appeared evident to me that the motion of the heart consists in a certain universal tension—both contraction in the line of its fibres, and constriction in every sense. It becomes erect, hard, and of diminished size during its action; the motion is plainly of the same nature as that of the muscles when they contract in the line of their sinews and fibres; for the muscles, when in action, acquire vigour and tenseness, and from soft become hard, prominent and thickened: in the same manner the heart.

We are therefore authorized to conclude that the heart, at the moment of its action, is at once constricted on all sides, rendered thicker in its parietes and smaller in its ventricles, and so made apt to project or expel its charge of blood. This, indeed, is made sufficiently manifest by the fourth observation preceding in which we have seen that the heart, by squeezing out the blood it contains becomes paler, and then when it sinks into repose and the ventricle is filled anew with blood, that the deeper crimson colour returns. But no one need remain in doubt of the fact, for if the ventricle be pierced the blood will be seen to be forcibly projected outwards upon each motion or pulsation when the heart is tense.

These things, therefore, happen together or at the same instant: the tension of the heart, the pulse of its apex, which is felt externally by its striking against the chest, the thickening of its parietes, and the forcible expulsion of the blood it contains by the constriction of its ventricles.

Hence the very opposite of the opinions commonly received, appears to be true; inasmuch as it is generally believed that when the heart strikes the breast and the pulse is felt without, the heart is dilated in its ventricles and is filled with blood; but the contrary of this is the fact, and the heart, when it contracts [and the shock is given], is emptied. Whence the motion which is generally regarded as the diastole of the heart, is in truth its systole. And in like manner the intrinsic motion of the heart is not the diastole but the systole; neither is it in the diastole that the heart grows firm and tense, but in the systole, for then only, when tense, is it moved and made vigorous.

Neither is it by any means to be allowed that the heart only moves in the line of its straight fibres, although the great Vesalius, giving this notion countenance, quotes a bundle of osiers bound into a pyramidal heap in illustration; meaning, that as the apex is approached to the base, so are the sides made to bulge out in the fashion of arches, the cavities to dilate, the ventricles to acquire the form of a cupping-glass and so to suck in the blood. But the true effect of every one of its fibres is to constringe the heart at the same time that they render it tense; and this rather with the effect of thickening and amplifying the walls and substance of the organ than enlarging its ventricles. And, again, as the fibres run from the apex to the base, and draw the apex towards the base, they do not tend to make the walls of the heart bulge out in circles, but rather the contrary; inasmuch as every fibre that is circularly disposed tends to become straight when it contracts; and is distended laterally and thickened, as in the case of muscular fibres in general, when they contract, that is when they are shortened longitudinally, as we see them in the bellies of the muscles of the body at large. To all this let it be added that not only are the ventricles contracted in virtue of the direction and condensation of their walls, but farther, that those fibres, or bands, styled nerves by Aristotle, which are so conspicuous in the ventricles of the larger animals, and contain all the straight fibers, (the parietes of the heart containing only circular ones,) when they contract simultaneously, by an admirable adjustment all the internal surfaces are drawn together, as if with cords, and so is the charge of blood expelled with force.

Neither is it true, as vulgarly believed, that the heart by any dilatation or motion of its own, has the power of drawing the blood into the ventricles; for when it acts and becomes tense, the blood is expelled; when it relaxes and sinks together it receives the blood in the manner and wise which will by and by be explained.

CHAPTER III

OF THE MOTIONS OF ARTERIES, AS SEEN IN THE DISSECTION OF LIVING ANIMALS

In connexion with the motions of the heart these things are further to be observed having reference to the motions and pulses of the arteries:

1. At the moment the heart contracts, and when the breast is struck, when in short the organ is in its state of systole, the arteries are dilated, yield a pulse, and are in the state of diastole. In like manner, when the right ventricle contracts and propels its charge of blood, the arterial vein [the pulmonary artery] is distended at the same time with the other arteries of the body.

2. When the left ventricle ceases to act, to contract, to pulsate, the pulse in the arteries also ceases; further, when this ventricle contracts languidly, the pulse in the arteries is scarcely perceptible. In like manner, the pulse in the right ventricle failing, the pulse in the vena arteriosa [pulmonary artery] ceases also.

3. Further, when an artery is divided or punctured, the blood is seen to be forcibly propelled from the wound at the moment the left ventricle contracts; and, again, when the pulmonary artery is wounded, the blood will be seen spouting forth with violence at the instant when the right ventricle contracts.

So also in fishes, if the vessel which leads from the heart to the gills be divided, at the moment when the heart becomes tense and contracted, at the same moment does the blood flow with force from the divided vessel.

In the same way, finally, when we see the blood in arteriotomy projected now to a greater, now to a less distance, and that the greater jet corresponds to the diastole of the artery and to the time when the heart contracts and strikes the ribs, and is in its state of systole, we understand that the blood is expelled by the same movement.

From these facts, it is manifest, in opposition to commonly received opinions, that the diastole of the arteries corresponds with the time of the heart's systole; and that the arteries are filled and distended by the blood forced into them by the contraction of the ventricles; the arteries, therefore, are distended, because they are filled like sacs or bladders, and are not filled because they expand like bellows. It is in virtue of one and the same cause, therefore, that all the arteries of the body pulsate, viz., the contraction of the left ventricle; in the same way as the pulmonary artery pulsates by the contraction of the right ventricle.

Finally, that the pulses of the arteries are due to the impulses of the blood from the left ventricle, may be illustrated by blowing into a glove, when the whole of the fingers will be found to become distended at one and the same time, and in their tension to bear some resemblance to the pulse. For in the ratio of the tension is the pulse of the heart, fuller, stronger, more frequent as that acts more vigorously, still preserving the rhythm and volume, and order of the heart's contractions. Nor is it to be expected that because of the motion of the blood, the time at which the contraction of the heart takes place, and that at which the pulse in an artery (especially a distant one) is felt, shall be otherwise than simultaneous: it is here the same as in blowing up a glove or bladder; for in a plenum (as in a drum, a long piece of timber, etc.) the stroke and the motion occur at both extremities at the same time. Aristotle,[1] too, has said, "the blood of all animals palpitates within their veins (meaning the arteries), and by the pulse is sent everywhere simultaneously." And further,[2] "thus do all the veins pulsate together and by successive strokes, because they all depend upon the heart; and, as it is always in motion, so are they likewise always moving together, but by successive movements." It is well to observe with Galen, in this place, that the old philosophers called the arteries veins.

---

[1]De Animal. iii, cap. 9.
[2]De Respirat. cap. 20.

I happened upon one occasion to have a particular case under my care, which plainly satisfied me of this truth: A certain person was affected with a large pulsating tumour on the right side of the neck, called an aneurism, just at that part where the artery descends into the axilla, produced by an erosion of the artery itself, and daily increasing in size: this tumour was visibly distended as it received the charge of blood brought to it by the artery, with each stroke of the heart: the connexion of parts was obvious when the body of the patient came to be opened after his death. The pulse in the corresponding arm was small, in consequence of the greater portion of the blood being diverted into the tumour and so intercepted.

Whence it appears that wherever the motion of the blood through the arteries is impeded, whether it be by compression or infarction, or interception, there do the remote divisions of the arteries beat less forcibly, seeing that the pulse of the arteries is nothing more than the impulse or shock of the blood in these vessels.

CHAPTER IV

OF THE MOTION OF THE HEART AND ITS AURICLES, AS SEEN IN THE BODIES OF LIVING ANIMALS

Besides the motions already spoken of, we have still to consider those that appertain to the auricles.

Caspar Bauhin and John Riolan,[1] most learned men and skilful anatomists, inform us from their observations, that if we carefully watch the movements of the heart in the vivisection of an animal, we shall perceive four motions distinct in time and place, two of which are proper to the auricles, two to the ventricles. With all deference to such authority I say, that there are four motions distinct in point of place, but not of time; for the two auricles move together, and so also do the two ventricles, in such wise that though the places be four, the times are only two. And this occurs in the following manner:

There are, as it were, two motions going on together; one of the auricles, another of the ventricles; these by no means taking place simultaneously, but the motion of the auricles preceding, that of the heart itself following; the motion appearing to begin from the auricles and to extend to the ventricles. When all things are becoming languid, and the heart is dying, as also in fishes and the colder blooded animals, there is a short pause between these two motions, so that the heart aroused, as it were, appears to respond to the motion, now more quickly, now more tardily; and at length, and when near to death, it ceases to respond by its proper motion, but seems, as it were, to nod the head, and is so obscurely moved that it appears to give signs of motion to the pulsating

[1]Bauhin, lib. ii, cap. 21. Riolan, lib. viii, cap. 1.

auricle, rather than actually to move. The heart, therefore, ceases to pulsate sooner than the auricles, so that the auricles have been said to outlive it, the left ventricle ceasing to pulsate first of all: then its auricle, next the right ventricle; and, finally, all the other parts being at rest and dead, as Galen long since observed, the right auricle still continues to beat; life, therefore, appears to linger longest in the right auricle. Whilst the heart is gradually dying, it is sometimes seen to reply, after two or three contractions of the auricles, roused as it were to action, and making a single pulsation, slowly, unwillingly, and with an effort.

But this especially is to be noted, that after the heart has ceased to beat, the auricles however still contracting, a finger placed upon the ventricles perceives the several pulsations of the auricles, precisely in the same way and for the same reason, as we have said, that the pulses of the ventricles are felt in the arteries, to wit, the distension produced by the jet of blood. And if at this time, the auricles alone pulsating, the point of the heart be cut off with a pair of scissors, you will perceive the blood flowing out upon each contraction of the auricles. Whence it is manifest how the blood enters the ventricles, not by any attraction or dilatation of the heart, but thrown into them by the pulses of the auricles.

And here I would observe, that whenever I speak of pulsations as occurring in the auricles or ventricles, I mean contractions: first the auricles *contract,* and then and subsequently the heart itself *contracts.* When the auricles contract they are seen to become whiter, especially where they contain but little blood; but they are filled as magazines or reservoirs of the blood, which is tending spontaneously and, by the motion of the veins, under pressure towards the centre; the whiteness indicated is most conspicuous towards the extremities or edges of the auricles at the time of their contractions.

In fishes and frogs, and other animals which have hearts with but a single ventricle, and for an auricle have a kind of bladder much distended with blood, at the base of the organ, you may very plainly perceive this bladder contracting first, and the contraction of the heart or ventricle following afterwards.

But I think it right to describe what I have observed of an opposite character: the heart of an eel, of several fishes, and even of some [of the higher] animals taken out of the body, beats without auricles; nay, if it be cut in pieces the several parts may still be seen contracting and relaxing; so that in these creatures the body of the heart may be seen pulsating, palpitating, after the cessation of all motion in the auricle. But is not this perchance peculiar to animals more tenacious of life, whose radical moisture is more glutinous, or fat and sluggish, and less readily soluble? The same faculty indeed appears in the flesh of eels, generally, which even when skinned and embowelled, and cut into pieces, are still seen to move.

Experimenting with a pigeon upon one occasion, after the heart had wholly ceased to pulsate, and the auricles too had become motionless, I kept my finger wetted with saliva and warm for a short time upon the heart, and observed, that under the influence of this fomentation it recovered new strength and life, so that both ventricles and auricles pulsated, contracting and relaxing alternately, recalled as it were from death to life.

Besides this, however, I have occasionally observed, after the heart and even its right auricle had ceased pulsating,—when it was in articulo mortis in short, that an obscure motion, an indulation or palpitation, remained in the blood itself, which was contained in the right auricle, this being apparent so long as it was imbued with heat and spirit. And indeed a circumstance of the same kind is extremely manifest in the course of the generation of animals, as may be seen in the course of the first seven days of the incubation of the chick: A drop of blood makes its appearance which palpitates, as Aristotle had already observed; from this, when the growth is further advanced and the chick is fashioned, the auricles of the heart are formed, which pulsating henceforth give constant signs of life. When at length, and after the lapse of a few days, the outline of the body begins to be distinguished, then is the ventricular part of the heart also produced; but it continues for a time white and apparently bloodless, like the rest of the animal; neither does it pulsate or give signs of motion. I have seen a similar condition of the heart in the human foetus about the beginning of the third month, the heart being then whitish and bloodless, although its auricles contained a considerable quantity of purple blood. In the same way in the egg, when the chick was formed and had increased in size, the heart too increased and acquired ventricles, which then began to receive and to transmit blood.

And this leads me to remark, that he who inquires very particularly into this matter will not conclude that the heart, as a whole, is the primum vivens, ultimum moriens—the first part to live, the last to die, but rather its auricles, or the part which corresponds to the auricles in serpents, fishes, etc., which both lives before the heart[1] and dies after it.

Nay, has not the blood itself or spirit an obscure palpitation inherent in it, which it has even appeared to me to retain after death? And it seems very questionable whether or not we are to say that life begins with the palpitation or beating of the heart. The seminal fluid of all animals—the prolific spirit, as Aristotle observed, leaves their body with a bound and like a living thing; and nature in death, as Aristotle[2] further remarks, retracing her steps, reverts to whence she had set out, returns at the end of her course to the goal whence she had started; and as animal

[1]The reader will observe that Harvey, when he speaks of the *heart,* always means the ventricles or ventricular portion of the organ [Willis, 1847].

[2]De Motu Animal. cap. 8.

generation proceeds from that which is not animal, entity from non-entity, so, by a retrograde course, entity, by corruption, is resolved into non-entity; whence that in animals, which was last created, fails first; and that which was first, fails last.

I have also observed, that almost all animals have truly a heart, not the larger creatures only and those that have red blood, but the smaller, and [seemingly] bloodless ones also, such as slugs, snails, scallops, shrimps, crabs, crayfish, and many others; nay, even in wasps, hornets and flies, I have, with the aid of a magnifying glass, and at the upper part of what is called the tail, both seen the heart pulsating myself, and shown it to many others.

But in the exsanguine tribes the heart pulsates sluggishly and deliberately, contracting slowly as in animals that are moribund, a fact that may readily be seen in the snail, whose heart will be found at the bottom of that orifice in the right side of the body which is seen to be opened and shut in the course of respiration, and whence saliva is discharged, the incision being made in the upper aspect of the body, near the part which corresponds to the liver.

This, however, is to be observed: that in winter and the colder season, exsanguine animals, such as the snail, show no pulsations; they seem rather to live after the manner of vegetables, or of those other productions which are therefore designated plant-animals.

It is also to be noted that all animals which have a heart, have also auricles, or something analogous to auricles; and further, that wherever the heart has a double ventricle there are always two auricles present, but not otherwise. If you turn to the production of the chick in ovo, however, you will find at first no more than a vesicle or auricle, or pulsating drop of blood; it is only by and by, when the development has made some progress, that the heart is fashioned: even so in certain animals not destined to attain to the highest perfection in their organization, such as bees, wasps, snails, shrimps, crayfish, etc., we only find a certain pulsating vesicle, like a sort of red or white palpitating point, as the beginning or principle of their life.[1]

We have a small shrimp in these countries, which is taken in the Thames and in the sea, the whole of whose body is transparent; this creature, placed in a little water, has frequently afforded myself and particular friends an opportunity of observing the motions of the heart with the greatest distinctness, the external parts of the body presenting no obstacle to our view, but the heart being perceived as though it had been seen through a window.

I have also observed the first rudiments of the chick in the course of the fourth or fifth day of the incubation in the guise of a little cloud, the

[1]The Editor begs here to be allowed to remark on Harvey's obvious perception of the correspondence between that permanent condition of an organ in the lower, and its transitory condition in the higher animals [Willis, 1847].

shell having been removed and the egg immersed in clear tepid water. In the midst of the cloudlet in question there was a bloody point so small that it disappeared during the contraction and escaped the sight, but in the relaxation it reappeared again, red and like the point of a pin; so that betwixt the visible and invisible, betwixt being and not being, as it were, it gave by its pulses a kind of representation of the commencement of life.[1]

CHAPTER V

OF THE MOTION, ACTION, AND OFFICE OF THE HEART

From these and other observations of the like kind, I am persuaded it will be found that the motion of the heart is as follows:

First of all, the auricle contracts, and in the course of its contraction throws the blood (which it contains in ample quantity as the head of the veins, the store-house and cistern of the blood) into the ventricle, which being filled, the heart raises itself straightway, makes all its fibres tense, contracts the ventricles, and performs a beat, by which beat it immediately sends the blood supplied to it by the auricle into the arteries; the right ventricle sending its charge into the lungs by the vessel which is called vena arteriosa, but which, in structure and function, and all things else, is an artery; the left ventricle sending its charge into the aorta, and through this by the arteries to the body at large.

These two motions, one of the ventricles, another of the auricles, take place consecutively, but in such a manner that there is a kind of harmony or rhythm preserved between them, the two concurring in such wise that but one motion is apparent, especially in the warmer blooded animals, in which the movements in question are rapid. Nor is this for any other reason than it is in a piece of machinery, in which, though one wheel gives motion to another, yet all the wheels seem to move simultaneously; or in that mechanical contrivance which is adapted to fire-arms, where the trigger being touched, down comes the flint, strikes against the steel, elicits a spark, which falling among the powder, is ignited, upon which the flame extends, enters the barrel, causes the explosion, propels the ball and the mark is attained—all of which incidents, by reason of the celerity with which they happen, seem to take place in the twinkling of an eye. So also in deglutition: by the elevation of the root of the tongue, and the compression of the mouth, the food or drink is pushed into the fauces, the larynx is closed by its own muscles, and the epiglottis, whilst the pharynx, raised and opened by its muscles no otherwise than is a sac that is to be filled, is lifted up, and its mouth dilated; upon which, the mouthful being received, it is forced downwards by the

[1]At the period Harvey indicates, a rudimentary auricle and ventricle exist, but are so transparent that unless with certain precautions their parietes cannot be seen. The filling and emptying of them, therefore, give the appearance of a speck of blood alternately appearing and disappearing [Willis, 1847].

transverse muscles, and then carried farther by the longitudinal ones. Yet are all these motions, though executed by different and distinct organs, performed harmoniously, and in such order, that they seem to constitute but a single motion and act, which we call deglutition.

Even so does it come to pass with the motions and action of the heart, which constitute a kind of deglutition, a transfusion of the blood from the veins to the arteries. And if any one, bearing these things in mind, will carefully watch the motions of the heart in the body of a living animal, he will perceive not only all the particulars I have mentioned, viz., the heart becoming erect, and making one continuous motion with its auricles; but farther, a certain obscure undulation and lateral inclination in the direction of the axis of the right ventricle [the organ], twisting itself slightly in performing its work. And indeed every one may see, when a horse drinks, that the water is drawn in and transmitted to the stomach at each movement of the throat, the motion being accompanied with a sound, and yielding a pulse both to the ear and the touch; in the same way it is with each motion of the heart, when there is the delivery of a quantity of blood from the veins to the arteries, that a pulse takes place, and can be heard within the chest.

The motion of the heart, then, is entirely of this description, and the one action of the heart is the transmission of the blood and its distribution, by means of the arteries, to the very extremities of the body; so that the pulse which we feel in the arteries is nothing more than the impulse of the blood derived from the heart.

Whether or not the heart, besides propelling the blood, giving it motion locally, and distributing it to the body, adds anything else to it,—heat, spirit, perfection,—must be inquired into by and by, and decided upon other grounds. So much may suffice at this time, when it is shown that by the action of the heart the blood is transfused through the ventricles from the veins to the arteries, and distributed by them to all parts of the body.

So much, indeed, is admitted by all [physiologists], both from the structure of the heart and the arrangement and action of its valves. But still they are like persons purblind or groping about in the dark; and then they give utterance to diverse, contradictory, and incoherent sentiments, delivering many things upon conjecture, as we have already had occasion to remark.

The grand cause of hesitation and error in this subject appears to me to have been the intimate connexion between the heart and the lungs. When men saw both the vena arteriosa [or pulmonary artery] and the arteriae venosae [or pulmonary veins] losing themselves in the lungs, of course it became a puzzle to them to know how or by what means the right ventricle should distribute the blood to the body, or the left draw it from the venae cavae. This fact is borne witness to by Galen, whose words, when writing against Erasistratus in regard to the origin and use of the veins and the coction of the blood, are the following:[1] "You will reply," he says, "that the effect is so; that the blood is prepared in the liver, and is thence transferred to the heart to receive its proper form and last perfection; a statement which does not appear devoid of reason; for no great and perfect work is ever accomplished at a single effort, or receives its final polish from one instrument. But if this be actually so, then show us another vessel which draws the absolutely perfect blood from the heart, and distributes it as the arteries do the spirits over the whole body." Here then is a reasonable opinion not allowed, because, forsooth, besides not seeing the true means of transit, he could not discover the vessel which should transmit the blood from the heart to the body at large!

But had any one been there in behalf of Erasistratus, and of that opinion which we now espouse, and which Galen himself acknowledges in other respects consonant with reason, to have pointed to the aorta as the vessel which distributes the blood from the heart to the rest of the body, I wonder what would have been the answer of that most ingenious and learned man? Had he said that the artery transmits spirits and not blood, he would indeed sufficiently have answered Erasistratus, who imagined that the arteries contained nothing but spirits; but then he would have contradicted himself, and given a foul denial to that for which he had keenly contended in his writings against this very Erasistratus, to wit, that blood in substance is contained in the arteries, and not spirits; a fact which he demonstrated not only by many powerful arguments, but by experiments.

But if the divine Galen will here allow, as in other places he does, "that all the arteries of the body arise from the great artery, and that this takes its origin from the heart; that all these vessels naturally contain and carry blood; that the three semilunar valves situated at the orifice of the aorta prevent the return of the blood into the heart, and that nature never connected them with this, the most noble viscus of the body, unless for some most important end"; if, I say, this father of physic admits all these things,—and I quote his own words,—I do not see how he can deny that the great artery is the very vessel to carry the blood, when it has attained its highest term of perfection, from the heart for distribution to all parts of the body. Or would he perchance still hesitate, like all who have come after him, even to the present hour, because he did not perceive the route by which the blood was transferred from the veins to the arteries, in consequence, as I have already said, of the intimate connexion between the heart and the lungs? And that this difficulty puzzled anatomists not a little, when in their dissections they found the pulmonary artery and left ventricle full of thick, black, and clotted blood, plainly appears, when they felt themselves compelled to

[1] De Placitis Hippocratis et Platonis, vi.

affirm that the blood made its way from the right to the left ventricle by sweating through the septum of the heart. But this fancy I have already refuted. A new pathway for the blood must therefore be prepared and thrown open, and being once exposed, no further difficulty will, I believe, be experienced by anyone in admitting what I have already proposed in regard to the pulse of the heart and arteries, viz. the passage of the blood from the veins to the arteries, and its distribution to the whole of the body by means of these vessels.

CHAPTER VI

OF THE COURSE BY WHICH THE BLOOD IS CARRIED FROM THE VENA CAVA INTO THE ARTERIES, OR FROM THE RIGHT INTO THE LEFT VENTRICLE OF THE HEART

Since the intimate connexion of the heart with the lungs, which is apparent in the human subject, has been the probable cause of the errors that have been committed on this point, they plainly do amiss who, pretending to speak of the parts of animals generally, as anatomists for the most part do, confine their researches to the human body alone, and that when it is dead. They obviously act no otherwise than he who, having studied the forms of a single commonwealth, should set about the composition of a general system of polity; or who, having taken cognizance of the nature of a single field, should imagine that he had mastered the science of agriculture; or who, upon the ground of one particular proposition, should proceed to draw general conclusions.

Had anatomists only been as conversant with the dissection of the lower animals as they are with that of the human body, the matters that have hitherto kept them in a perplexity of doubt would, in my opinion, have met them freed from every kind of difficulty.

And, first, in fishes, in which the heart consists of but a single ventricle, they having no lungs, the thing is sufficiently manifest. Here the sac, which is situated at the base of the heart, and is the part analogous to the auricle in man, plainly throws the blood into the heart, and the heart, in its turn, conspicuously transmits it by a pipe or artery, or vessel analogous to an artery; these are facts which are confirmed by simple ocular inspection, as well as by a division of the vessel, when the blood is seen to be projected by each pulsation of the heart.

The same thing is also not difficult of demonstration in those animals that have either no more, or, as it were, no more than a single ventricle to the heart, such as toads, frogs, serpents, and lizards, which, although they have lungs in a certain sense, as they have a voice (and I have many observations by me on the admirable structure of the lungs of these animals, and matters apertaining which, however, I cannot introduce in this place), still their anatomy plainly shows that the blood is transferred in them from the veins to the arteries in the same manner as in higher animals, viz., by the action of the heart; the way, in fact, is patent, open, manifest; there is no difficulty, no room for hesitating about it; for in them the matter stands precisely as it would in man, were the septum of his heart perforated or removed, or one ventricle made out of two; and this being the case, I imagine that no one will doubt as to the way by which the blood may pass from the veins into the arteries.

But as there are actually more animals which have no lungs than there are which be furnished with them, and in like manner a greater number which have only one ventricle than there are which have two, it is open to us to conclude, judging from the mass or multitude of living creatures, that for the major part, and generally, there is an open way by which the blood is transmitted from the veins through the sinuses or cavities of the heart into the arteries.

I have, however, cogitating with myself, seen further, that the same thing obtained most obviously in the embryos of those animals that have lungs; for in the foetus the four vessels belonging to the heart, viz., the vena cava, the vena arteriosa or pulmonary artery, the arteria venalis or pulmonary vein, and the arteria magna or aorta, are all connected otherwise than in the adult; a fact sufficiently known to every anatomist. The first contact and union of the vena cava with the arteria venosa or pulmonary veins, which occurs before the cava opens properly into the right ventricle of the heart, or gives off the coronary vein, a little above its escape from the liver, is by a lateral anastomosis; this is an ample foramen, of an oval form, communicating between the cava and the arteria venosa, or pulmonary vein, so that the blood is free to flow in the greatest abundance by that foramen from the vena cava into the arteria venosa or pulmonary vein, and left auricle, and from thence into the left ventricle; and farther, in this foramen ovale, from that part which regards the arteria venosa, or pulmonary vein, there is a thin tough membrane, larger than the opening, extended like an operculum or cover; this membrane in the adult blocking up the foramen, and adhering on all sides, finally closes it up, and almost obliterates every trace of it. This membrane, however, is so contrived in the foetus, that falling loosely upon itself, it permits a ready access to the lungs and heart, yielding a passage to the blood which is streaming from the cava, and hindering the tide at the same time from flowing back into that vein. All things, in short, permit us to believe that in the embryo the blood must constantly pass by this foramen from the vena cava into the arteria venosa, or pulmonary vein, and from thence into the left auricle of the heart; and having once entered there, it can never regurgitate.

Another union is that by the vena arteriosa, or pulmonary artery, and is effected when that vessel divides into two branches after its escape from the right ventricle of the heart. It is as if to the two trunks already mentioned a third were superadded, a kind of arterial canal, carried obliquely from the vena arteriosa, or pulmonary artery, to perforate and terminate in the arteria magna or aorta. In the embryo, consequently, there are, as it were, two aortas, or two roots of the arteria magna, springing from the heart. This canalis arteriosus shrinks gradually after birth, and is at length and finally almost entirely withered, and removed, like the Umbilical vessels.

The canalis arteriosus contains no membrane or valve to direct or impede the flow of the blood in this or in that direction: for at the root of the vena arteriosa, or pulmonary artery, of which the canalis arteriosus is the continuation in the foetus, there are three sigmoid or semilunar valves, which open from within outwards, and oppose no obstacle to the blood flowing in this direction or from the right ventricle into the pulmonary artery and aorta; but they prevent all regurgitation from the aorta or pulmonic vessels back upon the right ventricle; closing with perfect accuracy, they oppose an effectual obstacle to everything of the kind in the embryo. So that there is also reason to believe that when the heart contracts, the blood is regularly propelled by the canal or passage indicated from the right ventricle into the aorta.

What is commonly said in regard to these two great communications, to wit, that they exist for the nutrition of the lungs, is both improbable and inconsistent; seeing that in the adult they are closed up, abolished, and consolidated, although the lungs, by reason of their heat and motion, must then be presumed to require a larger supply of nourishment. The same may be said in regard to the assertion that the heart in the embryo does not pulsate, that it neither acts nor moves, so that nature was forced to make these communications for the nutrition of the lungs. This is plainly false; for simple inspection of the incubated egg, and of embryos just taken out of the uterus, shows that the heart moves precisely in them as in adults, and that nature feels no such necessity. I have myself repeatedly seen these motions, and Aristotle is likewise witness of their reality. "The pulse," he observes, "inheres in the very constitution of the heart, and appears from the beginning, as is learned both from the dissection of living animals, and the formation of the chick in the egg."[1] But we further observe, that the passages in question are not only pervious up to the period of birth in man, as well as in other animals, as anatomists in general have described them, but for several months subsequently, in some indeed for several years, not to say for the whole course of life; as, for example, in the goose, snipe, and various birds, and many of the smaller animals. And this circumstance it was, perhaps, that imposed upon Botallus, who thought he had discovered a new passage for the blood from the vena cava into the left ventricle of the heart; and I own that when I met with the same arrangement in one of the

[1]Lib. de Spiritu, cap. v.

larger members of the mouse family, in the adult state, I was myself at first led to something of a like conclusion.

From this it will be understood that in the human embryo, and in the embryos of animals in which the communications are not closed, the same thing happens, namely, that the heart by its motion propels the blood by obvious and open passages from the vena cava into the aorta through the cavities of both the ventricles; the right one receiving the blood from the auricle, and propelling it by the vena arteriosa, or pulmonary artery, and its continuation, named the ductus arteriosus, into the aorta; the left, in like manner, charged by the contraction of its auricle, which has received its supply through the foramen ovale from the vena cava, contracting, and projecting the blood through the root of the aorta into the trunk of that vessel.

In embryos, consequently, whilst the lungs are yet in a state of inaction, performing no function, subject to no motion any more than if they had not been present, nature uses the two ventricles of the heart as if they formed but one, for the transmission of the blood. The condition of the embryos of those animals which have lungs, whilst these organs are yet in abeyance and not employed, is the same as that of those animals which have no lungs.

So clearly, therefore, does it appear in the case of the foetus, viz., that the heart by its action transfers the blood from the vena cava into the aorta, and that by a route as obvious and open, as if in the adult the two ventricles were made to communicate by the removal of their septum. Since, then, we find that in the greater number of animals, in all, indeed, at a certain period of their existence, the channels for the transmission of the blood through the heart are so conspicuous, we have still to inquire wherefore in some creatures—those, namely, that have warm blood, and that have attained to the adult age, man among the number—we should not conclude that the same thing is accomplished through the substance of the lungs, which in the embryo, and at a time when the function of these organs is in abeyance, nature effects by the direct passages described, and which, indeed, she seems compelled to adopt through want of a passage by the lungs; or wherefore it should be better (for nature always does that which is best) that she should close up the various open routes which she had formerly made use of in the embryo and foetus, and still uses in all other animals; not only opening up no new apparent channels for the passage of the blood, therefore, but even entirely shutting up those which formerly existed.

And now the discussion is brought to this point, that they who inquire into the ways by which the blood reaches the left ventricle of the heart and pulmonary veins from the vena cava, will pursue the wisest course if they seek by dissection to discover the causes why in the larger and more perfect animals of mature age, nature has rather chosen to make the blood percolate the parenchyma of the lungs than as in other instances chosen a direct and obvious course—for I assume that no other path or mode of transit can be entertained. It must be either because the larger and more perfect animals are warmer, and when adult their heat greater —ignited, as I might say, and requiring to be damped or mitigated; therefore it may be that the blood is sent through the lungs, that it may be tempered by the air that is inspired, and prevented from boiling up, and so becoming extinguished, or something else of the sort. But to determine these matters, and explain them satisfactorily, were to enter on a speculation in regard to the office of the lungs and the ends for which they exist; and upon such a subject as well as upon what pertains to eventilation, to the necessity and use of the air, etc., as also to the variety and diversity of organs that exist in the bodies of animals in connexion with these matters, although I have made a vast number of observations, still, lest I should be held as wandering too wide of my present purpose, which is the use and motion of the heart, and be charged with speaking of things beside the question, and rather complicating and quitting than illustrating it, I shall leave such topics till I can more conveniently set them forth in a treatise apart. And now, returning to my immediate subject, I go on with what yet remains for demonstration, viz., that in the more perfect and warmer adult animals, and man, the blood passes from the right ventricle of the heart by the vena arteriosa, or pulmonary artery, into the lungs, and thence by the arteriae venosae, or pulmonary veins, into the left auricle, and thence into the left ventricle of the heart. And, first, I shall show that this may be so, and then I shall prove that it is so in fact.

CHAPTER VII

THE BLOOD PERCOLATES THE SUBSTANCE OF THE LUNGS FROM THE RIGHT VENTRICLE OF THE HEART INTO THE PULMONARY VEINS AND LEFT VENTRICLE

That this is possible, and that there is nothing to prevent it from being so, appears when we reflect on the way in which water percolating the earth produces springs and rivulets, or when we speculate on the means by which the sweat passes through the skin, or the urine through the parenchyma of the kidneys. It is well known that persons who use the Spa waters, or those of La Madonna, in the territories of Padua, or others of an acidulous or vitriolated nature, or who simply swallow drinks by the gallon, pass all off again within an hour or two by urine. Such a quantity of liquid must take some short time in the concoction: it must pass through the liver (it is allowed by all that the juices of the food we consume pass twice through this organ in the course of the day); it must flow through the veins, through the parenchyma of the kidneys, and through the ureters into the bladder.

To those, therefore, whom I hear denying that the blood, aye the whole mass of the blood may pass through the substance of the lungs, even as the nutritive juices percolate the liver, asserting such a proposition to be impossible, and by no means to be entertained as credible, I reply, with the poet, that they are of that race of men who, when they will, assent full readily, and when they will not, by no manner of means; who, when their assent is wanted, fear, and when it is not, fear not to give it.

The parenchyma of the liver is extremely dense, so is that of the kidney; the lungs, again, are of a much looser texture, and if compared with the kidneys are absolutely spongy. In the liver there is no forcing, no impelling power; in the lungs the blood is forced on by the pulse of the right ventricle, the necessary effect of whose impulse is the distension of the vessels and pores of the lungs. And then the lungs, in respiration, are perpetually rising and falling; motions, the effect of which must needs be to open and shut the pores and vessels, precisely as in the case of a sponge, and of parts having a spongy structure, when they are alternately compressed and again are suffered to expand. The liver, on the contrary, remains at rest, and is never seen to be dilated and constricted. Lastly, if no one denies the possibility of the whole of the ingested juices passing through the liver, in man, oxen, and the larger animals, generally, in order to reach the vena cava, and for this reason, that if nourishment is to go on, these juices must needs get into the veins, and there is no other way but the one indicated, why should not the same arguments be held of avail for the passage of the blood in adults through the lungs? Why not, with Columbus, that skillful and learned anatomist, maintain and believe the like, from the capacity and structure of the pulmonary vessels; from the fact of the pulmonary veins and ventricle corresponding with them, being always found to contain blood, which must needs have come from the veins, and by no other passage save through the lungs? Columbus, and we also, from what precedes, from dissections, and other arguments, conceive the thing to be clear. But as there are some who admit nothing unless upon authority, let them learn that the truth I am contending for can be confirmed from Galen's own words, namely, that not only may the blood be transmitted from the pulmonary artery into the pulmonary veins, then into the left ventricle of the heart, and from thence into the arteries of the body, but that this is effected by the ceaseless pulsation of the heart and the motion of the lungs in breathing.

There are, as every one knows, three sigmoid or semilunar valves situated at the orifice of the pulmonary artery, which effectually prevent the blood sent into the vessel from returning into the cavity of the heart. Now Galen, explaining the uses of these valves, and the necessity for them, employs the following language.[1] "There is everywhere a mutual anastomosis and inosculation of the arteries with the veins, and they severally transmit both blood and spirit, by certain invisible and undoubtedly very narrow passages. Now if the mouth of the vena arteriosa, or pulmonary artery, had stood in like manner continually open, and nature had found no contrivance for closing it when requisite, and opening it again, it would have been impossible that the blood could ever have passed by the invisible and delicate mouths, during the contractions of the thorax, into the arteries; for all things are not alike readily attracted or repelled; but that which is light is more readily drawn in, the instrument being dilated, and forced out again when it is contracted, than that which is heavy; and in like manner is anything drawn more rapidly along an ample conduit, and again driven forth, than it is through a narrow tube. But when the thorax is contracted, the pulmonary veins, which are in the lungs, being driven inwardly, and powerfully compressed on every side, immediately force out some of the spirit they contain, and at the same time assume a certain portion of blood by those subtile mouths; a thing that could never come to pass were the blood at liberty to flow back into the heart through the great orifice of the pulmonary artery. But its return through this great opening being prevented, when it is compressed on every side, a certain portion of it distils into the pulmonary veins by the minute orifices mentioned." And shortly afterwards, in the very next chapter, he says: "The more the thorax contracts, the more it strives to force out the blood, the more exactly do these membranes (viz., the sigmoid valves) close up the mouth of the vessel, and suffer nothing to regurgitate." The same fact he has also alluded to in a preceding part of the tenth chapter: "Were there no valves, a three-fold inconvenience would result, so that the blood would then perform this lengthened course in vain; it would flow inwards during the diastoles of the lungs, and fill all their arteries; but in the systoles, in the manner of the tide, it would ever and anon, like the Euripus, flow backwards and forwards by the same way, with a reciprocating motion, which would nowise suit the blood. This, however, may seem a matter of little moment; but if it meantime appear that the function of respiration suffer, then I think it would be looked upon as no trifle, etc." And again, and shortly afterwards: "And then a third inconvenience, by no means to be thought lightly of, would follow, were the blood moved backwards during the expirations, had not our Maker instituted those supplementary membranes [the sigmoid valves]." Whence, in the eleventh chapter, he concludes: "That they have all a common use (to wit, the valves), and that it is to prevent regurgitation or backward motion; each, however, having a proper function, the one set drawing matters from the heart, and preventing their return, the other drawing

[1] De Usu Partium, lib. vi, cap. 10.

matters into the heart, and preventing their escape from it. For nature never intended to distress the heart with needless labour, neither to bring aught into the organ which it had been better to have kept away, nor to take from it again aught which it was requisite should be brought. Since, then, there are four orifices in all, two in either ventricle, one of these induces, the other educes.'' And again he says: ''Farther, since there is one vessel, consisting of a simple tunic, implanted in the heart, and another, having a double tunic extending from it (Galen is here speaking of the right side of the heart. but I extend his observations to the left side also), a kind of reservoir had to be provided, to which both belonging, the blood should be drawn in by the one, and sent out by the other.''

This argument Galen adduces for the transit of the blood by the right ventricle from the vena cava into the lungs; but we can use it with still greater propriety, merely changing the terms, for the passage of the blood from the veins through the heart into the arteries. From Galen, however, that great man, that father of physicians, it clearly appears that the blood passes through the lungs from the pulmonary artery into the minute branches of the pulmonary veins, urged to this both by the pulses of the heart and by the motions of the lungs and thorax; that the heart, moreover, is incessantly receiving and expelling the blood by and from its ventricles, as from a magazine or cistern, and for this end is furnished with four sets of valves, two serving for the induction and two for the eduction of the blood, lest, like the Euripus, it should be incommodiously sent hither and thither, or flow back into the cavity which it should have quitted, or quit the part where its presence was required, and so the heart be oppressed with labour in vain, and the office of the lungs be interfered with.[1] Finally, our position that the blood is continually passing from the right to the left ventricle, from the vena cava into the aorta, through the porous structure of the lungs, plainly appears from this that since the blood is incessantly sent from the right ventricle into the lungs by the pulmonary artery, and in like manner is incessantly drawn from the lungs into the left ventricle, as appears from what precedes and the position of the valves, it cannot do otherwise than pass through continuously. And then, as the blood is incessantly flowing into the right ventricle of the heart, and is continually passed out from the left, as appears in like manner, and as is obvious both to sense and reason, it is impossible that the blood can do otherwise than pass continually from the vena cava into the aorta.

Dissection consequently shows distinctly what takes place [in regard to the transit of the blood] in the greater number of animals, and indeed in all, up to the period of their [foetal] maturity; and that the same thing occurs in adults is equally certain, both from Galen's words, and what has already been said on the subject, only that in the former

[1]See the Commentary of the learned Hofmann upon the Sixth Book of Galen, De Usu Partium, a work which I first saw after I had written what precedes.

the transit is effected by open and obvious passages, in the latter by the obscure porosities of the lungs and the minute inosculations of vessels. Whence it appears that, although one ventricle of the heart, the left to wit, would suffice for the distribution of the blood over the body, and its eduction from the vena cava, as indeed is done in those creatures that have no lungs, nature, nevertheless, when she ordained that the same blood should also percolate the lungs, saw herself obliged to add another ventricle, the right, the pulse of which should force the blood from the vena cava through the lungs into the cavity of the left ventricle. In this way, therefore, it may be said that the right ventricle is made for the sake of the lungs, and for the transmission of the blood through them, not for their nutrition; seeing it were unreasonable to suppose that the lungs required any so much more copious a supply of nutriment, and that of so much purer and more spiritous a kind, as coming immediately from the ventricle of the heart, than either the brain with its peculiarly pure substance, or the eyes with their lustrous and truly admirable structure, or the flesh of the heart itself, which is more commodiously nourished by the coronary artery.

CHAPTER VIII

OF THE QUANTITY OF BLOOD PASSING THROUGH THE HEART FROM THE VEINS TO THE ARTERIES; AND OF THE CIRCULAR MOTION OF THE BLOOD

Thus far I have spoken of the passage of the blood from the veins into the arteries, and of the manner in which it is transmitted and distributed by the action of the heart; points to which some, moved either by the authority of Galen or Columbus, or the reasonings of others, will give in their adhesion. But what remains to be said upon the quantity and source of the blood which thus passes, is of so novel and unheard of character, that I not only fear injury to myself from the envy of a few, but I tremble lest I have mankind at large for my enemies, so much doth wont and custom, that become as another nature, and doctrine once sown and that hath struck deep root, and respect for antiquity influence all men. Still the die is cast, and my trust is in my love of truth, and the candour that inheres in cultivated minds. And sooth to say, when I surveyed my mass of evidence, whether derived from vivisections, and my various reflections on them, or from the ventricles of the heart, and the vessels that enter into and issue from them, the symmetry and size of these conduits,—for nature doing nothing in vain, would never have given them so large a relative size without a purpose,—or from the arrangement and intimate structure of the valves in particular, and of the other parts of the heart in general, with many things besides, I frequently and seriously bethought me, and long revolved in my mind, what might be the quantity of blood which was transmitted, in how short a time its passage might be effected, and the like; and not finding it possible that this could be supplied by the juices of the ingested aliment without the veins on the one hand becoming drained, and the arteries on the other getting ruptured through the excessive charge of blood, unless the blood should somehow find its way from the arteries into the veins, and so return to the right side of the heart; I began to think whether there might not be A MOTION, AS IT WERE, IN A CIRCLE. Now this I afterwards found to be true; and I finally saw that the blood, forced by the action of the left ventricle into the arteries, was distributed to the body at large, and its several parts, in the same manner as it is sent through the lungs; impelled by the right ventricle into the pulmonary artery, and that it then passed through the veins and along the vena cava, and so round to the left ventricle in the manner already indicated. Which motion we may be allowed to call circular, in the same way as Aristotle says that the air and the rain emulate the circular motion of the superior bodies; for the moist earth, warmed by the sun, evaporates; the vapours drawn upwards are condensed, and descending in the form of rain, moisten the earth again; and by this arrangement are generations of living things produced; and in like manner too are tempests and meteors engendered by the circular motion, and by the approach and recession of the sun.

And so, in all likelihood, does it come to pass in the body, through the motion of the blood; the various parts are nourished, cherished, quickened by the warmer, more perfect, vaporous, spiritous, and, as I may say, alimentive blood; which, on the contrary, in contact with these parts becomes cooled, coagulated, and, so to speak, effete; whence it returns to its sovereign the heart, as if to its source, or to the inmost home of the body, there to recover its state of excellence or perfection. Here it resumes its due fluidity and receives an infusion of natural heat —powerful, fervid, a kind of treasury of life, and is impregnated with spirits, and it might be said with balsam; and thence it is again dispersed; and all this depends on the motion and action of the heart.

The heart, consequently, is the beginning of life; the sun of the microcosm, even as the sun in his turn might well be designated the heart of the world; for it is the heart by whose virtue and pulse the blood is moved, perfected, made apt to nourish, and is preserved from corruption and coagulation; it is the household divinity which, discharging its function, nourishes, cherishes, quickens the whole body, and is indeed the foundation of life, the source of all action. But of these things we shall speak more opportunely when we come to speculate upon the final cause of this motion of the heart.

Hence, since the veins are the conduits and vessels that transport the blood, they are of two kinds, the cava and the aorta; and this not by reason of there being two sides of the body, as Aristotle has it, but because of the difference of office; nor yet, as is commonly said, in consequence of any diversity of structure, for in many animals, as I have said, the vein does not differ from the artery in the thickness of its tunics, but solely in virtue of their several destinies and uses. A vein and an artery, both styled vein by the ancients, and that not undeservedly, as Galen has remarked, because the one, the artery to wit, is the vessel which carries the blood from the heart to the body at large, the other or vein of the present day bringing it back from the general system to the heart; the former is the conduit from, the latter the channel to, the heart; the latter contains the cruder, effete blood, rendered unfit for nutrition; the former transmits the digested, perfect, peculiarly nutritive fluid.

CHAPTER IX

THAT THERE IS A CIRCULATION OF THE BLOOD IS CONFIRMED FROM THE FIRST PROPOSITION

But lest anyone should say that we give them words only, and make mere specious assertions without any foundation, and desire to innovate without sufficient cause, three points present themselves for confirmation, which being stated, I conceive that the truth I contend for will follow necessarily, and appear as a thing obvious to all. First,—the blood is incessantly transmitted by the action of the heart from the vena cava to the arteries in such quantity, that it cannot be supplied from the ingesta, and in such wise that the whole mass must very quickly pass through the organ; second,—the blood under the influence of the arterial pulse enters and is impelled in a continuous, equable, and incessant stream through every part and member of the body, in much larger quantity than were sufficient for nutrition, or than the whole mass of fluids could supply; third, —the veins in like manner return this blood incessantly to the heart from all parts and members of the body. These points proved, I conceive it will be manifest that the blood circulates, revolves, propelled and then returning, from the heart to the extremities, from the extremities to the heart, and thus that it performs a kind of circular motion.

Let us assume either arbitrarily or from experiment, the quantity of blood which the left ventricle of the heart will contain when distended to be, say two ounces, three ounces, one ounce and a half—in the dead body I have found it to hold upwards of two ounces. Let us assume further, how much less the heart will hold in the contracted than in the dilated state; and how much blood it will project into the aorta upon each contraction;—and all the world allows that with the systole something is always projected, a necessary consequence demonstrated in the third chapter, and obvious from the structure of the valves; and let us suppose as approaching the truth that the fourth, or fifth, or sixth, or even but the eighth part of its charge is thrown into the artery at each contraction; this would give either half an ounce, or three drachms, or one drachm of blood as propelled by the heart at each pulse into the aorta; which quantity, by reason of the valves at the root of the vessel, can by no means return into the ventricle. Now in the course of half an hour, the heart will have made more than one thousand beats, in some as many as two, three, and even four thousand. Multiplying the number of drachms propelled by the number of pulses, we shall have either one thousand half ounces, or one thousand times three drachms, or a like proportional quantity of blood, according to the amount which we assume as propelled with each stroke of the heart, sent from this organ into the artery; a larger quantity in every case than is contained in the whole body! In the same way, in the sheep or dog, say that but a single scruple of blood passes with each stroke of the heart, in one-half hour we should have one thousand scruples, or about three pounds and a half of blood injected into the aorta; but the body of neither animal contains above four pounds of blood, a fact which I have myself ascertained in the case of the sheep.

Upon this supposition, therefore, assumed merely as a ground for reasoning, we see the whole mass of blood passing through the heart, from the veins to the arteries, and in like manner through the lungs.

But let it be said that this does not take place in half an hour, but in an hour, or even in a day; any way it is still manifest that more blood passes through the heart in consequence of its action, than can either be supplied by the whole of the ingesta, or than can be contained in the veins at the same moment.

Nor can it be allowed that the heart in contracting sometimes propels and sometimes does not propel, or at most propels but very little, a mere nothing, or an imaginary something: all this, indeed, has already been refuted; and is, besides, contrary both to sense and reason. For if it be a necessary effect of the dilatation of the heart that its ventricles become filled with blood, it is equally so that, contracting, these cavities should expel their contents; and this is not in any trifling measure, seeing that neither are the conduits small, nor the contractions few in number, but frequent, and always in some certain proportion, whether it be a third or sixth, or an eighth, to the total capacity of the ventricles, so that a like proportion of blood must be expelled, and a like proportion received with each stroke of the heart, the capacity of the ventricle contracted always bearing a certain relation to the capacity of the ventricle when dilated. And since in dilating, the ventricles cannot be supposed to get filled with nothing, or with an imaginary something; so in contracting they never expel nothing or aught imaginary, but always a certain something, viz., blood, in proportion to the amount of the contraction. Whence it is to be inferred that if at one stroke the heart in man, the ox or the sheep, ejects but a single drachm of blood, and there are one thousand strokes in half an hour, in this interval there will have been ten pounds five ounces expelled: were there with each stroke two drachms expelled, the quantity would of course amount to twenty pounds and ten ounces; were there half an ounce, the quantity would come to forty-one pounds and eight ounces; and were there one ounce it would be as much as eighty-three pounds and four ounces; the whole of which, in the course of one half-hour, would have been transfused from the veins to the arteries. The actual quantity of blood expelled at each stroke of the heart, and the circumstances under which it is either greater or less than ordinary, I leave for particular determination afterwards, from numerous observations which I have made on the subject.

Meantime this much I know, and would here proclaim to all, that the blood is transfused at one time in larger, at another in smaller quantity; and that the circuit of the blood is accomplished now more rapidly, now more slowly, according to the temperament, age, etc., of the individual, to external and internal circumstances, to naturals and non-naturals,—sleep, rest, food, exercise, affections of the mind, and the like. But indeed, supposing even the smallest quantity of blood to be passed through the heart and lungs with each pulsation, a vastly greater amount would still be thrown into the arteries and whole body, than could by any possibility be supplied by the food consumed; in short it could be furnished in no other way than by making a circuit and returning.

This truth, indeed, presents itself obviously before us when we consider what happens in the dissection of living animals; the great artery need not divide, but a very small branch only (as Galen even proves in regard to man), to have the whole of the blood in the body, as well that of the veins as of the arteries, drained away in the course of no long time—some half-hour or less. Butchers are well aware of the fact and can bear witness to it; for, cutting the throat of an ox and so dividing the vessels of the neck, in less than a quarter of an hour they have all the vessels bloodless—the whole mass of blood has escaped. The same thing also occasionally occurs with great rapidity in performing amputations and removing tumours in the human subject.

Nor would this argument lose any of its force, did any one say that in killing animals in the shambles, and performing amputations, the blood escaped in equal, if not perchance in larger quantity by the veins than by the arteries. The contrary of this statement, indeed, is certainly the truth; the veins, in fact, collapsing, and being without any propelling power, and further, because of the impediment of the valves, as I shall show immediately, pour out but very little blood; whilst the arteries spout it forth with force abundantly, impetuously, and as if it were propelled by a syringe. And then the experiment is easily tried of leaving the vein untouched, and only dividing the artery in the neck of a sheep or dog, when it will be seen with what force, in what abundance, and how quickly, the whole blood in the body, of the veins as well as of the arteries, is emptied. But the arteries receive blood from the veins in no other way than by transmission through the heart, as we have already seen; so that if the aorta be tied at the base of the heart, and the carotid or any other artery be opened, no one will now be surprised to find it empty, and the veins only replete with blood.

And now the cause is manifest, wherefore in our dissections we usually find so large a quantity of blood in the veins, so little in the arteries; wherefore there is much in the right ventricle, little in the left, circumstances which probably led the ancients to believe that the arteries (as their name implies) contained nothing but spirits during the life of an animal. The true cause of the difference is this perhaps: that as there is no passage to the arteries, save through the lungs and the heart, when an animal has ceased to breathe and the lungs to move, the blood in the pulmonary artery is prevented from passing into the pulmonary veins, and from thence into the left ventricle of the heart, just as we have already seen the same transit prevented in the embryo, by the want of movement in the lungs and the alternate opening and shutting of their minute orifices and invisible pores. But the heart not ceasing to act at the same precise moment as the lungs, but surviving them and continuing to pulsate for a time, the left ventricle and arteries go on distributing their blood to the body at large and sending it into the veins; receiving none from the lungs, however, they are soon exhausted, and left, as it were, empty. But even this fact confirms our views, in no trifling manner, seeing that it can be ascribed to no other than the cause we have just assumed.

Moreover it appears from this that the more frequently or forcibly the arteries pulsate, the more speedily will the body be exhausted in an hemorrhage. Hence, also, it happens, that in fainting fits and in states of alarm, when the heart beats more languidly and with less force, hemorrhages are diminished or arrested.

Still further, it is from this that after death, when the heart has ceased to beat, it is impossible by dividing either the jugular or femoral veins and arteries, by any effort to force out more than one-half of the whole mass of the blood. Neither could the butcher, did he neglect to cut the throat of the ox which he has knocked on the head and stunned, until the heart had ceased beating, ever bleed the carcass effectually.

CHAPTER X

THE FIRST POSITION: OF THE QUANTITY OF BLOOD PASSING FROM THE VEINS TO THE ARTERIES. AND THAT THERE IS A CIRCUIT OF THE BLOOD, FREED FROM OBJECTIONS, AND FARTHER CONFIRMED BY EXPERIMENT*

So far our first position is confirmed, whether the thing be referred to calculation or to experiment and dissection, viz., that the blood is incessantly infused into the arteries in larger quantities than it can be supplied by the food; so that the whole passing over in a short space of time, it is a matter of necessity that the blood perform a circuit, that it return to whence it set out.

But if any one shall here object that a large quantity may pass through and yet no necessity be found for a circulation, that all may come from the meat and drink consumed, and quote as an illustration the abundant supply of milk in the mammae—for a cow will give three, four, and even seven gallons and more in a day, and a woman, two or three pints whilst nursing a child or twins, which must manifestly be derived from the food consumed; it may be answered, that the heart by computation does as much and more in the course of an hour or two.

And if not yet convinced, he shall still insist, that when an artery is divided a preternatural route is, as it were, opened, and that so the blood escapes in torrents, but that the same thing does not happen in the healthy and uninjured body when no outlet is made; and that in arteries filled, or in their natural state, so large a quantity of blood cannot pass in so short a space of time as to make any return necessary;—to all this it may be answered, that from the calculation already made, and the reasons assigned, it appears that by so much as the heart in its dilated state contains in addition to its contents in the state of constriction, so much in a general way must it emit upon each pulsation, and in such quantity must the blood pass, the body being healthy and naturally constituted.

But in serpents, and several fishes, by tying the veins some way below the heart, you will perceive a space between the ligature and the heart speedily to become empty; so that, unless you would deny the evidence of your senses, you must needs admit the return of the blood to the heart. The same thing will also plainly appear when we come to discuss our second position.

---

*Proposition.—F. A. W., 1940.

Let us here conclude with a single example, confirming all that has been said, and from which every one may obtain conviction through the testimony of his own eyes.

If a live snake be laid open, the heart will be seen pulsating quietly, distinctly for more than an hour, moving like a worm, contracting in its longitudinal dimensions (for it is of an oblong shape) and propelling its contents; becoming of a paler colour in the systole, of a deeper tint in the diastole; and almost all things else by which I have already said that the truth I contend for is established, only that here everything takes place more slowly, and is more distinct. This point in particular may be observed more clearly than the noonday sun: the vena cava enters the heart at its lower part, the artery quits it at the superior part; the vein being now seized either with forceps or between the finger and thumb, and the course of the blood for some space below the heart interrupted, you will perceive the part that intervenes between the fingers and the heart almost immediately to become empty, the blood being exhausted by the action of the heart; at the same time the heart will become of a much paler colour, even in its state of dilatation, than it was before; it is also smaller than at first, from wanting blood; and then it begins to beat more slowly, so that it seems at length as if it were about to die. But the impediment to the flow of blood being removed, instantly the colour and the size of the heart are restored.

If, on the contrary, the artery instead of the vein be compressed or tied, you will observe the part between the obstacle and the heart, and the heart itself, to become inordinately distended, to assume a deep purple or even livid colour, and at length to be so much oppressed with blood that you will believe it about being choked; but the obstacle removed, all things immediately return to their pristine state—the heart to its colour, size, stroke, etc.

Here, then, we have evidence of two kinds of death: extinction from deficiency, and suffocation from excess. Examples of both have now been set before you, and you have had opportunity of viewing the truth contended for with your own eyes in the heart.

CHAPTER XI

THE SECOND POSITION IS DEMONSTRATED

That this may the more clearly appear to every one, I have here to cite certain experiments, from which it seems obvious that the blood enters a limb by the arteries, and returns from it by the veins; that the arteries are the vessels carrying the blood from the heart, and the veins the returning channels of the blood to the heart; that in the limbs and extreme parts of the body the blood passes either immediately by anastomosis from the arteries into the veins, or mediately by the pores of the flesh, or in both ways, as has already been said in speaking of the passage of the blood through the lungs: whence it appears manifest that in the circuit the blood moves from thence hither, and from hence thither; from the centre to the extremities, to wit; in from the extreme parts back again to the centre. Finally, upon the grounds of calculation, with the same elements as before, it will be obvious that the quantity can neither be accounted for by the ingesta, nor yet be held necessary to nutrition.

The same thing will also appear in regard to ligatures, and wherefore they are said to *draw;* though this is neither from the heat, nor the pain, nor the vacuum they occasion, nor indeed from any other cause yet thought of; it will also explain the uses and advantages to be derived from ligatures in medicine, the principle upon which they either suppress or occasion hemorrhage; how they induce sloughing and more extensive mortification in extremities; and how they act in the castration of animals and the removal of warts and fleshy tumours. But it has come to pass, from no one having duly weighed and understood the causes and rationale of these various effects, that though almost all, upon the faith of the old writers, recommend ligatures in the treatment of disease, yet very few comprehend their proper employment, or derive any real assistance from them in effecting cures.

Ligatures are either very tight or of middling tightness. A ligature I designate as tight or perfect when it is drawn so close about an extremity that no vessel can be felt pulsating beyond it. Such a ligature we use in amputations to control the flow of blood; and such also are employed in the castration of animals and the removal of tumours. In the latter instances, all afflux of nutriment and heat being prevented by the ligature, we see the testes and large fleshy tumours dwindle, and die, and finally fall off.

Ligatures of middling tightness I regard as those which compress a limb firmly all around, but short of pain, and in such a way as still suffers a certain degree of pulsation to be felt in the artery beyond them. Such a ligature is in use in blood letting, an operation in which the fillet applied above the elbow is not drawn so tight but that the arteries at the wrist may still be felt beating under the finger.

Now let any one make an experiment upon the arm of a man, either using such a fillet as is employed in blood letting, or grasping the limb lightly with his hand, the best subject for it being one who is lean, and who has large veins, and the best time after exercise, when the body is warm, the pulse is full, and the blood carried in larger quantity to the extremities, for all then is more conspicuous; under such circumstances let a ligature be thrown about the extremity, and drawn as tightly as can be borne, it will first be perceived that beyond the ligature, neither in the wrist nor anywhere else, do the arteries pulsate, at the same time that immediately above the ligature the artery begins to rise higher at each diastole, to throb more violently, and to swell in its vicinity with a kind of tide, as if it strove to break through and overcome the obstacle to its current; the artery here, in short, appears as if it were preternaturally full. The hand under such circumstances retains its natural colour and appearance; in the course of time it begins to fall somewhat in temperature, indeed, but nothing is *drawn* into it.

After the bandage has been kept on for some short time in this way, let it be slackened a little, brought to that state or term of middling tightness which is used in bleeding, and it will be seen that the whole hand and arm will instantly become deeply suffused and distended, and the veins show themselves tumid and knotted; after ten or fifteen pulses of the artery, the hand will be perceived excessively distended, injected, gorged with blood, *drawn,* as it is said, by this middling ligature, without pain, or heat, or any horror of a vacuum, or any other cause yet indicated.

If the finger be applied over the artery as it is pulsating by the edge of the fillet, at the moment of slackening it, the blood will be felt to glide through, as it were, underneath the finger; and he, too, upon whose arm the experiment is made, when the ligature is slackened, is distinctly conscious of a sensation of warmth, and of something, viz., a stream of blood suddenly making its way along the course of the vessels and diffusing itself through the hand, which at the same time begins to feel hot, and becomes distended.

As we had noted, in connexion with the tight ligature, that the artery above the bandage was distended and pulsated, not below it, so, in the case of the moderately tight bandage, on the contrary, do we find that the veins below, never above, the fillet, swell, and become dilated, whilst the arteries shrink; and such is the degree of distension of the veins here, that it is only very strong pressure that will force the blood beyond the fillet, and cause any of the veins in the upper part of the arm to rise.

From these facts it is easy for every careful observer to learn that the blood enters an extremity by the arteries; for when they are effectually compressed nothing is *drawn* to the member; the hand preserves its colour; nothing flows into it, neither is it distended; but when the pressure is diminished, as it is with the bleeding fillet, it is manifest that the blood is instantly thrown in with force, for then the hand begins to swell; which is as much as to say, that when the arteries pulsate the blood is flowing through them, as it is when the moderately tight ligature is applied; but where they do not pulsate, as, when a tight ligature is used, they cease from transmitting anything; they are only distended above the part where the ligature is applied. The veins again being compressed, nothing can flow through them; the certain indication of which is, that below the ligature they are much more tumid than above it, and than they usually appear when there is no bandage upon the arm.

It therefore plainly appears that the ligature prevents the return of the blood through the veins to the parts above it, and maintains those beneath it in a state of permanent distension. But the arteries, in spite of its pressure, and under the force and impulse of the heart, send on the blood from the internal parts of the body to the parts beyond the bandage. And herein consists the difference between the tight and the medium bandage, that the former not only prevents the passage of the blood in the veins, but in the arteries also; the latter, however, whilst it does not prevent the pulsific force from extending beyond it, and so propelling the blood to the extremities of the body, compresses the veins, and greatly or altogether impedes the return of the blood through them.

Seeing, therefore, that the moderately tight ligature renders the veins turgid, and the whole hand full of blood, I ask, whence is this? Does the blood accumulate below the ligature coming through the veins, or through the arteries, or passing by certain secret pores? Through the veins it cannot come; still less can it come by any system of invisible pores; it must needs arrive by the arteries, then, in conformity with all that has been already said. That it cannot flow in by the veins appears plainly enough from the fact that the blood cannot be forced towards the heart unless the ligature be removed; when on a sudden all the veins collapse, and disgorge themselves of their contents into the superior parts, the hand at the same time resuming its natural pale colour,—the tumefaction and the stagnating blood have disappeared.

Moreover, he whose arm or wrist has thus been bound for some little time with the medium bandage, so that it has not only got swollen and livid but cold, when the fillet is undone is aware of something cold making its way upwards along with the returning blood, and reaching the elbow or the axilla. And I have myself been inclined to think that this cold blood rising upwards to the heart was the cause of the fainting that often occurs after bloodletting: fainting frequently supervenes even in robust subjects, and mostly at the moment of undoing the fillet, as the vulgar say, from the turning of the blood.

Farther, when we see the veins below the ligature instantly swell up and become gorged, when from extreme tightness it is somewhat relaxed, the arteries meantime continuing unaffected, this is an obvious indication that the blood passes from the arteries into the veins, and not from the veins into the arteries, and that there is either an anastomosis of the two orders of vessels, or pores in the flesh and solid parts generally that are permeable to the blood. It is farther an indication that the veins have frequent communications with one another, because they all become turgid together, whilst under the medium ligature applied above the elbow; and if any single small vein be pricked with a lancet, they all speedily shrink, and disburthening themselves into this they subside almost simultaneously.

These considerations will enable any one to understand the nature of the attraction that is exerted by ligatures, and perchance of fluxes generally; how, for example, the veins when compressed by a bandage of medium tightness applied above the elbow, the blood cannot escape, whilst it still continues to be driven in, to wit, by the forcing power of the heart, by which the parts are by necessity filled, gorged with blood. And how should it be otherwise? Heat and pain and the *vis vacui* draw, indeed; but in such wise only that parts are filled, not preternaturally distended or gorged, not so suddenly and violently overwhelmed with the charge of blood forced in upon them, that the flesh is lacerated and the vessels ruptured. Nothing of the kind as an effect of heat, or pain, or the vacuum force, is either credible or demonstrable.

Besides, the ligature is competent to occasion the afflux in question without either pain, or heat, or *vis vacui*. Were pain in any way the cause, how should it happen that, with the arm bound above the elbow, the hand and fingers should swell below the bandage, and their veins become distended? The pressure of the bandage certainly prevents the blood from getting there by the veins. And then, wherefore is there neither swelling nor repletion of the veins, nor any sign or symptom of attraction or afflux, above the ligature? But this is the obvious cause of the preternatural attraction and swelling below the bandage, and in the hand and fingers, that the blood is entering abundantly, and with force, but cannot pass out again.

Now is not this the cause of all tumefaction, as indeed Avicenna has it, and of all oppressive redundancy in parts, that the access to them is open, but the egress from them is closed? Whence it comes that they are gorged and tumefied. And may not the same thing happen in local inflammations, where, so long as the swelling is on the increase, and has not reached its extreme term, a full pulse is felt in the part, especially when the disease is of the more acute kind, and the swelling usually takes place most rapidly. But these are matters for after discussion. Or does this, which occurred in my own case, happen from the same cause. Thrown from a carriage upon one occasion, I struck my forehead a blow upon the place where a twig of the artery advances from the temple, and immediately, within the time in which twenty beats could have been made, I felt a tumour the size of an egg developed, without either heat or any great pain: the near vicinity of the artery had caused the blood to be effused into the bruised part with unusual force and quickness.

And now, too, we understand wherefore in phlebotomy we apply our fillet above the part that is punctured, not below it; did the flow come from above, not from below, the bandage in this case would not only be of no service, but would prove a positive hinderance; it would have to be applied below the orifice, in order to have the flow more free, did the blood descend by the veins from superior to inferior parts; but as it is elsewhere forced through the extreme arteries into the extreme veins, and the return in these last is opposed by the ligature, so do they fill and swell, and being thus filled and distended, they are made capable of projecting their charge with force, and to a distance, when any of them is suddenly punctured; but the fillet being slackened, and the returning channels thus left open, the blood forthwith no longer escapes, save by drops; and, as all the world knows, if in performing phlebotomy the bandage be either slackened too much or the limb be bound too tightly, the blood escapes without force, because in the one case the returning channels are not adequately obstructed; in the other the channels of influx, the arteries, are impeded.

CHAPTER XII

THAT THERE IS A CIRCULATION OF THE BLOOD IS SHOWN FROM THE SECOND POSITION DEMONSTRATED

If these things be so, another point which I have already referred to, viz., the continual passage of the blood through the heart, will also be confirmed. We have seen, that the blood passes from the arteries into the veins, not from the veins into the arteries; we have seen, farther, that almost the whole of the blood may be withdrawn from a puncture made in one of the cutaneous veins of the arm if a bandage properly applied be used; we have seen, still farther, that the blood flows so freely and rapidly that not only is the whole quantity which was contained in the arm beyond the ligature, and before the puncture was made, discharged, but the whole which is contained in the body, both that of the arteries and that of the veins.

Whence we must admit, first, that the blood is sent along with an impulse, and that it is urged with force below the fillet; for it escapes with force, which force it receives from the pulse and power of the heart; for the force and motion of the blood are derived from the heart alone. Second, that the afflux proceeds from the heart, and through the heart by a course from the great veins [into the aorta]; for it gets into the parts below the ligature through the arteries, not through the veins; and the arteries nowhere receive blood from the veins, nowhere receive blood save and except from the left ventricle of the heart. Nor could so large a quantity of blood be drawn from one vein (a ligature having been duly applied), nor with such impetuosity, such readiness, such celerity, unless through the medium of the impelling power of the heart.

But if all things be as they are now represented, we shall feel ourselves at liberty to calculate the quantity of the blood, and to reason on its circular motion. Should any one, for instance, in performing phlebotomy, suffer the blood to flow in the manner it usually does, with force and freely, for some half hour or so, no question but that the greatest part of the blood being abstracted, faintings and syncopes would ensue, and that not only would the arteries but the great veins also be nearly emptied of their contents. It is only consonant with reason to conclude that in the course of the half hour hinted at, so much as has escaped has also passed from the great veins through the heart into the aorta. And further, if we calculate how many ounces flow through one arm, or how many pass in twenty or thirty pulsations under the medium ligature, we shall have some grounds for estimating how much passes through the other arm in the same space of time; how much through both lower extremities, how much through the neck on either side, and through all the other arteries and veins of the body, all of which have been supplied with fresh blood, and as this blood must have passed through the lungs and ventricles of the heart, and must have come from the great veins,—we shall perceive that a circulation is absolutely necessary, seeing that the quantities hinted at cannot be supplied immediately from the ingesta, and are vastly more than can be requisite for the mere nutrition of the parts.

It is still further to be observed, that the truths contended for are sometimes confirmed in another way; for having tied up the arm properly, and made the puncture duly, still, if from alarm or any other causes, a state of faintness supervenes, in which the heart always pulsates more languidly, the blood does not flow freely, but distils by drops only. The reason is, that with the somewhat greater than usual resistance offered to the transit of the blood by the bandage, coupled with the weaker action of the heart, and its diminished impelling power, the stream cannot make its way under the fillet; and farther, owing to the weak and languishing state of the heart, the blood is not transferred in such quantity as wont from the veins to the arteries through the sinuses of that organ. So also, and for the same reasons, are the menstrual fluxes of women, and indeed hemorrhages of every kind, controlled. And now, a contrary state of things occurring, the patient getting rid of his fear and recovering his courage, the pulsific power is increased, the arteries begin again to beat with greater force, and to drive the blood even into the part that is bound; so that the blood now springs from the puncture in the vein, and flows in a continuous stream.

CHAPTER XIII

THE THIRD POSITION IS CONFIRMED: AND THE CIRCULATION OF THE BLOOD IS DEMONSTRATED FROM IT

Thus far we have spoken of the quantity of blood passing through the heart and the lungs in the centre of the body, and in like manner from the arteries into the veins in the peripheral parts and the body at large. We have yet to explain, however, in what manner the blood finds its way back to the heart from the extremities by the veins, and how and in what way these are the only vessels that convey the blood from the external to the central parts; which done, I conceive that the three fundamental propositions laid down for the circulation of the blood will be so plain, so well established, so obviously true, that they may claim general credence. Now the remaining position will be made sufficiently clear from the valves which are found in the cavities of the veins themselves, from the uses of these, and from experiments cognizable by the senses.

The celebrated Hieronymus Fabricius of Aquapendente, a most skilful anatomist, and venerable old man, or, as the learned Riolan will have it, Jacobus Sylvius, first gave representations of the valves in the veins, which consist of raised or loose portions of the inner membranes of these vessels, of extreme delicacy, and a sigmoid or semilunar shape. They are situated at different distances from one another, and diversely in different individuals; they are connate at the sides of the veins; they are directed upwards or towards the trunks of the veins; the two—for there are for the most part two together—regard each other, mutually touch, and are so ready to come into contact by their edges, that if anything attempt to pass from the trunks into the branches of the veins, or from the greater vessels into the less, they completely prevent it; they are farther so arranged, that the horns of those that succeed are opposite the middle of the convexity of those that precede, and so on alternately.

The discoverer of these valves did not rightly understand their use, nor have succeeding anatomists added anything to our knowledge: for their office is by no means explained when we are told that it is to hinder the blood, by its weight, from all flowing into inferior parts; for the edges of the valves in the jugular veins hang downwards, and are so contrived that they prevent the blood from rising upwards; the valves, in a word, do not invariably look upwards, but always towards the trunks of the veins, invariably towards the seat of the heart. I, and indeed others, have sometimes found valves in the emulgent veins, and in those of the mesentery, the edges of which were directed towards the vena cava and vena portae. Let it be added that there are no valves in the arteries [save at their roots], and that dogs, oxen, etc., have invariably valves at the divisions of their crural veins, in the veins that meet towards the top of the os sacrum, and in those branches which come from the haunches, in which no such effect of gravity from the erect position was to be apprehended. Neither are there valves in the jugular veins for the purpose of guarding against apoplexy, as some have said; because in sleep the head is more apt to be influenced by the contents of the carotid arteries. Neither are the valves present, in order that the blood may be retained in the divarications or smaller trunks and minuter branches, and not to be suffered to flow entirely into the more open and capacious channels; for they occur where there are no divarications; although it must be owned that they are most frequent at the points where branches join. Neither do they exist for the purpose of rendering the current of blood more slow from the centre of the body, for it seems likely that the blood would be disposed to flow with sufficient slowness of its own accord, as it would have to pass from larger into continually smaller vessels, being separated from the mass and fountain head, and attaining from warmer into colder places.

But the valves are solely made and instituted lest the blood should pass from the greater into the lesser veins, and either rupture them or cause them to become varicose; lest, instead of advancing from the extreme to the central parts of the body, the blood should rather proceed along the veins from the centre to the extremities; but the delicate valves, while they readily open in the right direction, entirely prevent all such contrary motion, being so situated and arranged, that if anything escapes, or is less perfectly obstructed by the cornua of the one above, the fluid passing, as it were, by the chinks between the cornua, it is immediately received on the convexity of the one beneath, which is placed transversely with reference to the former, and so is effectually hindered from getting any farther.

And this I have frequently experienced in my dissections of the veins: if I attempted to pass a probe from the trunk of the veins into one of the smaller branches, whatever care I took I found it impossible to introduce it far any way, by reason of the valves; whilst, on the contrary, it was most easy to push it along in the opposite direction, from without inwards, or from the branches towards the trunks and roots. In many places two valves are so placed and fitted, that when raised they come exactly together in the middle of the vein, and are there united by the contact of their margins; and so accurate is the adaptation, that neither by the eye nor by any other means of examination can the slightest chink along the line of contact be perceived. But if the probe be now introduced from the extreme towards the more central parts, the valves, like the floodgates of a river, give way, and are most readily pushed aside. The effect of this arrangement plainly is to prevent all motion of the blood from the heart and vena cava, whether it be upwards towards the head, or downwards towards the feet, or to either side towards the arms, not a drop can pass; all motion of the blood, beginning in the larger and tending towards the smaller veins, is opposed and resisted by them; whilst the motion that proceeds from the lesser to end in the larger branches is favoured, or, at all events, a free and open passage is left for it.

But that this truth may be made the more apparent, let an arm be tied up above the elbow as if for phlebotomy (A, A, Fig. 1). At intervals in the course of the veins, especially in labouring people and those whose veins are large, certain knots or elevations (B, C, D, E, F) will be perceived, and this not only at the places where a branch is received (E, F), but also where none enters (C, D): these knots or risings are all formed by valves, which thus show themselves externally. And now if you press the blood from the space above one of the valves, from H to O (Fig. 2), and keep the point of a finger upon the vein inferiorly, you will see no influx of blood from above; the portion of the vein between the point of the finger and the valve O will be obliterated; yet will the vessel continue sufficiently distended above that valve (O, G). The blood being thus pressed out, and the vein emptied, if you now apply a finger of the other hand upon the distended part of the vein above the valve O

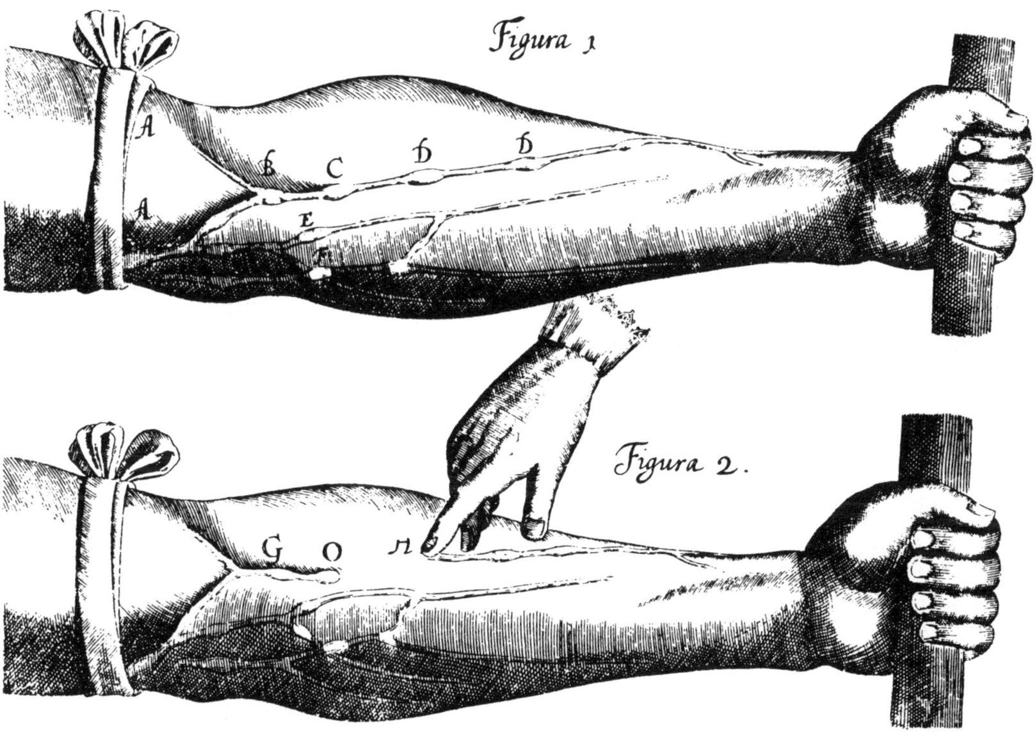

(Fig. 3), and press downwards, you will find that you cannot force the blood through or beyond the valve; but the greater effort you use, you will only see the portion of vein that is between the finger and the valve become more distended, that portion of the vein which is below the valve remaining all the while empty (H, O, Fig. 3).

It would therefore appear that the function of the valves in the veins is the same as that of the three sigmoid valves which we find at the commencement of the aorta and pulmonary artery, viz., to prevent all reflux of the blood that is passing over them.

Farther, the arm being bound as before, and the veins looking full and distended, if you press at one part in the course of a vein with the point of a finger (L, Fig. 4), and then with another finger streak the blood upwards beyond the next valve (N), you will perceive that this portion of the vein continues empty (L N), and that the blood cannot retrograde, precisely as we have already seen the case to be in Fig. 2; but the finger first applied (H, Fig. 2, L, Fig. 4), being removed, immediately the vein is filled from below, and the arm becomes as it appears at D C, Fig. 1. That the blood in the veins therefore proceeds from inferior or more remote to superior parts, and towards the heart, moving in these vessels in this and not in the contrary direction, appears most obviously. And although in some places the valves, by not acting with such perfect accuracy, or where there is but a single valve, do not seem totally to prevent the passage of the blood from the centre, still the greater number of them

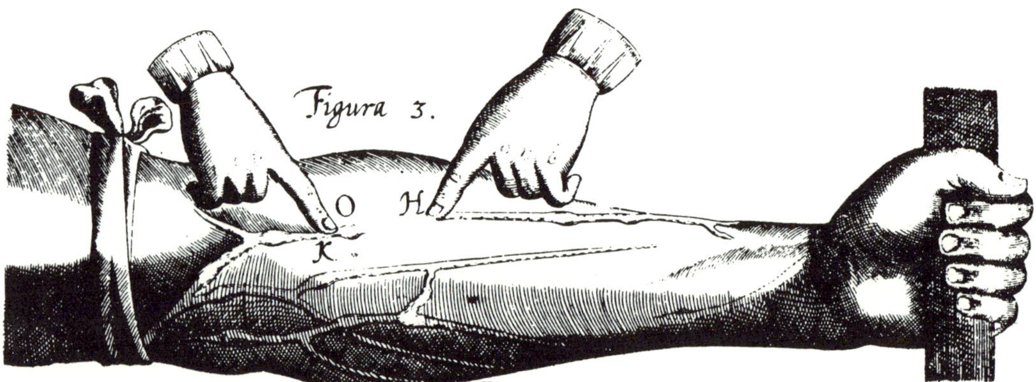

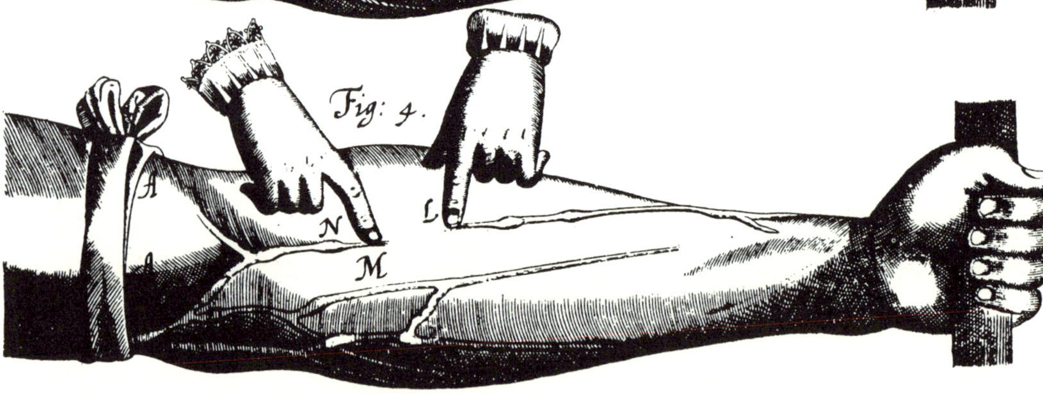

plainly do so; and then, where things appear contrived more negligently, this is compensated either by the more frequent occurrence or more perfect action of the succeeding valves or in some other way: the veins, in short, as they are the free and open conduits of the blood returning *to* the heart, so are they effectually prevented from serving as its channels of distribution *from* the heart.

But this other circumstance has to be noted: The arm being bound, and the veins made turgid, and the valves prominent, as before, apply the thumb or finger over a vein in the situation of one of the valves in such a way as to compress it, and prevent any blood from passing upwards from the hand; then, with a finger of the other hand, streak the blood in the vein upwards till it has passed the next valve above, the vessel now remains empty; but the finger being removed for an instant, the vein is immediately filled from below; apply the finger again, and having in the same manner streaked the blood upwards, again remove the finger below, and again the vessel becomes distended as before; and this repeat, say a thousand times, in a short space of time. And now compute the quantity of blood which you have thus pressed up beyond the valve, and then multiplying the assumed quantity by one thousand, you will find that so much blood has passed through a certain portion of the vessel; and I do now believe that you will find yourself convinced of the circulation of the blood, and of its rapid motion. But if in this experiment you say that a violence is done to nature, I do not doubt but that, if you proceed in the same way, only taking as great a length of vein as possible, and merely remark with what rapidity the blood flows upwards, and fills the vessel from below, you will come to the same conclusion.

CHAPTER XIV

CONCLUSION OF THE DEMONSTRATION OF THE CIRCULATION

And now I may be allowed to give in brief my view of the circulation of the blood, and to propose it for general adoption.

Since all things, both argument and ocular demonstration, show that the blood passes through the lungs and heart by the action of the [auricles and] ventricles, and is sent for distribution to all parts of the body, where it makes its way into the veins and pores of the flesh, and then flows by the veins from the circumference on every side to the centre, from the lesser to the greater veins, and is by them finally discharged into the vena cava and right auricle of the heart, and this in such a quantity or in such a flux and reflux thither by the arteries, hither by the veins, as cannot possibly be supplied by the ingesta, and is much greater than can be required for mere purposes of nutrition; it is absolutely necessary to conclude that the blood in the animal body is impelled in a circle, and is in a state of ceaseless motion; that this is the act or function which the heart performs by means of its pulse; and that it is the sole and only end of the motion and contraction of the heart.

CHAPTER XV

THE CIRCULATION OF THE BLOOD IS FURTHER CONFIRMED BY PROBABLE REASONS

It will not be foreign to the subject if I here show further, from certain familiar reasonings, that the circulation is matter both of convenience and necessity. In the first place, since death is a corruption which takes place through deficiency of heat[1] and since all living things are warm, all dying things cold, there must be a particular seat and fountain, a kind of home and hearth, where the cherisher of nature, the original of the native fire, is stored and preserved; whence heat and life are dispensed to all parts as from a fountain head; whence sustenance may be derived; and upon which concoction and nutrition, and all vegetative energy may depend. Now, that the heart is this place, that the heart is the principle of life, and that all passes in the manner just mentioned, I trust no one will deny.

The blood, therefore, required to have motion, and indeed such a motion that it should return again to the heart; for sent to the external parts of the body far from its fountain, as Aristotle says, and without motion, it would become congealed. For we see motion generating and keeping up heat and spirits under all circumstances, and rest allowing them to escape and be dissipated. The blood, therefore, become thick or congealed by the cold of the extreme and outward parts, and robbed of its spirits, just as it is in the dead, it was imperative that from its fount and origin, it should again receive heat and spirits, and all else requisite to its preservation—that, by returning, it should be renovated and restored.

We frequently see how the extremities are chilled by the external cold, how the nose and cheeks and hands look blue, and how the blood, stagnating in them as in the pendent or lower parts of a corpse, becomes of a dusky hue; the limbs at the same time getting torpid, so that they can scarcely be moved, and seem almost to have lost their vitality. Now they can by no means be so effectually, and especially so speedily restored to heat and colour and life, as by a new afflux and appulsion of heat from its source. But how can parts attract in which the heat and life are almost extinct? Or how should they whose passages are filled with condensed and frigid blood, admit fresh aliment—renovated blood—unless they had first got rid of their old contents? Unless the heart were truly that fountain where life and heat are restored to the refrigerated fluid, and whence new blood, warm, imbued with spirits, being sent out by the arteries, that which has become cooled and effete is forced on, and all the particles recover their heat which was failing, and their vital stimulus well-nigh exhausted.

Hence it is that if the heart be unaffected, life and health may be restored to almost all the other parts of the body; but the heart being chilled, or smitten with any serious disease, it seems matter of necessity that the whole animal fabric should suffer and fall into decay. When the source is corrupted, there is nothing, as Aristotle says,[2] which can be of service either to it or aught that depends on it. And hence, by the way, it may perchance be wherefore grief, and love, and envy, and anxiety, and all affections of the mind of a similar kind are accompanied with emaciation and decay, or with cacochemy and crudity, which engender all manner of

[1]Aristotle's De Respiratione, lib. ii et iii: De Part. Animal. et alibi.
[2]De Part. Animal. iii.

diseases and consume the body of man. For every affection of the mind that is attended with either pain or pleasure, hope or fear, is the cause of an agitation whose influence extends to the heart, and there induces change from the natural constitution, in the temperature, the pulse and the rest, which impairing all nutrition in its source and abating the powers at large, it is no wonder that various forms of incurable disease in the extremities and in the trunk are the consequence, inasmuch as in such circumstances the whole body labours under the effects of vitiated nutrition and a want of native heat.

Moreover, when we see that all animals live through food concocted in their interior, it is imperative that the digestion and distribution be perfect; and, as a consequence, that there be a place and receptacle where the aliment is perfected and whence it is distributed to the several members. Now this place is the heart, for it is the only organ of the body which contains blood for the general use; all the others receive it merely for their peculiar or private advantage, just as the heart also has a supply for its own especial behoof in its coronary veins and arteries; but it is of the store which the heart contains in its auricles and ventricles that I here speak; and then the heart is the only organ which is so situated and constituted that it can distribute the blood in due proportion to the several parts of the body, the quantity sent to each being according to the dimensions of the artery which supplies it, the heart serving as a magazine or fountain ready to meet its demands.

Further, a certain impulse or force, as well as an impeller or forcer, such as the heart, was required to effect this distribution and motion of the blood; both because the blood is disposed from slight causes, such as cold, alarm, horror, and the like, to collect in its source, to concentrate like parts to a whole, or the drops of water spilt upon a table to the mass of liquid; and then because it is forced from the capillary veins into the smaller ramifications, and from these into the larger trunks by the motion of the extremities and the compression of the muscles generally. The blood is thus more disposed to move from the circumference to the centre than in the opposite direction, were there even no valves to oppose its motion; whence that it may leave its source and enter more confined and colder channels, and flow against the direction to which it spontaneously inclines, the blood requires both force and an impelling power. Now such is the heart and the heart alone, and that in the way and manner already explained.

CHAPTER XVI

THE CIRCULATION OF THE BLOOD IS FURTHER PROVED FROM CERTAIN CONSEQUENCES

There are still certain phenomena, which, taken as consequences of this truth assumed as proven, are not without their use in exciting belief, as it were, *a posteriore;* and which, although they may seem to be involved in much doubt and obscurity, nevertheless readily admit of having reasons and causes assigned for them. The phenomena alluded to are those that present themselves in connexion with contagious, poisoned wounds, the bites of serpents and rabid animals, lues venerea and the like. We sometimes see the whole system contaminated, though the part first infected remains sound; the lues venerea has occasionally made its attack with pains in the shoulders and head, and other symptoms, the genital organs being all the while unaffected; and then we know that the wound made by the rabid dog having healed, fever and a train of disastrous symptoms nevertheless supervene. Whence it appears that the contagion impressed upon or deposited in a particular part, is by and by carried by the returning current of blood to the heart, and by that organ is sent to contaminate the whole body.

In tertian fever, the morbific cause seeking the heart in the first instance, and hanging about the heart and lungs, renders the patient shortwinded, disposed to sighing, indisposed to exertion; because the vital principle is oppressed and the blood forced into the lungs and rendered thick, does not pass through their substance (as I have myself seen in opening the bodies of those who had died in the beginning of the attack), when the pulse is always frequent, small, and occasionally irregular; but the heat increasing, the matter becoming attenuated, the passages forced, and the transit made, the whole body begins to rise in temperature, and the pulse becomes fuller, stronger—the febrile paroxysm is fully formed, whilst the preternatural heat kindled in the heart, is thence diffused by the arteries through the whole body along with the morbific matter, which is in this way overcome and dissolved by nature.

When we perceive, further, that medicines applied externally exert their influence on the body just as if they had been taken internally, the truth we are contending for is confirmed. Colocynth and aloes [applied externally] move the belly, cantharides excites the urine, garlic applied to the soles of the feet assists expectoration, cordials strengthen, and an infinite number of examples of the same kind might be cited. It will not, therefore, be found unreasonable perchance, if we say that the veins, by means of their orifices, absorb some of the things that are applied externally and carry this inwards with the blood, not otherwise, it may be, than those of the mesentery imbibe the chyle from the intestines and carry it mixed with the blood to the liver. For the blood entering the mesentery by the coeliac artery, and the superior and inferior mesenterics, proceeds to the intestines, from which, along with the chyle that has been attracted into the veins, it returns by their numerous ramifications into the vena portae of the liver, and from this into the vena cava, and this in such wise that the blood in these veins has the same colour and consistency as in other veins, in opposition to what many believe to be the fact. Nor indeed can we imagine two contrary motions in any capillary system—the chyle upwards, the blood downwards. This could scarcely take place, and must be held as altogether improbable. But is not the thing rather arranged as it is by the consummate providence of nature? For were the chyle mingled with the blood, the crude with the concocted, in equal proportions, the result would not be concoction, transmutation, and sanguification, but rather, and because they are severally active and passive, a mixture or combination, or medium compound of the two, precisely as happens when wine is mixed with water and syrup. But when a very minute quantity of chyle is mingled with a very large quantity of circulating blood, a quantity of chyle that bears no kind of proportion to the mass of blood, the effect is the same, as Aristotle says, as when a drop of water is added to a cask of wine, or the contrary; the mass does not then present itself as a mixture, but is still sensibly either wine or water. So in the mesenteric veins of an animal we do not find either chyme or chyle and blood, blended together or distinct, but only blood, the same in colour, consistency, and other sensible properties, as it appears in the veins generally. Still as there is a certain though small and inappreciable proportion of chyle or unconcocted matter mingled with this blood, nature has interposed the liver, in whose meandering channels it suffers delay and undergoes additional change, lest arriving prematurely and crude at the heart, it should oppress the vital principle. Hence in the embryo, there is almost no use for the liver, but the umbilical vein passes directly through, a foramen or anastomosis existing from the vena portae, so that the blood returns from the intestines of the foetus, not through the liver, but into the umbilical vein mentioned, and flows at once into the heart, mingled with the natural blood which is returning from the placenta; whence also it is that in the development of the foetus the liver is one of the organs that is last formed; I have observed all the members perfectly marked out in the human foetus, even the genital organs, whilst there was yet scarcely any trace of the liver. And indeed at the period when all the parts, like the heart itself in the beginning, are still white, and save in the veins there is no appearance of redness, you shall see nothing in the seat of the liver but a shapeless collection, as it were, of extravasated blood, which you might take for the effects of a contusion or ruptured vein.

But in the incubated egg there are, as it were, two umbilical vessels, one from the albumen passing entire through the liver, and going straight to the heart; another from the yelk, ending in the vena portae; for it appears that the chick, in the first instance, is entirely formed and nourished by the white; but by the yelk after it has come to perfection and is excluded from the shell; for this part may still be found in the abdomen of the check many days after its exclusion, and is a substitute for the milk to other animals.

But these matters will be better spoken of in my observations on the formation of the foetus, where many propositions, the following among the number, will be discussed: Wherefore is this part formed or perfected first, that last?—and of the several members: what part is the cause of another? And many points having special reference to the heart, such as: Wherefore does it first acquire consistency, and appear to possess life, motion, sense, before any other part of the body is perfected? as Aristotle says in his third book, *De Partibus Animalium*. And so also of the blood: Wherefore does it precede all the rest? And in what way does it possess the vital and animal principle? And show a tendency to motion, and to be impelled hither and thither, the end for which the heart appears to be made? In the same way, in considering the pulse: Wherefore one kind of pulse should indicate death, another recovery? And so of all the other kinds of pulse, what may be the cause and indication of each. So also in the consideration of crises and natural critical discharges; of nutrition, and especially the distribution of the nutriment; and of defluxions of every description. Finally, reflecting on every part of medicine, physiology, pathology, semeiotics, therapeutics, when I see how many questions can be answered, how many doubts resolved, how much obscurity illustrated, by the truth we have declared, the light we have made to shine, I see a field of such vast extent in which I might proceed so far, and expatiate so widely, that this my tractate would not only swell out into a volume, which was beyond my purpose, but my whole life, perchance, would not suffice for its completion.

In this place, therefore, and that indeed in a single chapter, I shall only endeavour to refer the various particulars that present themselves in the dissection of the heart and arteries to their several uses and causes; for so I shall meet with many things which receive light from the truth I have been contending for, and which, in their turn, render it more obvious. And indeed I would have it confirmed and illustrated by anatomical arguments above all others.

There is but a single point which indeed would be more correctly placed among our observations on the use of the spleen, but which it will not be altogether impertinent to notice in this place incidentally. From the splenic branch which passes into the pancreas, and from the upper part, arise the posterior coronary, gastric, and gastroepiploic veins, all of which are distributed upon the stomach in numerous branches and twigs, just as the mesenteric vessels are upon the intestines; in like manner, from the inferior part of the same splenic branch, and along the back of the colon and rectum proceed the hemorrhoidal veins. The blood returning by these veins, and bringing the cruder juices along with it, on the one hand from the stomach, where they are thin, watery, and not yet perfectly chylified; on the other thick and more earthy, as derived from the faeces, but all poured into this splenic branch, are duly tempered by the admixture of contraries; and nature mingling together these two kinds of juices, difficult of coction by reason of most opposite defects, and then diluting them with a large quantity of warm blood (for we see that the quantity returned from the spleen must be very large when we contemplate the size of its arteries), they are brought to the porta of the liver in a state of higher preparation; the defects of either extreme are supplied and compensated by this arrangement of the veins.

CHAPTER XVII

THE MOTION AND CIRCULATION OF THE BLOOD ARE CONFIRMED FROM THE PARTICULARS APPARENT IN THE STRUCTURE OF THE HEART, AND FROM THOSE THINGS WHICH DISSECTION UNFOLDS

I do not find the heart as a distinct and separate part in all animals; some indeed, such as the zoophytes, have no heart; this is because these animals are coldest, of no great bulk, of soft texture or of a certain uniform sameness or simplicity of structure; among the number I may instance grubs and earthworms, and those that are engendered of putrefaction and do not preserve their species. These have no heart, as not requiring any impeller of nourishment into the extreme parts; for they have bodies which are connate and homogeneous, and without limbs; so that by the contraction and relaxation of the whole body they assume and expel, move and remove the aliment. Oysters, mussels, sponges, and the whole genus of zoophytes or plant-animals have no heart; for the whole body is used as a heart, or the whole animal is a heart. In a great number of animals, almost the whole tribe of insects, we cannot see distinctly by reason of the smallness of the body; still in bees, flies, hornets, and the like, we can perceive something pulsating with the help of a magnifying glass; in pediculi, also, the same thing may be seen, and as the body is transparent, the passage of food through the intestines, like a black spot or stain, may be perceived by the aid of the same magnifying glass.

In some of the bloodless[1] and colder animals, further, as in snails, whelks, shrimps, and shell-fish, there is a part which pulsates—a kind of vesicle or auricle without a heart—slowly indeed, and not to be perceived save in the warmer season of the year. In these creatures this part is so

[1]I.e., not having red blood [Willis, 1847].

contrived that it shall pulsate, as there is here a necessity for some impulse to distribute the nutritive fluid by reason of the variety of organic parts, or of the density of the substance; but the pulsations occur infrequently, and sometimes in consequence of the cold not at all, an arrangement the best adapted to them as being of a doubtful nature, so that sometimes they appear to live, sometimes to die; sometimes they show the vitality of an animal, sometimes of a vegetable. This seems also to be the case with the insects which conceal themselves in winter, and lie, as it were, defunct, or merely manifesting a kind of vegetative existence. But whether the same thing happens in the case of certain animals that have red blood, such as frogs, tortoises, serpents, swallows, may be made a question without any kind of impropriety.

In all the larger and warmer, because [red-] blooded animals, there was need of an impeller of the nutritive fluid, and that perchance possessing a considerable amount of power. In fishes, serpents, lizards, tortoises, frogs, and others of the same kind there is a heart present, furnished with both an auricle and a ventricle, whence it is perfectly true, as Aristotle has observed,[1] that no [red-] blooded animal is without a heart, by the impelling power of which the nutritive fluid is forced, both with greater vigour and rapidity to a greater distance; it is not merely agitated by an auricle as it is in lower forms. And then in regard to animals that are yet larger, warmer, and more perfect, as they abound in blood, which is ever hotter and more spirituous, and possess bodies of greater size and consistency, they require a larger, stronger, and more fleshy heart, in order that the nutritive fluid may be propelled with yet greater force and celerity. And further, inasmuch as the more perfect animals require a still more perfect nutrition, and a larger supply of native heat, in order that the aliment may be thoroughly concocted and acquire the last degree of perfection, they required both lungs and a second ventricle, which should force the nutritive fluid through them.

Every animal that has lungs has therefore two ventricles to its heart, one right, and another left; and wherever there is a right, also is there a left ventricle; but the contrary of this does not hold good: where there is a left there is not always a right ventricle. The left ventricle I call that which is distinct in office, not in place from the other, that one namely which distributes the blood to the body at large, not to the lungs only. Hence the left ventricle seems to form the principal part of the heart; situated in the middle, more strongly marked, and constructed with greater care, the heart seems formed for the sake of the left ventricle, and the right but to minister to it; for the right neither reaches to the apex of the heart, nor is it nearly of such strength, being three times thinner in its walls, and in some sort jointed on to the left, (as Aristotle says;) though

[1]De Part. Animal., lib. iii.

indeed it is of greater capacity, inasmuch as it has not only to supply material to the left ventricle, but likewise to furnish aliment to the lungs.

It is to be observed, however, that all this is otherwise in the embryo, where there is not such a difference between the two ventricles; but as in a double nut, they are nearly equal in all respects, the apex of the right reaching to the apex of the left, so that the heart presents itself as a sort of double-pointed cone. And this is so, because in the foetus, as already said, whilst the blood is not passing through the lungs from the right to the left cavities of the heart, but flowing by the foramen ovale and ductus arteriosus, directly from the vena cava into the aorta, whence it is distributed to the whole body, both ventricles have in fact the same office to perform, whence their equality of constitution. It is only when the lungs come to be used, and it is requisite that the passages indicated should be blocked up, that the difference in point of strength and other things between the two ventricles begins to be apparent: in the altered circumstances the right has only to throw the blood through the lungs, whilst the left has to impel it through the whole body.

There are further within the heart numerous braces, so to speak, fleshy columns and fibrous bands, which Aristotle, in his third book on Respiration, and the Parts of Animals, entitles nerves. These are variously extended, and are either distinct or contained in grooves in the walls and partition, where they occasion numerous pits or depressions. They constitute a kind of small muscles, which are superadded and supplementary to the heart, assisting it to execute a more powerful and perfect contraction, and so proving subservient to the complete expulsion of the blood. They are in some sort like the elaborate and artful arrangement of ropes in a ship, bracing the heart on every side as it contracts, and so enabling it more effectually and forcibly to expel the charge of blood from its ventricles. This much is plain, at all events, that some animals have them strongly marked, others have them less so; and, in all that have them, they are more numerous and stronger in the left than in the right ventricle; and whilst some have them in the left, there are yet none present in the right ventricle. In the human subject, again, these fleshy columns and braces are more numerous in the left than in the right ventricle, and they are more abundant in the ventricles than in the auricles; occasionally, indeed, in the auricles there appear to be none present whatsoever. In large, more muscular and hardier bodies, as of countrymen, they are numerous; in more slender frames and in females they are fewer.

In those animals in which the ventricles of the heart are smooth within, and entirely without fibres or muscular bands, or anything like foveae, as in almost all the smaller birds, the partridge and the common fowl, serpents, frogs, tortoises, and also fishes, for the major part, there are no chordae tendinae, nor bundles of fibres, neither are there any tricuspid valves in the ventricles.

Some animals have the right ventricle smooth internally, but the left provided with fibrous bands, such as the goose, swan, and larger birds; and the reason here is still the same as elsewhere: as the lungs are spongy, and loose, and soft, no great amount of force is required to force the blood through them; hence the right ventricle is either without the bundles in question, or they are fewer and weaker, not so fleshy or like muscles; those of the left ventricle, however, are both stronger and more numerous, more fleshy and muscular, because the left ventricle requires to be stronger, inasmuch as the blood which it propels has to be driven through the whole body. And this, too, is the reason why the left ventricle occupies the middle of the heart, and has parietes three times thicker and stronger than those of the right. Hence all animals—and among men it is not otherwise—that are endowed with particularly strong frames, and that have large and fleshy limbs at a great distance from the heart, have this central organ of greater thickness, strength, and muscularity. And this is both obvious and necessary. Those, on the contrary, that are of softer and more slender make have the heart more flaccid, softer, and internally either sparely or not at all fibrous. Consider farther the use of the several valves, which are all so arranged, that the blood once received into the ventricles of the heart shall never regurgitate, once forced into the pulmonary artery and aorta shall not flow back upon the ventricles. When the valves are raised and brought together they form a three cornered line, such as is left by the bite of a leech; and the more they are forced, the more firmly do they oppose the passage of blood. The tricuspid valves are placed, like gate-keepers, at the entrance into the ventricles from the venae cavae and pulmonary veins, lest the blood when most forcibly impelled should flow back; and it is for this reason that they are not found in all animals; neither do they appear to have been constructed with equal care in all the animals in which they are found; in some they are more accurately fitted, in others more remissly or carelessly contrived and always with a view to their being closed under a greater or a slighter force of the ventricle. In the left ventricle, therefore, and in order that the occlusion may be the more perfect against the greater impulse, there are only two valves, like a mitre, and produced into an elongated cone, so that they come together and touch to their middle; a circumstance which perhaps led Aristotle into the error of supposing this ventricle to be double, the division taking place transversely. For the same reason, indeed, and that the blood may not regurgitate upon the pulmonary veins, and thus the force of the ventricle in propelling the blood through the system at large come to be neutralized, it is that these mitral valves excel those of the right ventricle in size and strength, and exactness of closing. Hence, too, it is essential that there can be no heart without a ventricle, since this must be the source and storehouse of the blood. The same law does not hold good in reference to the brain. For almost no genus of birds has a ventricle in the brain, as is obvious in the goose and swan, the brains of which nearly equal that of a rabbit in size; now rabbits have ventricles in the brain, whilst the goose has none. In like manner, wherever the heart has a single ventricle, there is an auricle appended, flaccid, membranous, hollow, filled with blood; and where there are two ventricles, there are likewise two auricles. On the other hand, however, some animals have an auricle without any ventricle; or at all events they have a sac analogous to an auricle; or the vein itself dilated at a particular part, performs pulsations, as is seen in hornets, bees, and other insects, which certain experiments of my own enable me to demonstrate have not only a pulse, but a respiration in that part which is called the tail, whence it is that this part is elongated and contracted now more rarely, now more frequently, as the creature appears to be blown and to require a larger quantity of air. But of these things, more in our Treatise on Respiration.

It is in like manner evident that the auricles pulsate, contract, as I have said before, and throw the blood into the ventricles; so that wherever there is a ventricle an auricle is necessary, not merely that it may serve, according to the general belief, as a source and magazine for the blood: for what were the use of its pulsations had it nothing to do save to contain? No; the auricles are prime movers of the blood, especially the right auricle, which is "the first to live, the last to die;" as already said; whence they are subservient to sending the blood into the ventricle, which, contracting incontinently, more readily and forcibly expels the blood already in motion; just as the ball-player can strike the ball more forcibly and further if he takes it on the rebound than if he simply threw it. Moreover, and contrary to the general opinion, since neither the heart nor anything else can dilate or distend itself so as to draw aught into its cavity during the diastole, unless, like a sponge, it has been first compressed, and as it is returning to its primary condition; but in animals all local motion proceeds from, and has its original in the contraction of some part: it is consequently by the contraction of the auricles that the blood is thrown into the ventricles, as I have already shown, and from thence, by the contraction of the ventricles, it is propelled and distributed. Which truth concerning local motions, and how the immediate moving organ in every motion of an animal primarily endowed with a motive spirit (as Aristotle has it[1]) is contractile; and how Aristotle was acquainted with the muscles, and did not unadvisedly refer all motion in animals to the nerves, or to the contractile element, and therefore called those little bands in the heart nerves—all this, if I am permitted to proceed in my purpose of making a particular demonstration of the organs of motion in animals from observations in my possession, I trust I shall be able to make sufficiently plain.

But that we may go on with the subject we have in hand, viz., the use of the auricles in filling the ventricles: we should expect that the more

[1]In the book, De Spiritu, and elsewhere.

dense and compact the heart, the thicker its parietes, the stronger and more muscular must be the auricle to force and fill it, and vice versa. Now this is actually so: in some the auricle presents itself as a sanguinolent vesicle, as a thin membrane containing blood, as in fishes, in which the sac that stands in lieu of the auricle, is of such delicacy and ample capacity, that it seems to be suspended or to float above the heart; in those fishes in which the sac is somewhat more fleshy, as in the carp, barbel, tench, and others, it bears a wonderful and strong resemblance to the lungs.

In some men of sturdier frame and stouter make, the right auricle is so strong, and so curiously constructed within of bands and variously interlacing fibres, that it seems to equal the ventricle of the heart in other subjects; and I must say that I am astonished to find such diversity in this particular in different individuals. It is to be observed, however, that in the foetus the auricles are out of all proportion large, which is because they are present before the heart [the ventricular portion] makes its appearance or suffices for its office even when it has appeared, and they therefore have, as it were, the duty of the whole heart committed to them, as has already been demonstrated. But what I have observed in the formation of the foetus as before remarked (and Aristotle had already confirmed all in studying the incubated egg) throws the greatest light and likelihood upon the point. Whilst the foetus is yet in the guise of a soft worm, or, as is commonly said, in the milk, there is a mere bloody point or pulsating vesicle, a portion apparently of the umbilical vein, dilated at its commencement or base; by and by, when the outline of the foetus is distinctly indicated, and it begins to have greater bodily consistence, the vesicle in question having become more fleshy and stronger, and changed its position, passes into the auricles, over or upon which the body of the heart begins to sprout, though as yet it apparently performs no duty; but when the foetus is farther advanced, when the bones can be distinguished from the soft parts, and movements take place, then it has also a heart internately which pulsates, and, as I have said, throws blood by either ventricle from the vena cava into the arteries.

Thus nature, ever perfect and devine, doing nothing in vain, has neither given a heart where it was not required, nor produced it before its office had become necessary; but by the same stages in the development of every animal, passing through the constitutions of all, as I may say (ovum, worm, foetus), it acquires perfection in each. These points will be found elsewhere confirmed by numerous observations on the formation of the foetus.

Finally, it was not without good grounds that Hippocrates, in his book, *De Corde,* intitles it as a muscle; as its action is the same, so is its function, viz., to contract and move something else, in this case, the charge of the blood.

Farther, as in muscles at large, so can we infer the action and use of the heart from the arrangement of its fibres and its general structure. All anatomists admit with Galen that the body of the heart is made up of various courses of fibres running straight, obliquely, and transversely, with reference to one another; but in a heart which has been boiled the arrangement of the fibres is seen to be different: all the fibres in the parietes and septum are circular, as in the sphincters; those, again, which are in the columnae extend lengthwise, and are oblique longitudinally; and so it comes to pass, that when all the fibres contract simultaneously, the apex of the cone is pulled towards its base by the columnae, the walls are drawn circularly together into a globe, the whole heart in short is contracted, and the ventricles narrowed; it is therefore impossible not to perceive that, as the action of the organ is so plainly contraction, its function is to propel the blood into the arteries.

Nor are we the less to agree with Aristotle in regard to the sovereignty of the heart; nor are we to inquire whether it receives sense and motion from the brain? whether blood from the liver? whether it be the origin of the veins and of the blood? and more of the same description. They who affirm these propositions against Aristotle, overlook, or do not rightly understand the principal argument, to the effect that the heart is the first part which exists, and that it contains within itself blood, life, sensation, motion, before either the brain or the liver were in being, or had appeared distinctly, or, at all events, before they could perform any function. The heart, ready furnished with its proper organs of motion, like a kind of internal creature, is of a date anterior to the body: first formed, nature willed that it should afterwards fashion, nourish, preserve, complete the entire animal, as its work and dwelling place: the heart, like the prince in a kingdom, in whose hands lie the chief and highest authority, rules over all; it is the original and foundation from which all power is derived, on which all power depends in the animal body.

And many things having reference to the arteries farther illustrate and confirm this truth. Why does not the arteria venosa pulsate, seeing that it is numbered among the arteries? Or wherefore is there a pulse in the vena arteriosa? Because the pulse of the arteries is derived from the impulse of the blood. Why does an artery differ so much from a vein in the thickness and strength of its coats? Because it sustains the shock of the impelling heart and streaming blood. Hence, as perfect nature does nothing in vain, and suffices under all circumstances, we find that the nearer the arteries are to the heart, the more do they differ from the veins in structure; here they are both stronger and more ligamentous, whilst in extreme parts of the body, such as the feet and hands, the brain, the mesentery, and the testicles, the two orders of vessels are so much alike that it is impossible to distinguish between them with the eye. Now this is for the following very sufficient reasons: for the more remote vessels are from the heart, with so much the less force are they impinged upon by the stroke of the heart, which is broken by the great distance at which it is given. Add to this, that the impulse of the heart exerted upon the mass of blood, which must needs fill the trunks and branches of the arteries, is diverted, divided, as it were, and diminished at every subdivision; so that the ultimate capillary divisions of the arteries look like veins, and this not merely in constitution but in function; for they have either no perceptible pulse, or they rarely exhibit one, and never save where the heart beats more violently than wont, or at a part where the minute vessel is more dilated or open than elsewhere. Hence it happens that at times we are aware of a pulse in the teeth, in inflammatory tumours, and in the fingers; at another time we feel nothing of the sort. Hence, too, by this single symptom I have ascertained for certain that young persons, whose pulses are naturally rapid, were labouring under fever; in like manner, on compressing the fingers in youthful and delicate subjects during a febrile paroxysm, I have readily perceived the pulse there. On the other hand, when the heart pulsates more languidly, it is often impossible to feel the pulse not merely in the fingers, but at the wrist, and even at the temple; this is the case in persons afflicted with lipothymiae and asphyxia, and hysterical symptoms, as also in persons of very weak constitution and in the moribund.

And here surgeons are to be advised that, when the blood escapes with force in the amputation of limbs, in the removal of tumors, and in wounds, it constantly comes from an artery; not always per saltum, however, because the smaller arteries do not pulsate, especially if a tourniquet has been applied.

And then the reason is the same wherefore the pulmonary artery has not only the structure of an artery, but wherefore it does not differ so widely in the thickness of its tunics from the veins as the aorta: the aorta sustains a more powerful shock from the left ventricle than the pulmonary artery does from the right; and the tunics of this last vessel are thinner and softer than those of the aorta in the same proportion as the walls of the right ventricle of the heart are weaker and thinner than those of the left ventricle; and in like manner, in the same degree in which the lungs are softer and laxer in structure than the flesh and other constituents of the body at large, do the tunics of the branches of the pulmonary artery differ from the tunics of the vessels derived from the aorta. And the same proportion in these several particulars is universally preserved. The more muscular and powerful men are, the firmer their flesh, the stronger, thicker, denser, and more fibrous their heart, in the same proportion are the auricles and arteries in all respects thicker, closer, and stronger. And again, and on the other hand, in those animals the ventricles of whose heart are smooth within, without villi or valves, and the walls of which are thinner, as in fishes, serpents, birds, and very many genera of animals, in all of them the arteries differ little or nothing in the thickness of their coats from the veins.

Farther, the reason why the lungs have such ample vessels, both arteries and veins (for the capacity of the pulmonary veins exceeds that of both the crural and jugular vessels), and why they contain so large a quantity of blood, as by experience and ocular inspection we know they do, admonished of the fact indeed by Aristotle, and not led into error by the appearances found in animals which have been bled to death,—is, because the blood has its fountain, and storehouse, and the workshop of its last perfection in the heart and lungs. Why, in the same way we find in the course of our anatomical dissections the arteria venosa and left ventricle so full of blood, of the same black colour and clotted character, too, as that with which the right ventricle and pulmonary artery are filled, inasmuch as the blood is incessantly passing from one side of the heart to the other through the lungs. Wherefore, in fine, the pulmonary artery or vena arteriosa has the constitution of an artery, the pulmonary veins or arteriae venosae have the structure of veins; because, in sooth, in function and constitution, and everything else, the first is an artery, the others are veins, in opposition to what is commonly believed; and why the pulmonary artery has so large an orifice, because it transports much more blood than is requisite for the nutrition of the lungs.

All these appearances, and many others, to be noted in the course of dissection, if rightly weighed, seem clearly to illustrate and fully to confirm the truth contended for throughout these pages, and at the same time to stand in opposition to the vulgar opinion; for it would be very difficult to explain in any other way to what purpose all is constructed and arranged as we have seen it to be.

1640

PIERRE GASSENDI

A BRIEF NOTE UPON A DEMONSTRATION OF THE EXISTENCE OF THE FORAMEN OVALE IN THE ADULT

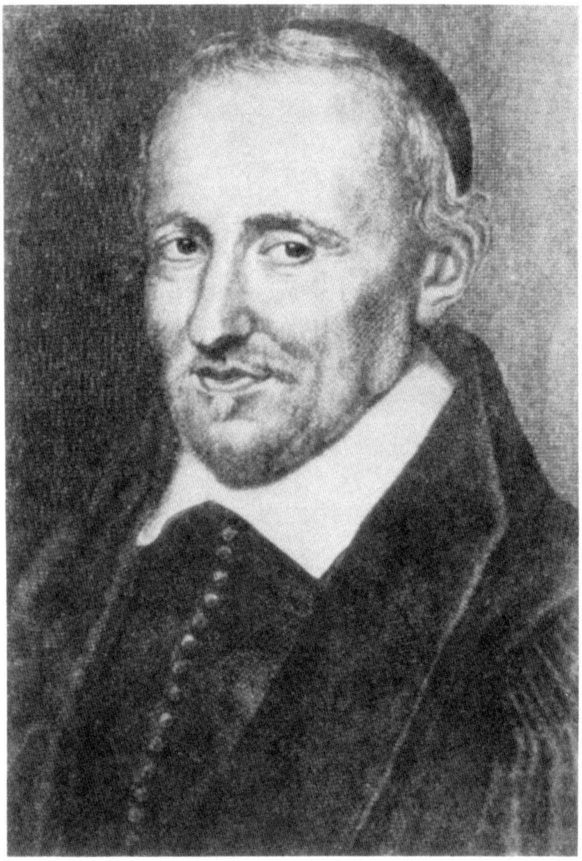

PIERRE GASSENDI

(Courtesy Zeitschrift für die gesamte Naturwissenschaft.)

PIERRE GASSENDI

(1592-1655)

PIERRE GASSENDI was born at Champtercier, near Digne, in Provence, France. His uncle, the curé of Champtercier, noticed that Gassendi had a remarkable ability for learning, and through his efforts Gassendi was sent to the college at Digne. When he was nineteen years of age, Gassendi matriculated at the University at Aix, where he studied philosophy under Fesaye. A year later (1612) he was recalled to the college at Digne to lecture on theology. In 1616 he received the degree of Doctor of Theology at Avignon and in the following year he was ordained. Following the acceptance of holy orders, he was invited to the University at Aix to occupy the chair of philosophy, which he accepted.

At Aix he became interested in anatomy, physics, and astronomy, and he once remarked that he frequently observed dissections in the anatomic amphitheater at Aix. He became more and more critical of the pedagogic reliance on the orthodox Aristotelio-scholastic teachings, and for this reason, presumably, he was asked to leave Aix in 1622. He next became a canon at Grenoble. In 1624 at Grenoble was published his "Exercitationes paradoxicae adversus Aristoteleos." This quarto volume contained his several arguments against the teachings of Aristotle.

In 1625, Gassendi was appointed to be provost of the Cathedral of Digne, but the appointment was not confirmed until 1634. During the interim he traveled first to Paris and later to Flanders and Holland. During these years he published attacks against Robert Fludd, the English physician who expounded mystical philosophy. From 1641 to 1646 in a series of writings he quarreled with Descartes regarding his metaphysical conceptions.

Through the influence of Richelieu, Gassendi was appointed by Louis XIV to the chair of mathematics in the Collège Royal. While he was in Paris, Gassendi became interested in Epicurean philosophy and later published three works on this subject.

Gassendi suffered from a disease of the thorax and in 1648 left Paris to seek a milder climate in southern France. In 1653, he returned to Paris but his health did not improve and after interminable bleedings by his physicians he died on October 24, 1655.

In 1640, Gassendi had published, in a volume (by himself and three other authors) entitled "De foetus formatione," a brief note on a demonstration of the existence of the vestigial foramen ovale in the adult. This was not Gassendi's discovery but merely a note or report of an anatomic dissection he had witnessed during his professorship at Aix. It is, however, an observation of great moment, and because the question of the perviousness of the septum of the heart was an important anatomic consideration vitally necessary to the establishment of the fact of the circulation of the blood, we have chosen to reproduce it.

A NICE OBSERVATION OF THE PERVIOUSNESS OF THE SEPTUM OF THE HEART*

By

PETER GASSENDI

I SHALL describe what I myself have seen.

While I was residing in Aix, whenever a dissection was being performed I was present frequently in the anatomical amphitheatre. Now for many years I had observed invariably that dissectors, taking the heart in their hands, would test the perviousness of its septum with a blunt instrument which they call a spatula, and would conclude, as physicians have concluded, that the transmission of blood from the right chamber to the left must occur by insensible transudation.

Now when this problem came to be discussed by the professors of anatomy, eight years ago, there came among the disputants a diligent surgeon, Payanus by name, who wanted to demonstrate to us onlookers that the facts were otherwise. So, taking up the spatula, he undertook to penetrate the mediastinum of the heart. But he did not attempt to push the instrument straight through, as the others had done, but having introduced its tip (for the tissue of the septum presents a thousand little openings) pushed onward with utmost gentleness, turning the instrument with the greatest patience up and down and from side to side, seeking always a farther ingress. And at last the instrument was seen entering the left chamber. But then, because we alleged that he had made an artificial opening, he himself requested one of us to incise the septum down to his instrument, with a sharp scalpel. When the incision had been made we found that no tissue anywhere had been injured, and we saw that only the meatus, or canal, notwithstanding the fact that it was a very winding passage, was lined with a very thin and glistening membrane.

These, then, are the passages which I mentioned to Fludd (who acknowledged clearly that he had been ignorant of their existence too); and I said that since they really do exist they cannot be without some function, and therefore it should be evident that there is a real percolation of blood from the right chamber into the left. And I maintained that the arterial blood was derived in this way.

**Elegans de septo cordis pervio observatio,* 1640. Translated by G. Kasten Tallmadge, Bull. Hist. Med. 7: 429-457, 1939.

Indeed, it seems probable that the more subtle part of the blood is, so to speak, sucked through this septum, or forced through by compression. But the grosser part of the blood, with the heavy vapours which it contains, enters the patent pulmonary artery and pervades and nourishes the tissues of the lungs. Then, after expiration has carried off the heavy breath and the heavy vapours, the more subtle residue of this blood is gathered into the pulmonary vein so that, together with the purer air which was inhaled in breathing, it may flow into the left ventricle, either drop by drop, as the general notion says it must, or in large spurts, as Harvey's opinion seems to have it.

1661

MARCELLO MALPIGHI

ON THE CAPILLARIES

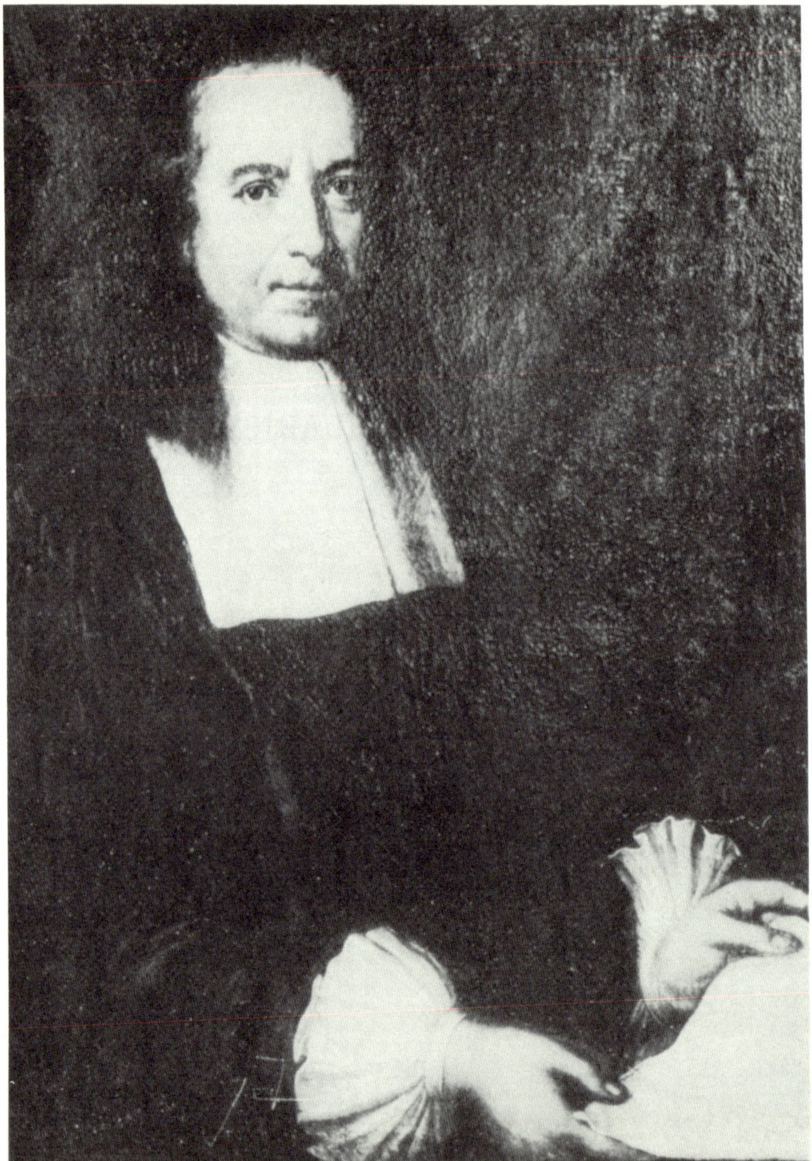

MARCELLO MALPIGHI

Portrait by unknown artist

(Courtesy Charles C Thomas.)

MARCELLO MALPIGHI

(1628-1694)

"I see with my eyes, a great, certain thing."

—Malpighi, paraphrasing Homer.

MARCELLO MALPIGHI is generally referred to as being the first histologist. The better to understand his several contributions to this subject, especially his discovery of the capillaries, mention should be made of the development of the compound microscope, on which his and the subsequent discoveries of his followers depended.

According to Henker,[1] there is reason to believe that the magnifying power of transparent media having convex surfaces was known very early, because a convex lens of rock crystal was found by Layard among the ruins of the palace at Nimrud. Seneca also described hollow spheres of glass filled with water as being commonly used for magnifiers. The perfect gem cutting of the ancients could not have been attained without the use of magnifiers, and it can be assumed that these artificers made their own magnifiers. Convex glass lenses were first generally used to assist ordinary vision as spectacles. The spectacle-makers were not only the first to produce glass magnifiers, but they were also the inventors of the telescope and the compound microscope. During the Thirty Years' War (1618-1648) the simple microscope was widely known, and Descartes in his "Dioptrique," published in 1637, described microscopes wherein a concave mirror was used in connection with a lens for illuminating the object. Antony van Leeuwenhoek (1632-1723), who added to Malpighi's initial description of the capillaries, appears to be the first to succeed in grinding and polishing lenses of such short focus and perfect figure as to render to the simple microscope a better object.

The early opticians contended that a compound microscope—that is, one having two lenses so that small objects can be magnified—would never produce images as good as those viewed by means of an instrument of the simple type, but this contention has proved to be erroneous. Although the simple microscope may be improved, it has relatively feeble powers of magnification, and to obtain stronger magnifications the compound form is necessary.

Soon after the discovery of the telescope, the compound microscope was invented. The inventors were probably the Middelburg lens-grinders, Johann and Zacharias Janssen; the time, about 1590. The microscope had a negative eyepiece. It was not greatly improved until 1646, when Fontana described a microscope which had a positive eyepiece. This produced much better images and was, most likely, the type of apparatus that Malpighi worked with. With it, he was able to describe the capillary circulation, the existence of which Harvey, because of his inferior equipment, was able only to postulate.

Marcello Malpighi was born at Crevalcuore, near Bologna. He was the son of well-to-do parents. In 1645 he entered the University of Bologna as a student of philosophy. He was forced to interrupt his studies in 1649 because of the sudden deaths of his father, mother, and his father's mother. Being the eldest son of the

[1]Henker, Otto: Microscope, The Encyclopaedia Britannica, ed. 11, vol. 18, pp. 392-407.

family, he was called upon to make settlement of the estate. This was rendered difficult by reason of a dispute concerning boundaries which had arisen between his family and the possessors of an adjoining property, the family of Sbaraglia. This dispute continued to the end of Malpighi's days and was a constant source of irritation. The Sbaraglia family not only brought political pressure to bear to obstruct professorial appointments, but also privately heckled Malpighi and his wife.

It was not until 1651 that Malpighi resumed his studies, this time with the idea of studying medicine. One of his professors, Bartolommeo Massari, to disseminate the new work of Harvey and the new learning of the English philosophers, occasionally gathered some of the instructors and more mature students at his home. This group eventually formed itself into a club, limited its membership to nine, the number of the Muses, and adopted the name, ''Corus anatomicus.'' Stimulated by Harvey's new viewpoint of learning by means of actual observation, members of this club not only met for discussion but soon were dissecting bodies and experimenting on living animals. Young Malpighi was soon admitted to the club, and therein learned the foundations for his future work. He was making remarkable progress in his studies and in 1653 achieved his doctorate in medicine and philosophy.

In 1654 Malpighi married Francesca, the sister of his learned professor, Massari. She bore him no children. In 1656 Malpighi, who had been busy in medical practice, obtained a chair at the University of Bologna and was made a professor of medicine. Meanwhile, in the same year, Ferdinand II, Grand Duke of Tuscany, offered him a post in theoretical medicine at the University of Pisa. Malpighi accepted the offer and for three years taught at Pisa. There, under the guidance of Duke Ferdinand, a brilliant intellectual activity was stimulated and sincere efforts were made by the entire staff at the university to broaden the bonds of natural knowledge.

It was at Pisa that Malpighi met Giovanni Borelli and much was to come of their friendship, which lasted many years. Borelli also had come to the university in 1656 to fill the position of professor of mathematics at the request of Duke Ferdinand. Borelli was twenty years Malpighi's senior and taught him the new mathematics and physics of the school of Galileo. Malpighi reciprocated and interested Borelli in anatomic and biologic problems to such an extent that soon Borelli was combining his mathematic talents in the study of the phenomena of living things. Borelli's great work, ''De motu animalium,'' published after his death (1680 or 1681) shows the influence of Malpighi. Although in later years Malpighi's private life was embittered by the coarse personal attacks of Borelli, they remained close friends for many years. Whenever a new idea occurred to Malpighi or whenever he made a new discovery, he always desired Borelli's opinion regarding it.

In 1659, because of some difficulties regarding the paternal estates, Malpighi resigned his post at Pisa and returned to Bologna. There he was again appointed professor of medicine, and in 1660 he was able to announce privately to Borelli, in two letters, his discovery of the structure of the lung. These two letters were printed in 1661 and constituted Malpighi's first published work. In these brief epistles, two discoveries of fundamental importance were announced. In the first letter he described the vesicular nature of the lung, showing how the divisions of the trachea terminated in the dilated air vesicles. He was the first, therefore, to supply an anatomic basis for the true conception of the respiratory process.

The second letter contained the first observation of the capillaries and supplied the missing link in the rationale of the circulation of the blood. Without the aid of a microscope, Harvey had discovered and proved the existence of the circulation. He had further predicted the possibility ''that in the limbs and extreme parts of the body the blood passes either immediately by anastomosis from the arteries into the veins or mediately from the pores of the flesh, or in both ways. . . .'' Malpighi, by histologic demonstration, proved the existence of capillary anastomosis between the arteries and veins.

In 1665, in a little tract, ''De omento pinguedine, et adiposis ductibus,'' Malpighi came upon another discovery concerning the blood, the demonstration of the red corpuscles. This he failed to interpret properly. Under the microscope he observed flat red cells in the mesenteric blood vessels of the hedgehog. Apparently, he mistook the red blood corpuscles for globules of fat passing from fatty tissues into the current of the blood. This observation was later clarified by van Leeuwenhoek who, in 1674 in the ''Philosophical Transactions'' of the Royal Society, gave the first accurate description of the red corpuscles.

Besides discovering the capillaries and being the first to observe, if not to describe accurately, the red blood corpuscles, Malpighi worked unceasingly on the structure of the glands and glandular organs. He is also regarded as the founder of descriptive embryology, because of his investigations of the chick embryo. He also discovered the ''rete mucosum'' or the Malpighian layer of the skin and further proved that the papillae of the tongue are organs of taste (Garrison, p. 255).

In his monumental work on the structure of the viscera (''De viscerum structura, Exercitatio anatomica,'' published at Bonn in 1666), Malpighi did much to advance the understanding of the physiology of the liver, spleen, and kidneys. In this volume, moreover, is contained the first account of the general enlargement of the lymphatic vessels with nodules in the spleen, more fully described by Thomas Hodgkin in 1832. During his later years, Malpighi spent much of his time in researches on the anatomy of the silkworm and the morphology of plants, in which latter endeavor he is equally famous in association with his researches in physiology. In 1684, he had a great misfortune. His house in Bologna burned. His microscopes were ruined and many of his precious manuscripts were destroyed.

In 1691, the new pope, Innocent XII, invited Malpighi to come to Rome as his personal physician. He at first refused, but after being urged by the pontiff, Malpighi, being an old friend, accepted. He continued to work in that capacity, but soon after his arrival at Rome he became ill. In July 1694, he suffered a mild apoplectic attack and on November 28th he suffered a second attack. On the following day he passed away.

EPISTLE II*:—ABOUT THE LUNGS†

To that very famous and learned Man

ALPHONSUS BORELLIUS

Celebrated Professor of Science at Pisa

By

MARCELLUS MALPIGHIUS

Professor of Medicine at Bologna

THERE is this difficulty and obscurity to be met with in natural things, that there seems to be something in them that is not to be determined altogether by our senses. And so, steadfastly working with very great labour, we may contemplate Nature showing herself in her beginnings, as it were in a volume elaborated through mysteries. And when we try to unravel the obscure things in the viscera of animals, at length by our efforts, and only with great weariness, we conclude that the truth of our observations is made out. We borrow illumination, as if by degrees, from dissection, sometimes of insects, sometimes of perfect animals. For Nature is accustomed to rehearse with certain large, perhaps baser, and all classes of wild (animals), and to place in the imperfect the rudiments of the perfect animals.

And now, most famous man, I will handle the matter more closely. There were two things which, in my epistle about observation on the lungs, I left as doubtful and to be investigated with more exact study.

(1) The first was what may be the network described therein, where certain bladders and sinuses are bound together in a certain way in the lungs.

(2) The other was whether the vessels of the lungs are connected by mutual anastomosis, or gape into the common substance of the lungs and sinuses.

The solution of these problems may prepare the way for greater things and will place the operations of Nature more clearly before the eyes. For the unloosing of these knots I have destroyed almost the whole race of frogs, which does not happen in that savage Batrachomyomachia of Homer. For

*In his second letter to Borellius, Malpighi describes his discovery of the capillary circulation.—F. A. W., 1940.

†*De pulmonibus observationes anatomiae*, Bologna, 1661. Translated by James Young, M.D., Proc. Roy. Soc. Med. (Part I)- 23: 7-11, 1929-1930.

in the anatomy of frogs, which, by favour of my very excellent colleague, D. Carolo Fracassato, I had set on foot in order to become more certain about the membranous substance of the lungs, it happened to me to see such things that not undeservedly I can better make use of that (saying) of Homer for the present matter—

"I see with my eyes a work trusty and great."

For in this (frog anatomy), owing to the simplicity of the structure, and the almost complete transparency of the vessels which admits the eye into the interior, things are more clearly shown, so that they will bring the light to other more obscure matters.

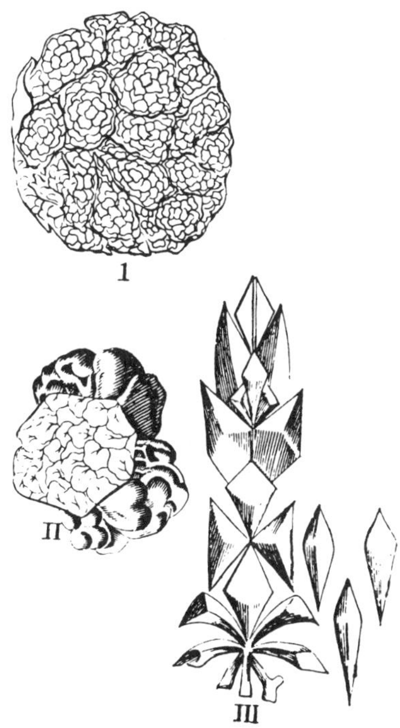

TABULA I

Fig. I. Outermost piece of dried lung showing the rete.

Fig. II. Interior vesicles and sinuses sketched with portion of the interstitium in the upper part. The beginning and complete prolongation could not be exhibited to the eye by the picture.

Fig. III. Adaptation over the trachea and the pulmonary vessels which also, parted from their usual site, are shown for easier understanding.

In the frog, therefore, the abdomen being laid open lengthwise, the lungs, adhering on each side to the heart, come forth. They are not slack as in other animals, but remain tense for the animal's requirements. They are nothing more than a membranous bladder, which at first sight seems to be spattered with very small spots, arranged in order after the fashion of the skin of the dogfish—commonly called Sagrino. In form and surface protuberances it resembles the cone of a pine: but internally and externally a certain texture of vessels diversely prolonged is connected together, which, by the pulse, by contrary movement, and the insertion of the vein, are pulmonary arteries. In the concave and interior part of this (bladder) it almost fades into an empty space devoted to the reception of air, but it is not everywhere smooth but is interrupted by the occurrence of alveoli. These are produced by membranous walls raised to a little height. They are not all of this shape, but when the walls are produced out in length and width and connected together, the bays (sinuses) are formed almost into hexagons; and bent at the corners of the sinuses the membrane is extended a little as an infundibulum is constituted; and thus the lungs of the smaller frogs are fashioned. But in those which are larger, the walls are raised higher, and from the middle of the enclosed floor three come out very visibly increasing. The partitions in the smaller frogs are almost unobservable, but those in the bigger ones are bound into three other sinuses as they divide the greater sinus very much. The area, or the floor of the sinuses, admits the vessels spoken of above, and the artery itself sometimes ends inconspicuously, fork-like in the middle, but

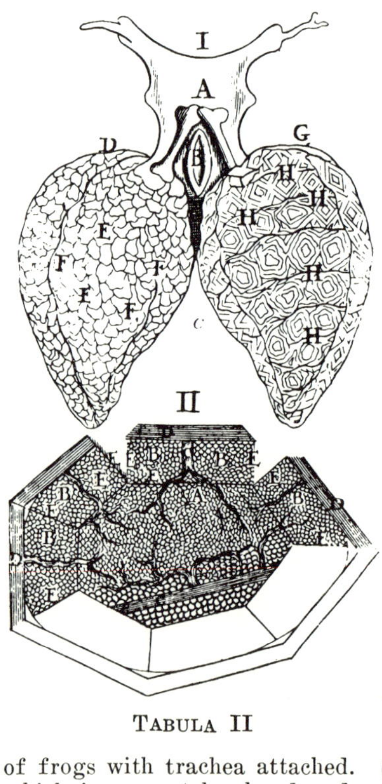

TABULA II

Fig. I. Showing lungs of frogs with trachea attached. (A) Larynx, which is semi-cartilaginous. (B) Rima, which is accurately closed and opened at the animal's need. Air being enclosed, it keeps the lungs expanded. (C) Site of the heart. (D) External part of the lung. (E) Prolonged rete of the cells. (F) Prolongation of the pulmonary artery. (G) Concave part of the lung divided through the middle. (H) Prolongation of the pulmonary vein running through the apices.

Fig. II. Containing the most simple cell without the intermediate walls (magnified). (A) Interior floor of the cell. (B) Parietes separated and bent. (C) Trunk of pulmonary artery with attached branches, as if ending in a network. (D) Trunk of pulmonary vein wandering with its branches over the slopes of the walls. (E) Vessel in the bottom and corners of the walls with the ramifications of the rete continued.

further on is spread out at the greater passage and sometimes manifestly produces another branch, but the vein glides down the inner slopes of the walls and is mingled with these, and, the branches having been sent down through the walls, at length runs into the area.

Observation by means of the microscope will reveal more wonderful things than those viewed in regard to mere structure and connection: for while the heart is still beating, the contrary (i.e., in opposite directions in the different vessels) movement of the blood is observed in the vessels,—though with difficulty,—so that the circulation of the blood is clearly exposed. This is more clearly recognized in the mesentery and in the other greater veins contained in the abdomen.

Thus, by this impulse, the blood is driven in very small (streams) through the arteries like a flood into the several cells, one or other branch clearly passing through or ending there. Thus the blood, much divided, puts off its red colour, and, carried round in a winding way, is poured out on all sides till at length it may reach the walls, the angles, and the absorbing branches of the veins. The power of the eye could not be extended further in the opened living animal, hence I had believed that this body of the blood breaks into the empty space, and is collected again by a gaping vessel and by the structure of the walls. The tortuous and diffused motion of the blood in divers directions, and its union at a determinate place offered a handle to this. But the dried lung of the frog made my belief dubious. This lung had, by chance, preserved the redness of the blood in (what afterwards proved to be) the smallest vessels, where by means of a more perfect lens, no more there met the eye the points forming the skin called Sagrino, but vessels mingled annularly. And, so great is the divarication of these vessels as they go out, here from a vein, there from an artery, that order is no longer preserved, but a network appears made up of the prolongations of both vessels. This network occupies not only the whole floor, but extends also to the walls, and is attached to the outgoing vessel, as I could see with greater difficulty but more abundantly in the oblong lung of a tortoise, which is similarly membranous and transparent. Here it was clear to sense that the blood flows away through the tortuous vessels, that it is not poured into spaces but always works through tubules, and is dispersed by the multiplex winding of the vessels. Nor is it a new practice of Nature to join together the extremities of vessels, since the same holds in the intestines and other parts; nay, what seems more wonderful, she joins the upper and the lower ends of veins to one another by visible anastomosis, as the most learned Fallopius has very well observed.

But in order that you may more easily get hold of what I have said, and follow it with your own sight, tie with a thread, just where it joins the heart, the projecting swollen lung of an opened frog while it is bathed on every side with abundant blood. This, when dried, will preserve the vessels turgid with blood. You will see this very well if you examine it by the microscope of one lens against the horizontal sun. Or you may institute another method of seeing these things. Place the lung on a crystal plate illuminated below through a tube by a lighted candle. To it bring a microscope of two lenses, and thus the vessels distributed in a ring-like fashion will be disclosed to you. By the same arrangement of the instruments and light, you will observe the movement of the blood through the vessels in question. You will yourself be able to contrive it by different degrees of light, which escape description by the pen. About the movement of the blood, however, one thing shows itself, worthy of your speculation. The auricle and the heart being ligatured, and thus deprived of motion and the impulse which might be derived from the heart into the connected vessels, the blood is still moved by the veins toward the heart so that it distends the vessels by its effort and copious flow. This lasts several hours. At the end, however, especially if it is exposed to the solar rays, it is agitated, not by the same continued motion, but, as if impelled by changing impulses, it advances and recedes fluctuating along the same way. This takes place when the heart and auricle are removed from the body.

From these things, therefore as to the first problems to be solved, from analogy and the simplicity which Nature uses in all her operations, it can be inferred that that network which formerly I believed to be nervous in nature, mingled in the bladders and sinuses, is (really) a vessel carrying the body of blood thither or carrying it away. Also that, although in the lungs of perfect animals the vessels seem sometimes to gape and end in the midst of the network of rings, nevertheless, it is likely that, as in the cells of frogs and tortoises, that vessel is prolonged further into very small vessels in the form of a network, and these escape the senses on account of their exquisite smallness.

Also from these things can be solved with the greatest probability the question of the mutual union and anastomosis of the vessels. For if Nature turns the blood about in vessels, and combines the ends of the vessels in a network, it is likely that in other cases an anastomosis joins them; this is clearly recognized in the bladder of frogs swollen with urine, in which the above described motion of the blood is observed through the transparent vessels joined together by anastomosis, and not that those vessels have received that connection and course which the veins or fibres mark out in the leaves of nearly all trees.

To what purpose all these things may be made, beyond those which I dealt with in the last letter concerning the pulmonary mixing of the blood, you yourself seemed to recognize readily, nor is the opinion to be lessened by your very famous device, because by your kindness you have entrusted me with elaborate letters in which you philosophised subtly by observing the strange portents of Nature in vegetables, when we wonder that apples hang from trunks not their own, and that by grafting of plants the processes have produced bastards in happy association with legitimates. We see that one and the same tree has assumed diverse fashions in its branches,—while here the hanging fruits please the taste by a grateful acidity, there they fulfill every desire by their nectar-like sweetness, and you furnish credibility to the truth at which you wondered when in Rome, that the vine and the jasmine had come forth from the bole of the Massilian apple. He who cultivated the gardens with a light inserted fork made these clever things with bigger branches, and he taught the unreluctant trees the bringing forth of divers things. About this matter Virgil in the Georgics fitly sang:—

> "They ingraft the sprout from the alien tree
> And teach it to grow from the moist inner bark."

You lay bare the secret of this wonderful result by your philosophising method, for we might consider the acid juice of the Massilian apple sweetens to the nature of pure wine as far as the particles of that juice may run through the small openings of the trunk proper, but not in the same way can they come up into the continued tubules of the vine. Here, stirred by their own motion, and torn away beyond their usual order by the impulse of those following after, and broken up, they must conform themselves to the superinduced form of the passage, and put on the new nature by which the vine or jasmine is brought forth. Nature pursues a like mode of operation in the lungs, for the turbid blood returns from the ambit of the body, widowed elsewhere of particles, to which a new humour from the subclavian vein is added to be perfected by the further action of Nature. This happens in order that it may be arranged and prepared into the nature of particles of flesh, bone, nerve, etc., while it enters the myriad vessels of the lungs. It is conducted into divers very small threads. Thus a new form, situation, and motion is prepared for the particles of the blood, from which flesh, bone, and spirits may be formed. The trustworthiness of your saying is increased by the like structure of the seminal vessels as if a certain nutrition of the living animal were also its regeneration.

I have put these few little observations into a letter that I might increase the things found out about the lungs. If I have set in motion all the point of my observations I have owed the addition to the frog. You will bring out the truth and dignity of these matters by your authority and contrivance. Meantime, apply yourself happily to philosophy, and may you go on to render me altogether happy by increasing a little my very unimportant thoughts of your writings "De Animalium Motu."

Farewell!

Bologna, 1661.

1664

NIELS STENSEN

ON THE MUSCULAR NATURE OF THE HEART

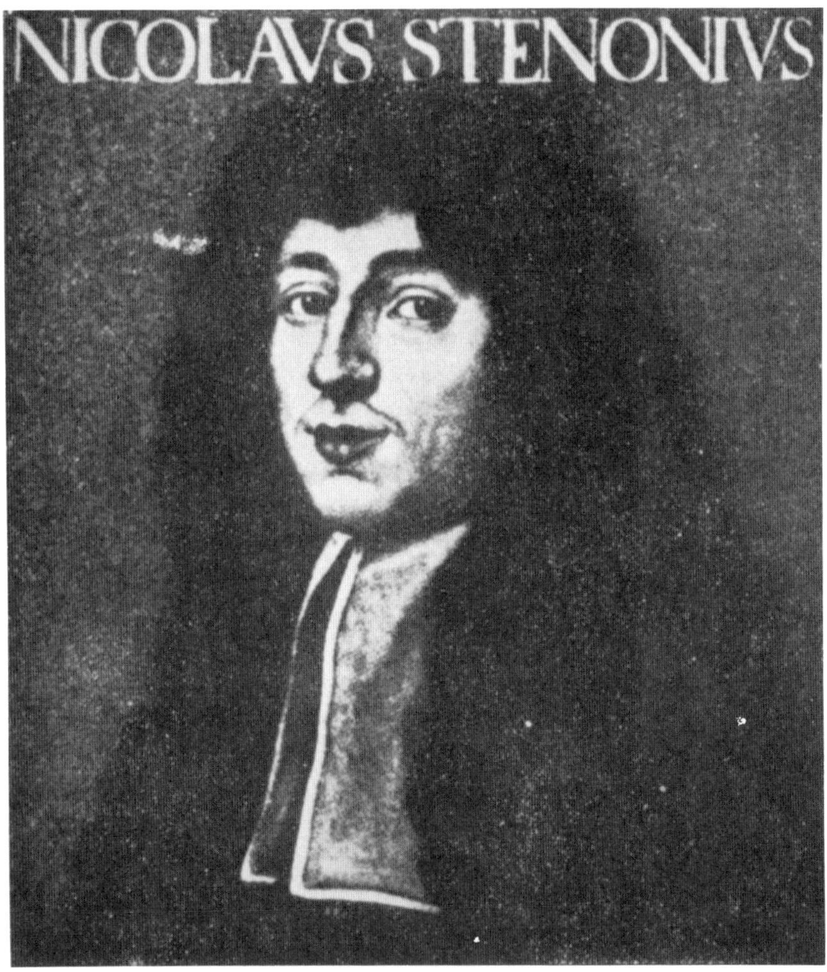

NIELS STENSEN

(Courtesy Annals of Medical History.)

NIELS STENSEN

(1638-1686)

NIELS STENSEN or "Nicholas Steno,"[1] as he was also called, was born on January 20, 1638, in Copenhagen, Denmark. His father, Steen Pedersen,[2] was a goldsmith who died before Niels was six years of age. When his mother remarried, the boy was sent to live with his grandparents and it may be assumed that they provided him with a tutor in order that he might qualify for training at a university.

In 1656 Stensen entered the University of Copenhagen. For his preceptor, who also was to act in the capacity of adviser, he chose Thomas Bartholin (1616-1680), the esteemed professor of anatomy. He not only studied anatomy but also devoted much time to the mathematical sciences. At the university he learned Hebrew, which was to be a great asset to him in later years when he became affiliated with the Roman Catholic Church. His later published works also show that he was proficient in Greek, Latin, French, German, Dutch, Italian, and English.

In 1658 the classes of the University of Copenhagen were interrupted by the Swedish invasion of Denmark. The Swedes besieged Copenhagen. Stensen, in the short war, held the commission of corporal in the student regiment, with eighty-six scholars under his charge.

After spending three years at the University of Copenhagen, Stensen went to Amsterdam, where he studied anatomy under Professor Gerhard Blasius (1626-1682). During his first year at Amsterdam, Stensen discovered the duct that bears his name, the secretory duct of the parotid gland, which he found in the head of a sheep he had dissected. Not long afterward, Stensen communicated his discovery to his preceptor, Bartholin, in a letter written from Leyden on April 22, 1661.

The letter provoked a quarrel with Blasius who claimed the discovery as his own. There is no evidence to support the claim of Blasius, and Jean van Hoorne (1621-1670) of Leyden named the duct after Stensen. Because of this quarrel, Stensen left the University of Amsterdam to continue his studies at the University of Leyden, where he worked under Van Hoorne and the celebrated Frenchman, François de la Boe Sylvius (1614-1672). Not long afterward Sylvius was able to demonstrate Stensen's duct in man.

Stensen next began to investigate the glands of the eye, and in the latter part of 1661 he published an account of the glands of the eye and the vessels of the nose.

From 1662 to 1663 Stensen was busy investigating the muscles. In 1664 the death of his stepfather called him home to Copenhagen. When he returned to his native city, he published a most important work: "De musculis et glandulis observationum specimen, cum epistolis duabus anatomicis" (Hafniae, Lit. M. Godieceniis, 1664). He dedicated this work to King Friedrich III of Denmark, to whom he had been recommended by Bartholin.

The observation, recorded in the aforementioned work, that the heart was composed chiefly of muscle fibers was one of the great anatomic discoveries of his era, and we consider it a special privilege to be able to present Stensen's description of the heart in translation.

---

[1]Other variations of Stensen: Stenon, Stènone, Stenonis, Stenonius.

[2]Lutz spelled this name "Peterson"; Miller, "Pedersen."

The importance of this discovery, according to Miller, was noted in 1665 by a contemporary, de Hedovvile, who said of it, ''This observation overthrew a system to which medicine clung most tenaciously,'' and Albrecht von Haller (1708-1777),[3] the great physiologist, in 1774, referred to this work as a golden book which contained the rich seed for new discoveries.

Lutz referred to Kurt Sprengel (1766-1833) as recording that Giovanni Borelli (1608-1679) claimed in 1680 that he had observed the structure of the heart in 1657, while he was working with Malpighi. The only other person to consider the heart a muscle before Stensen was an unknown Alexandrian who wrote a book on the heart which is placed among the Hippocratic works. Following Stensen, Richard Lower (1631-1691), in 1669, also demonstrated the muscular nature of the heart.

In 1665, Stensen went to Paris, where he continued his anatomical work and also performed dissections at the École de Médecine. During this year, Stensen gave a lecture on the anatomy of the brain. According to some authorities, modern neurologic observations received their impetus from Stensen's observations which are found in his lecture on the brain.

Stensen traveled to Southern France in the latter part of 1665 and spent the following spring in Italy. In Italy, he was kindly received and Grand Duke Ferdinand III, who, as we have noticed in our account of Malpighi, had done many things for the cause of science, appointed Stensen one of his physicians and gave him a pension and a residence. Stensen then followed the court which moved to the surrounding Italian cities. In 1667, at Florence, he published an extensive work on the muscles, ''Elementorum Myologiae specimen seu musculorum descriptio geometrica.''

On November 2, 1667, Stensen, who had given the matter considerable thought, was converted from Lutheranism to Roman Catholicism. In December of that year the Danish King, Friedrich III, offered him a professorship at the University of Copenhagen. Stensen wrote to the King asking him if he was willing to accept his new religious preference. He received no reply and on February 2, 1670, the King, who had been very ill, died. In 1672 the new King, Christian V, commanded Stensen to return to Denmark to assume his professorship, which he did. His position as a Roman Catholic professor in a Lutheran university was precarious. For some reason, probably his growing attachment to the Roman Catholic Church, he resigned his professorship in 1674. He then returned to Italy and devoted himself exclusively to the work of the church.

In addition to his anatomic discoveries, Stensen made many interesting geologic observations. He compared fossil teeth found in the Tuscany deposits with the teeth of the living shark. He compared deposits of rocks wherein fossils could be found with deposits wherein no fossils could be found, and came to the conclusion that the earth was at one time completely submerged in water. Stensen also laid the foundation for structural geology, believing from his studies that the movements of the earth were the cause of origin of vertical strata of rock which once had been horizontal.

When Stensen returned to Italy he assumed charge of the education of the son of Grand Duke Cosimo III.

In 1675, Stensen was ordained a priest, and, in 1677, he was consecrated Bishop of Titiopolis. Jean Frederick, Prince of Brunswick, called him to his court shortly thereafter. Pope Innocent XI allowed him to leave Italy appointing him ''Apostolic Vicar for the Northern Missions.'' Stensen spent the remainder of his life partly at the court of Jean Frederick and partly in visiting Roman Catholic missions in Germany. He died at Schwerin on November 25, 1686, and is buried in the Basilica of Saint Lawrence in Florence, Italy.

---

[3]See page 167, biographic sketch of Albrecht von Haller.

NICOLAI STENONIS

DE

MUSCULIS

ET

GLANDULIS

Observationum Specimen.

Cum.

Epistolis duabus Anatomicis

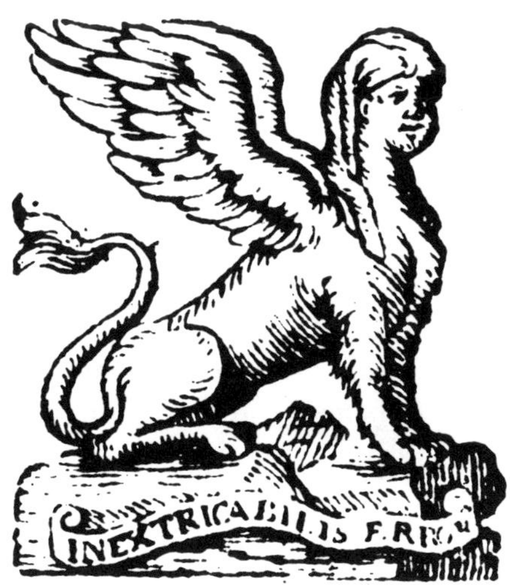

AMSTELODAMI.

Apud PETRUM le GRAND, 10[illegible]

ON THE MUSCULAR NATURE OF THE HEART*†

IF ONE desires to apply the word muscle to the heart, one must first demonstrate the proposition that *the heart is truly a muscle.* This is deduced from more detailed facts which I shall shortly present.

In all the substance of the heart there occurs nothing except *arteries, veins, nerves, fibers and membranes.* And in the muscle, except the above mentioned, there occur no others. I omit fat and bone, because all hearts do not have this, and no muscle has it. Whoever of the anatomists should demonstrate fibers distinctly in the parenchyma should attribute it not to the senses but to genius. I saw in certain splendid preparations linear structures running on the surface of the heart, which however were not lymphatics, but dissection showed them to be truly nerves. A nervous plexus was demonstrated by Fallopius at autopsy, who believed that they were dispersed not only over the surface but that they penetrated into the interior.

Among none of the fibers of the heart does one meet, in examination, fibers of which the center is not fleshy, and both extremes tendinous; this moreover is common to all the fibers of the muscle. . . .

And thus everything is in agreement, and truly muscle may be attributed to the heart, nor can it be otherwise; *truly the heart merits the name of muscle, because it has tendons and flesh and nerves.*

This the great Hippocrates appears to directly oppose . . . nevertheless his words when compared with ours would seem to be in intimate agreement; he said truly that the strength of a muscle was not in the tendon but in the flesh. Whatever really was the opinion of this author, his words are only slightly different from ours. . . .

If it be true, and the truth of an observation is dependent upon its correctness, that in the heart nothing is lacking which would make it a muscle, and not denying that muscle has been demonstrated in the heart, the heart thus is not a substance *sui generis,* and so cannot generate certain substances as heat (fire), innate warmth, the seat of the soul; nor can it produce certain humors as blood, certain spirits or vitality. But however that may be, I am examining solely the substance; thus, from the fibers proceeds all movement of the heart, occurring as a phenomenon of its own . . . , which subject, however, I wish to largely omit at present and defer a consideration of it until a later time. . . .

*Stensen, Niels: *De musculis et glandulis observationum specimen, cum epistolis duabus anatomicis,* Amstelodanum, OP. Le Grand, 1664, 90 pp. Translated by Maurice N. Walsh, M.D., Mayo Clinic.

†Only such a portion of Stensen's book as deals with the *musculature* of the heart has been translated.—Translator.

1705

WILLIAM COWPER

DESCRIPTION OF AORTIC INSUFFICIENCY

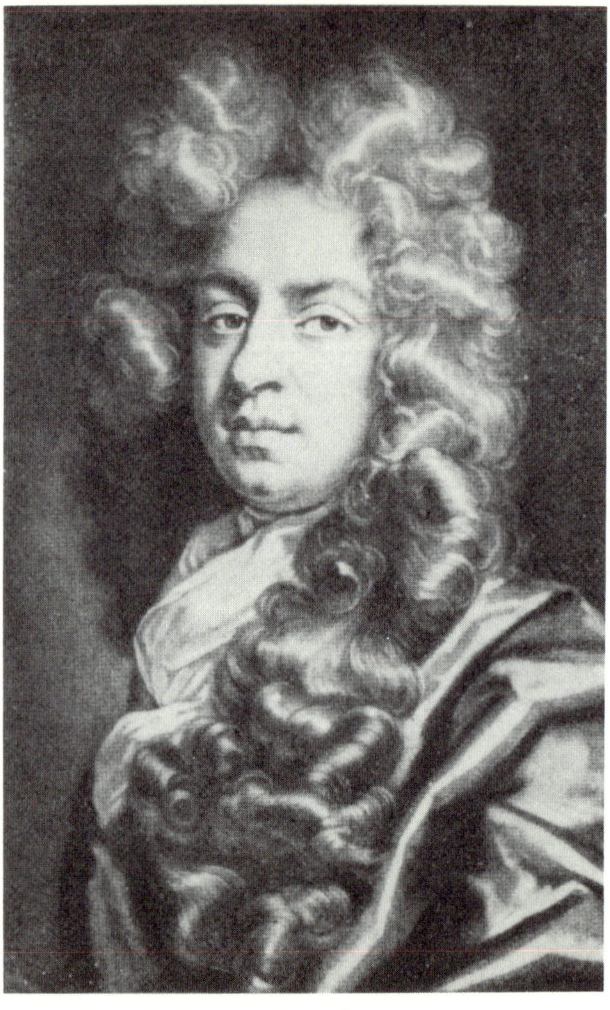

WILLIAM COWPER

(Courtesy Charles C Thomas.)

WILLIAM COWPER

(1666-1709)

WILLIAM COWPER, sometimes written as Cooper, was born in Petersfield, Sussex, England, in 1666. He was the youngest son of Richard Cowper. Young Cowper at the age of sixteen was apprenticed to William Bignall, an English surgeon who resided in London. At a later date, it is known, he continued his apprenticeship under John Fletcher.

In March, 1691, Cowper became free of the Company of Barber Surgeons of London. He settled in London, devoted himself to the study of anatomy, and three years later he published a work entitled ''Myotomia Reformata; or a New Administration of the Muscles of the Human Bodies, wherein the true uses of the muscles are explained, the errors of former anatomists concerning them confuted and several muscles not hitherto taken notice of described: to which are subjoined a graphical description of the bones and other anatomical observations'' [London, 1694].

This was a cleverly executed work and no doubt was one of the reasons that led to Cowper's election to a fellowship of the Royal Society in 1696.

In 1698 Cowper published a beautiful atlas with an original English text and the following long explanatory title page: ''The Anatomy of the Human Bodies, with figures drawn after the life by some of the best masters in Europe, and curiously engraven in one hundred and fourteen copper plates, illustrated with large explications, containing many new anatomical discoveries and chirurgical observations. To which is added an introduction explaining the animal oeconomy with a copious index by William Cowper. Oxford Printed at the Theater, for Sam-Smith and Benj. Walford, printers to the Royal Society, at the Princess Arms in St. Paul's Church Yard, London, MDCXCVIII.''

The publication of this work brought a storm of protests from Godfrey Bidloo, the famous Dutch anatomist. Bidloo in no uncertain terms asserted that this work was a plagiarism of his ''Anatomia corporis humani, centum et quinque tabulis ad vivum delineatis.'' Bidloo had originally published this work at Amsterdam in 1685. In 1700, with much bitterness, he called the attention of the medical profession to Cowper's illegal use of his work in a fifty-four-page pamphlet, ''Gulielmus Cowper criminus literarii citatus corum tribunali.''

In the following year, Cowper replied with his satirical pamphlet, ''Eucharistia,'' in which he stated that the figures for the atlas originally had been drawn for Swammerdam, that the English publishers had purchased the impressions and that he had written entirely new descriptions for the English edition.

The truth of the matter was that either Cowper or the publisher had pirated the 105 plates from Bidloo's anatomy. Cowper had supplied nine additional plates. He had increased the usefulness of Bidloo's plates by adding several references to them. The original drawings had been made by the famous Belgian artist, Gerard de Lairesse (1641-1711). A controversy exists concerning the identity of the engraver of the copper plates, but usually he is considered to have been Lairesse. Cowper, however, had supplied an original English text, and in an obscure place in a long preface he had said that the engravings ''were sometime since Published by Dr. Bidloo, now Professor of Anatomy in the University of Leyden.''

In spite of the quarrel, Cowper maintained his prestige. He was the outstanding British anatomist of his era and among other things became the teacher of the famous surgeon and anatomist, William Cheselden (1688-1752). In 1702 Cowper published his description of the two glands whose ducts, in man, open into the membranous urethra. Although these glands are now known as ''Cowper's glands,'' they were originally described by Jean Méry (1645-1722) in 1684.

Cowper contributed several interesting papers to the ''Philosophical Transactions'' of the Royal Society. In 1687 he confirmed Malpighi's demonstration (1661) of the capillary function of the pulmonary arteries and veins by demonstrating the capillary circulation in the dog and cat. Cowper was the first (1705) to describe aortic insufficiency and he paid particular attention, in his description of it, to the slow pulse that accompanies the condition. This most interesting account we are reproducing herein. As we shall later note, Vieussens in 1715 also described it and Corrigan in 1832 published his classic account of the condition.

Cowper suffered from asthma and dropsy in the last years of his life, so that he finally retired from the strain and strife of London to Bishop Sutton in Hampshire to conserve his health and strength. Yet his success was only fleeting, for he died a comparatively young man at forty-three, on the eighth of March, 1709. A stone, placed in the wall of the little church at Bishop Sutton by his widow, remains to guard his memory.

OF OSSIFICATION OR PETRIFACTIONS IN THE COATS OF ARTERIES, PARTICULARLY IN THE VALVES OF THE GREAT ARTERY*

By

WILLIAM COWPER

Surgeon, and F.R.S.

HOW FAR anatomical inquiries inform us respecting the true seats and causes of diseases, which have been ascribed to the want of spirits in some, and of radical moisture in aged people, etc., may be in some measure seen by two observations, among others, published in the Trans. No. 280: the first there mentioned is of a young gentlewoman, in whom the parietes, or membranes, that compose the trunks of the arteries of the arm near the axilla, being very much thickened, so that the diameter of its bore was lessened to more than a third part of its natural size; insomuch that a part of the trunk of the artery cut transversely, very much resembled a bit of the stem of a tobacco-pipe, its sides were so thick, and its bore consequently so much lessened: the other was of the trunks of the arteries of the leg, that were obstructed by petrifactions or ossifications, in a person about the age of 67. Since which, I have met with several of the like instances in aged people, particularly in the legs of an old gentleman; whose toes and foot were sphacelated, in which the ossifications diminishing their channels in some places, and totally obstructing them in others, is made very evident.

The dissections of morbid bodies not only instruct us in the seats and causes of diseases, but very often inform us in the true use of parts, as will appear by the following instances. The ossification or petrifaction in the great artery, at its rise from the heart, has been so commonly found, that some think it is constant; how it may be in some animals I cannot be certain, but in human bodies I am well assured that whenever it happens, it is a disease, and in some measure incommodes those parts in the due execution of their office, as the following cases will evince: but that this paper may be of some use, I shall set down the symptoms before death, which may help our conjectures when the like offers again. A thin man about 30, who languished with an ulcer in the thigh, attended with a caries, or rottenness of that bone, at its articulation with the tibia and patella, called the knee, where all those bones were affected, at length fell into a

*Trans. No. 299, p. 1970. Phil. Tr. Roy. Soc. London 5: 215-219, 1703-1712 (abridged 1809).

true phthisis, and coughed up no small quantity of pus; some months before his death I frequently saw him, when he would often offer me his wrist, to feel his unequal pulse, which was wont to amuse him; the artery there missing sometimes one, sometimes two strokes in six or seven; at first he told me he observed it missed but one in ten, but at length those stops became more frequent, especially on any agitation of the body or

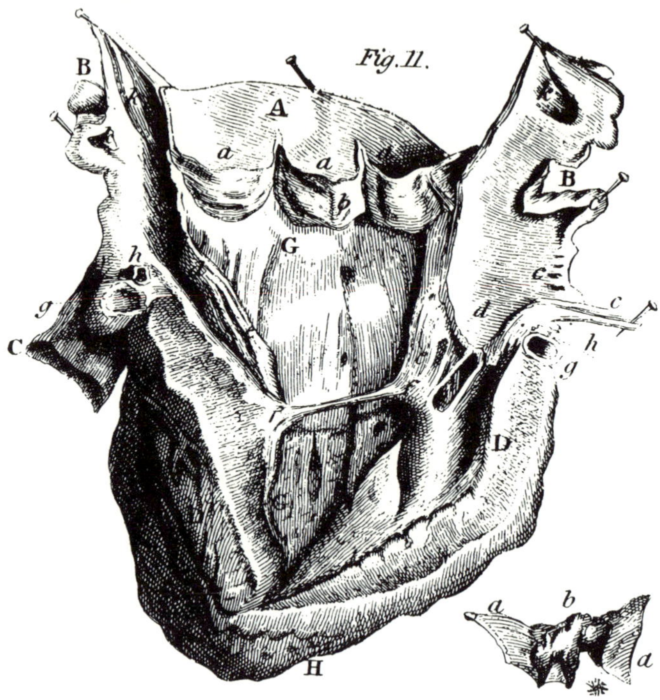

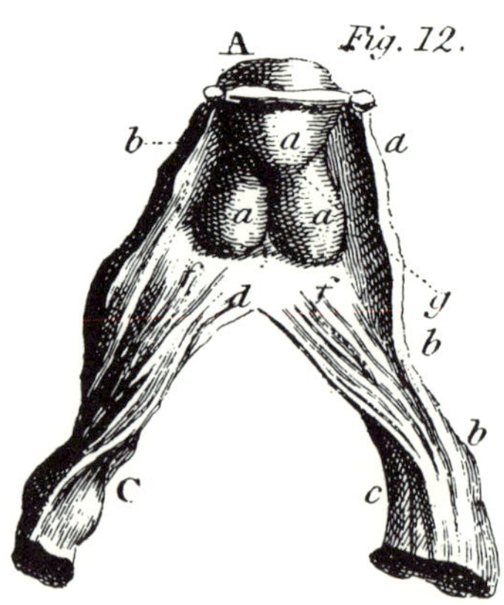

mind, though a polypus in any of the great vessels about the heart may induce that symptom, yet its continuance so long before death, shows it owing to some other cause, as appeared, on opening the heart and great artery of this person.

Fig. 11 represents the trunk of the great artery opened and displayed; *aaa,* the three semilunar valves of the aorta, which hinder the blood from

Fig. 13.

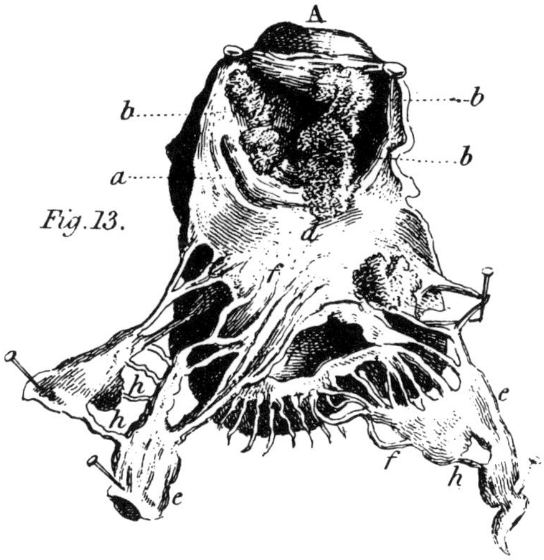

Fig. 14.

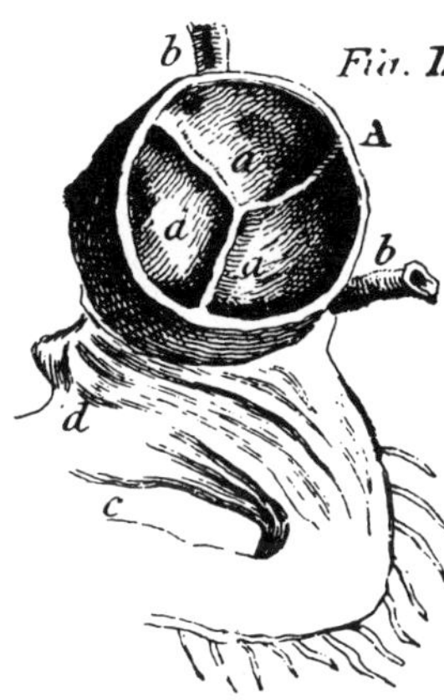

Fig. 15.

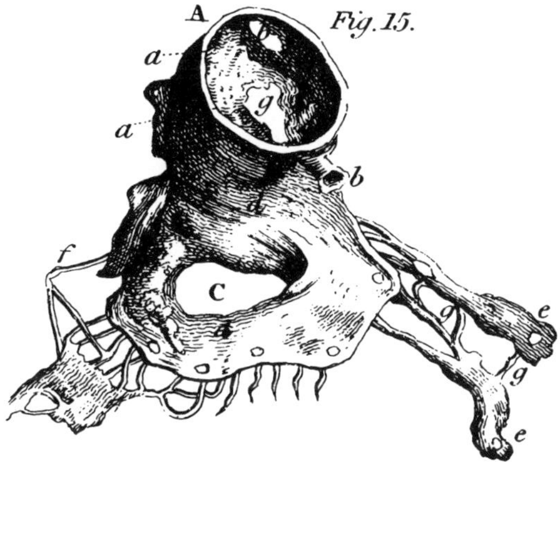

returning to the heart after it is expelled thence by its systole or contraction; these valves in this case were somewhat thicker, and not so pliable as naturally, and did not so adequately apply to each other; as is expressed by *aaa,* Fig. 14. Whence it happened sometimes that the blood in the great artery (A, Fig. 11) would recoil, and interrupt the heart in its systole. But this stubbornness of these valves was owing to a bony or stony substance, marked in the said figure, which appeared much plainer when the valves were dry, as represented in the figure beneath, marked with an *; *aa,* the two valves pinned out and dried; *b,* the petrifaction or stony body at their junction. In this instance I observed the left ventricle of the heart, expressed at GG, DD, *ee, ff,* to be a little dilated from its natural size, but was not, by two parts in three, so large as the left ventricle of the heart of a subject I have dissected. The symptoms, some years before the death of this person, who was about 40 years of age, were extraordinary shortness of breath, especially on any fatigue, with an intermission of one stroke in three of the pulse; the posture of sitting up was more eligible than any other; he complained of great faintness, and now and then pain about the heart, the extreme parts often cold, which towards his death increased more and more on him; his legs and arms being mortified some hours before. On opening the chest, the heart, particularly its left ventricle, was found larger than that of an ordinary ox, and filled with coagulated blood; the valves of the great artery *aaa,* Fig. 11, were petrified, insomuch that they could not approach each other, as expressed in Figs. 12 and 14; but an orifice, represented at Fig. 15, remained always open by the petrifactions *bb,* Fig. 13, and *aa,* Fig. 15, which had clogged these valves, and hindered their application to each other, as in a natural state is represented in Figs. 12 and 14, *aaa.*

The explication of the symptoms in both these cases is obvious enough: for though the person in the first instance did not die of the same disease as the other, yet the symptoms in his illness plainly showed what must follow from the disorders of these valves, as they are rendered more or less useless; for as their office is to prevent the return of the blood into the heart, in its diastole, by exactly shutting up the passage of the aorta, like the valves in water engines, so if by any accident they are hindered from doing their duty, as they were by the petrifactions mentioned, the consequences must be, not only a regurgitation of blood into the heart, but they baulk its impulsive force, when the muscular fibres in these valves cannot contract, to prepare the passage for the blood of the left ventricle, when it is to be expelled into the aorta. Hence the intermissions of the pulse in the first instance may be accounted for. In the latter instance, these valves were wholly useless, and the circulation became more difficult, as appeared by the refrigeration of the extreme parts, the mortifications, etc. In both these cases, the left ventricle of the heart was dilated proportionably to the bad constitution of these valves, which plainly shows these valves give such assistance to the heart, as it cannot be without, and that it gradually suffers according to their indisposition.

Before these papers were sent to the press, I had an opportunity of observing a like instance of that first mentioned, in an elderly gentleman, about 72, who sometimes had intermissions in his pulse several years before his death, in whom I found divers petrifactions in the mitral and semilunar valves of the left ventricle of the heart.

The Explanation of the Figures.—Fig. 11 represents the left ventricle of the heart opened, etc., AAA, the inside of the aorta slit open to the left ventricle; BB, the bulbous trunk of the vena pulmonalis divided through, and pinned aside; to show *aaa* the three semilunar valves of the aorta, which hinder the blood from returning to the heart; *b*, a small stony substance at the conjunction of two of the semilunar valves, expressed at the * below this figure: *aa*, parts of the two valves dried; *b*, the petrifaction, as it appears in the dried valves; C, part of the lower trunk of the vena cava, cut off immediately above the liver; *ccc*, the left auricle opened and pinned out; DD, the sides of the left ventricle divided and drawn aside, to show its inside *dd, ee, ff,* GG; *dd,* the mitral valves of the left ventricle of the heart, or arteria pulmonica, divided and turned aside; *ee,* the carneae columnae, whence spring the tendons fastened to the valves, *dd,* expressed by *df* in Fig. 13; *ff,* a transverse cord or tendon, by which the columnae carneae are drawn nearer each other in the systole, or contraction of the heart, when the blood is expelled into the aorta; by which the tendons expressed *ff,* Figs. 13 and 15, draw the mitral valve laterally; by which means its orifice, *gc* in the said figure, is not only closed to prevent the return of the blood by the vena pulmonalis, but at the same time it opens a passage for the blood of the arteria magna, by withdrawing the mitral valve *d,* Fig. 12, from the orifice of the aorta, *aaag;* GG, the internal surface of the left ventricle, where it is somewhat smoother as it leads to the aorta; *gg,* the trunk of the coronary vein divided when filled with wax; *hh,* the coronary artery in like manner divided; *i,* one of the trunks of the vena pulmonalis; *kkk;* the three orifices of the trunks of the vena pulmonalis, as they open into the bulbous trunk, expressed at BB; H, the cone of the heart.

In Fig. 12, A is part of the aorta next the heart; *aaa,* the three semilunar valves, as they appear next the heart in a natural state, when the heart is in diastole, and the blood hindered by these valves from returning to its left ventricle; *bb,* part of the basis of the heart cut off; *ee,* the two columnae carneae of the left ventricle; *d,* the mitral valve; *ff,* the tendons springing from the carneae columnae, and inserted into the upper and middle parts of the valve, as well as to its lower margin; which is better expressed in the following figure; *g,* the orifice of the aorta completely closed by the application of these three valves to each other.

Fig. 13 shows the same parts as in the preceding figure, as they appeared when the valves of the aorta were petrified, excepting *a,* which represents a part of one of the valves that was not covered with the petrifaction; *bbb,* the petrifactions on the rest of the valves; † a small petrifaction on the mitral valve; *hhh,* some of the transverse tendons, which draw the carneae columnae to each other, when the heart is in systole, for the more effectual closing the orifice of the mitral valve, expressed here at *g.*

Figs. 14 and 15 show the same parts represented in the two preceding figures, as they appear viewed towards the heart, when dried and displayed; AA, the trunk of the aorta; *aaa,* Fig. 14, the semilunar valves in a natural state, when the blood in the arteries presses them close to each other; *bbbb,* the trunks of the two coronary arteries cut off; *aa,* Fig. 15, the semilunar valves petrified; *c,* the orifice of the mitral valve next the vena pulmonalis; *ddd,* the internal surface of the mitral valve leading into the left ventricle; *eee,* the columnae carneae; *ff,* their tendons; *gg,* the transverse tendons, which draw the fleshy columns to each other, when the heart is in systole.

1708

ANTONY VAN LEEUWENHOEK

HIS CONCEPTION OF "THAT MOTION WHICH WE CALL THE PULSE"

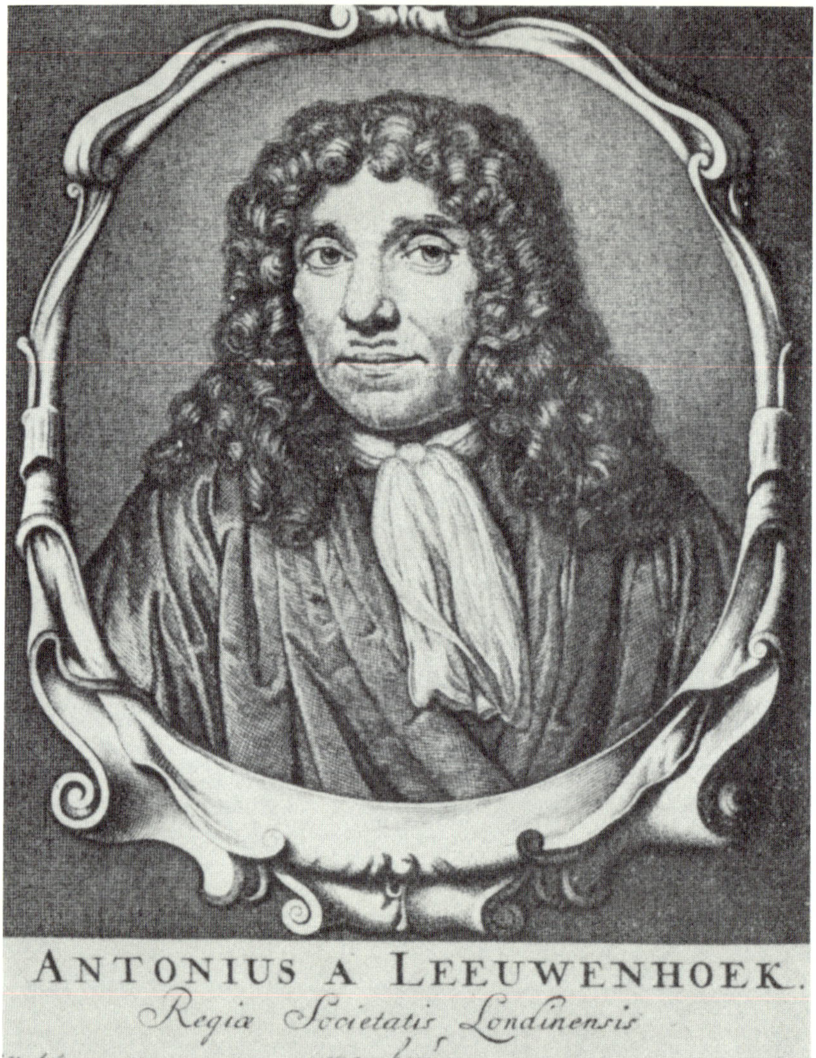

ANTONY VAN LEEUWENHOEK

(Courtesy Charles C Thomas.)

ANTONY VAN LEEUWENHOEK

(1632-1723)

"The Delphic Oracle"

—Molineux on Leeuwenhoek.

ANTONY VAN LEEUWENHOEK did not have the advantages of a university training, but early in life devoted himself diligently to the task of perfecting the single lens microscope. He succeeded in making this instrument reflect a clearer and more accurate picture than did the compound microscope of his era.

With his newly perfected instrument, he studied most assiduously during the long period of his life, making many noteworthy observations. Leeuwenhoek has been accused of making several errors in his discoveries, and it is true that he deceived himself in many of his observations. However, considering that he was, in many ways, a pioneer in the vast uncharted field in which he worked, and taking into account the inferiority of his equipment as judged by the excellence of today's microscope, there yet remains a remarkable general truth in many of his observations.

Leeuwenhoek was born in Delft, Holland, on October 24, 1632. He came of good Dutch stock. Some of his relatives were burghers who manufactured baskets and operated local breweries. His father died early and young Antony was sent to school to study for a government appointment. He left school at the age of sixteen, however, to become an assistant in a dry goods store in Amsterdam. There he remained six years, advancing to the position of cashier and bookkeeper. At the age of twenty-two he married a young woman named Barbe de Mey and settled in his native town Delft. Five children were born of this marriage; only one of them survived Leeuwenhoek. His wife died and he remarried, but no children were born from this second marriage. Not much is known concerning Leeuwenhoek for the next twenty years except that he was appointed to the post of chamberlain of the sheriffs of the town of Delft which seemed to be a glorified name for janitor of the City Hall. We can assume that much of this time was spent in polishing and in otherwise perfecting lenses for his many microscopes, of which the frames also were made by his own hands.

At a later date, Regnier de Graaf, who had immortalized his name by his discovery of the graafian follicle of the ovary, and who was also a native of Delft, became acquainted with Leeuwenhoek and his microscopic discoveries. De Graaf, a corresponding member of the Royal Society of London, realizing the importance of Leeuwenhoek's observations, communicated with the members of the society and suggested that they ask Leeuwenhoek to write them concerning his observations. Shortly afterward (1673), Leeuwenhoek sent them his first contribution. It was written in Dutch, for he knew no other language. His first paper was entitled "Some Observations made by a Microscope contrived by Mr. Leeuwenhoek in Holland, lately communicated by Dr. Regnerus de Graaf." In that paper he wrote about his microscopic studies of mould of the skin, the flesh, the sting of a bee, the anatomy of the bee, and also the anatomy of the louse. During the next fifty years he sent the society about 200 letters regarding his observations, and many of these subsequently were published in the "Philosophical Transactions." We have chosen to reproduce Leeuwenhoek's paper, "On the Circulation of the Blood in Fishes," which he published in the Transactions in 1708. In this paper is found his quaint conception of the pulse, a conception which of course was inaccurate, for he believed that the veins had pulsations and the arteries none.

In 1674 Leeuwenhoek first observed living protozoa. In the following years he described many species which he had demonstrated in well water, in canal water, in infusions of pepper, ginger, and nutmeg, and elsewhere. In 1675 he discovered bacteria of various kinds. In 1680 he discovered anaerobic bacteria in infusions of pepper, and in a letter describing them he recorded the first microscopic observations ever made on the yeasts in beer. That same year he was elected a member of the Royal Society. In 1681, this untiring worker discovered the bacteria of the human mouth and intestines, including the spirochetes.

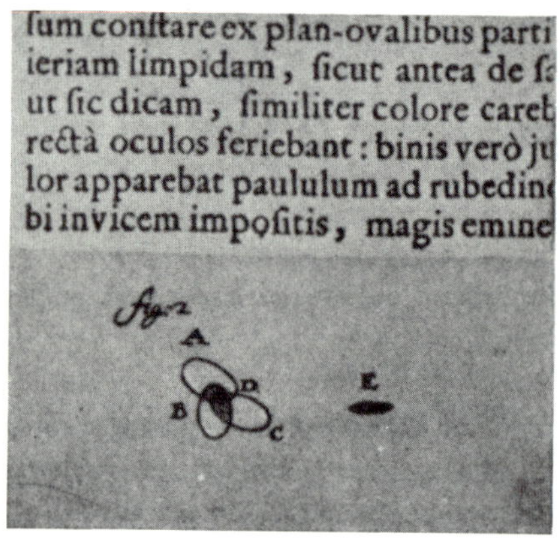

The erythrocytes as Leeuwenhoek saw them in 1696;
from his Arcana Naturae

(Courtesy Ciba Symposia.)

Leeuwenhoek confirmed Malpighi's discovery of the capillary system. He recognized, further, the part the heart played in the circulation. Plimmer wrote that Leeuwenhoek said, "I never looked upon the Heart as the maker of the Blood, but only as an Engine that caused the Blood to circulate, driving it forcibly in to the Arteries, and by its opening, giving way for the Blood to come in again out of the Veins."

Malpighi, as we have mentioned, was the first to demonstrate the blood corpuscles, but he mistook them for fat cells. Leeuwenhoek was the first to give corpuscles an accurate description. He also was the first to mention the leucocytes.

Leeuwenhoek also did some remarkable work on spermatozoa, his studies causing him to become a strong opponent of the theory of spontaneous generation.

Among his many investigations he produced the first true account of the structure of the optic nerve. He also was the first to describe the fibrillated structure of muscle.

Interestingly enough, he was the first to use the microscope in a medicolegal inquiry. Some material was sent to him which was said to be hair voided from the bladder of a woman. He found that it was wool from a stocking.

In 1697 Leeuwenhoek was elected a corresponding member of the Académie des Sciences of France, and he made twenty-six communications to that society.

Leeuwenhoek was visited in Delft by many royal personages including, in all probability, Charles II of England, who founded the Royal Society, Frederick I of Prussia, Queen Mary of Orange, to whom he gave two of his microscopes, and Peter the Great of Russia.

Leeuwenhoek lived to the fine old age of ninety-one. He died on August 26, 1723, and was buried in the Oude Kerk in Delft. At his decease he bequeathed a collection of twenty-six of his microscopes to the Royal Society.

ON THE CIRCULATION OF THE BLOOD IN FISHES, ETC.*

By

MR. LEUWENHOECK,† F.R.S.

I VIEWED the hearts of several fishes, particularly that of the large silver eel, the motion of which lasted near 4 hours, after it was taken out of the body of the fish, which motion was very regular; for when the blood is protruded out of the heart, it is not carried into the great arteries with the same velocity, which, in that case, would be overcharged with the great quantity of blood: but the blood thus coming from the heart, is forced into a small white vessel, almost of the shape of a pear, and which one would take for a kind of bladder; one orifice of which was united to the great artery, and the other to the heart; in the latter orifice is a valve, the use of which is, to prevent the blood, protruding from the heart into the said vessel, from running back again into it: which vessel having been cut across, I observed the inside of it to be furnished with a great many small particles, so that it was in a manner filled with them; and the design of these internal particles I conceive to be, that when the blood is protruded into the vessel, by dilating and contracting itself, it may presently force the same into the great artery. So that the blood is almost always running with an easy and constant course; though at every protrusion it must be in some manner quickened, yet that is so insensibly, that it cannot be observed or felt. And the case is probably the same in beasts and other large animals.

I have formerly communicated some discoveries relating to the circulation of the blood in eels; viz., that the blood, coming out of a great many small vessels in the tail of an eel, is united in one greater blood-vessel, where the fish-bones begin, and where the blood runs through a valve; for I observed that the blood-vein was not only moved in that part where the valve is, but also the parts about it, of the breadth of 4 or 5 hairs breadth; from whence it appeared, that at every protrusion of blood into the heart through the valve, the blood stood still for an instant of time, and then falling through the valve, it ran with great swiftness, and was thickest just at its protrusion out of the valve, but ran thinner or slenderer like the figure of a pear; and the vein that received this protruded blood,

*Trans. No. 319, p. 250. Phil. Tr. Roy. Soc. London 5: 461-464, 1703-1712 (abridged 1809).

†Spelling of name same as in the original article. Note variations from accepted usage.—F. A. W., 1940.

was not entirely filled with it, but seemed for a small space to be as it were empty, and its parts contracted; and further observing it, I saw the blood run slowly and leisurely along the same vessel.

From this observation I imagined, that the same thing happens in the heart of a human creature, viz., that there is a gentle and slow protrusion of the blood out of the heart into that vessel, called the artery; and consequently that there is no such motion there, as is called a pulse, and which is felt in the extreme parts of the body; but that the pulses are only caused by the protrusion of the blood through the valves in the veins; for I never observed any violent or swift protrusion of the blood into the arteries, as often as I have viewed its circulation: and though the blood, by the contraction of the heart, be suddenly and hastily protruded out of it, yet it is slowly carried into the artery; whereas, on the contrary, it runs into the heart from the veins with a violent and swift course; from whence it happens, I suppose, that the remaining part of the blood in the veins, being unable to follow with so swift a motion, is, as it were, violently and per saltum drawn or forced through the valves, and that it is this sort of motion which we take for pulses in the arteries.

To satisfy myself, in the above observations, I have often viewed that sort of motion in my arm, called the pulse, at the time when my body was without motion and warm; and I judged that the motion, which we perceived in the blood vessel, was not derived from the heart to the hand, but contrariwise from the hand to the arm, and so to the heart: from whence I concluded, that, like as in the tail of an eel, there are no valves in the blood vessels, as far as I could perceive, and that a great many small blood vessels, are, as it were, united in that part where the fish bones begin, and make one large blood vessel, where the first valve is, in the same manner in human bodies, a great many single blood vessels running out of the hand, are joined in the arm, where likewise the first valve is, through which the blood at each protrusion falls into the heart, producing what we call the pulse.

I have several times observed in the exceedingly small veins or capillary vessels, a little rising or swelling occasioned by a stronger motion of the blood, which I now firmly conclude, to proceed only from the sudden motion or running of the blood through the valves: I have also observed, that in sudden frights, and otherwise, one feels such motions at the end of one's fingers, just as if there were valves likewise in them, through which the blood gushes; but these sort of motions, I suppose, do only depend on that quick motion made by the blood, when it runs through the valve in the arm by the hand, to which we give the name of a pulse.

In the month of September, having opened an eel, the diameter or thickness of which was about an inch and a half; and having laid open the heart, I could not discover that part which receives the blood out of the great vein in order to bring it into the heart. But that I might the better discover that part, I prepared a little glass tube, and put it into the great vein at a little distance from the heart, and then blew some air into the said vein, as much as might take up the space of about half a pea: this air passed through the great vein into a little bladder that lay on the side of the heart, and no sooner was the air got into that bladder, but it first contracted, and then dilated itself, so regularly, and in such a manner that when the heart contracted itself, just as if it were going to protrude its blood, the said little bladder with air in it was dilated, and continued in such a motion above 5 full hours together: though indeed in the last hour it was so faint, that one could but just perceive it; and as for the heart, its motion was discontinued.

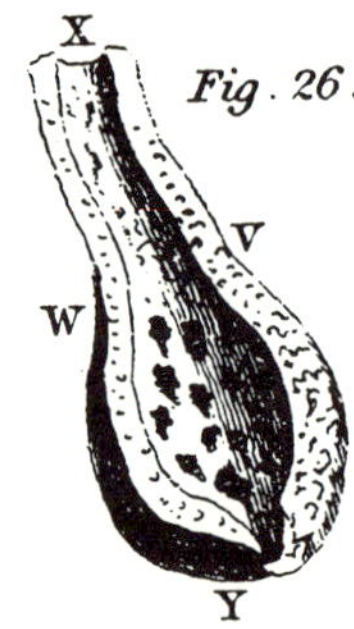

Fig. 26.

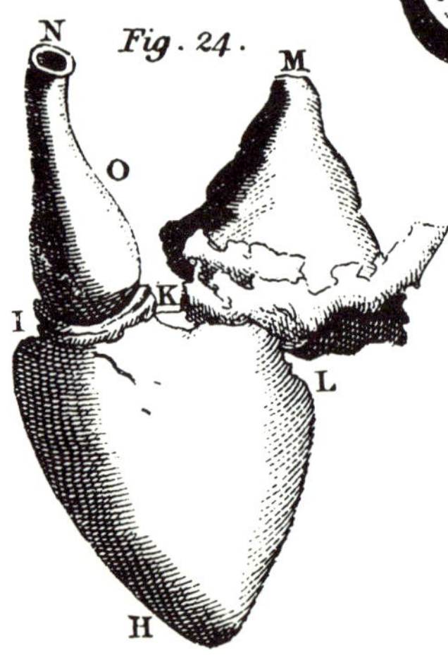

Fig. 24.

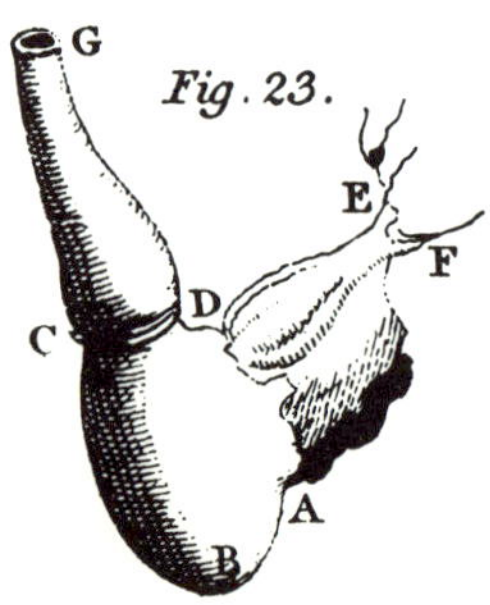

Fig. 23.

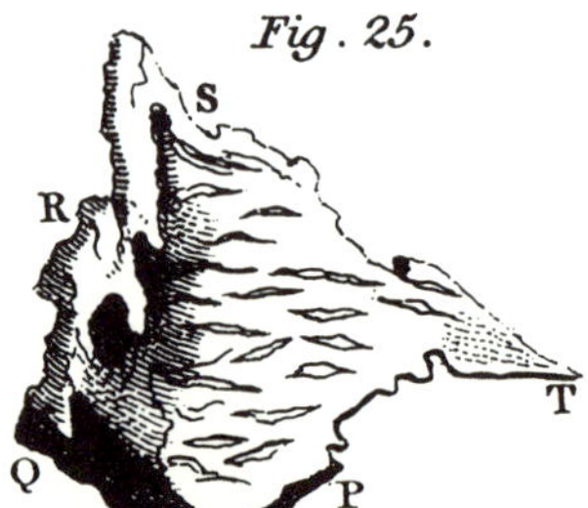

Fig. 25.

I also took a pike-fish, about 2 feet long, and opened it immediately while it was in its full strength of life, and observed not only the motion of the heart, and the regular motion of that part which receives the blood, and brings it into the heart, but also the motion of that other part, which receives the protruded blood from the heart, and carries it gently into the arteries.

Fig. 23, shows the heart of a pike; DEFA represents that part into which the blood is brought from the veins; and CDG, that other part which receives the blood from the heart, to carry into the arteries. Now when the heart receives the blood which is conveyed into it, it dilates to its utmost roundness; and then that vessel represented by ADEF at that very instant collapses; and discharging its blood into the vessel, CDG, this becomes distended by the sudden pouring in of the blood; and no sooner is it so dilated, but it contracts again, that it may force the blood into the arteries. In short, when ADEF is contracted, and throws the blood into the heart, this is dilated; and when the heart contracts and discharges the blood, CDG is dilated: and these three several motions happen in so short a time, and are performed so regularly, that it is quite surprising: and from hence we cannot but conclude, that such a motion as this could not be brought about, unless the vessel ADEF had a valve at AD, where it is joined to the heart, which valve is to prevent the blood, that is thrown into the heart, from returning the same way. And so likewise there must necessarily be another valve at CD, to prevent the blood, that is protruded from the heart, from flowing back again.

Also Fig. 24 represents the heart of a salmon, where KLM shows that instrument or vessel that was represented in Fig. 23, by ADEF, as INO shows the same as CDG in the said figure.

Also the instrument KLM being cut open, to discover with the naked eye, the sinewy parts and their branches; these appeared as in Fig. 25, in which QR is the part that was joined to the heart, and is the same that in Fig. 24 is represented by KL; in the said Fig. 25, we may observe how the sinewy parts and their branches run from QR to T. This instrument, or vessel, is very soft in its parts, and it seemingly is not strong.

Fig. 26 is that vessel dissected, which in Fig. 24 is represented by ION; which vessel is exceedingly thick and strong, and like that represented in Fig. 25, provided with strong sinewy parts, that when the parts are extended by the blood poured into them, they may be able both in roundness and length to convey the blood into the arteries: these parts, by reason of their great numbers, cannot be delineated in such manner as they ought to be.

From the whole I conclude, that the heart protrudes the blood gently into the arteries; and that the blood, which flows from the veins into the heart, causes that sudden revulsion, called the pulse; both because it cannot so immediately pass through the valves, and because the veins in that part are a little narrower, by which means there is a kind of stop or intermission in the circulation of the blood: and this I conceive is the cause of that motion which we call the pulse.*

---

*It is scarcely necessary to remark, that Mr. L.'s conjectures respecting the cause and nature of the pulse are extremely erroneous and absurd.

The above footnote probably was written by either Dr. George Shaw or Dr. Richard Pearson, who with Charles Hutton abridged the *Philosophical Transactions* in the edition (1809) from which we have reprinted Leeuwenhoek's communication.—F. A. W., 1940.

1733

STEPHEN HALES

EARLY EXPERIMENTS ON BLOOD PRESSURE AND BLOOD VELOCITY

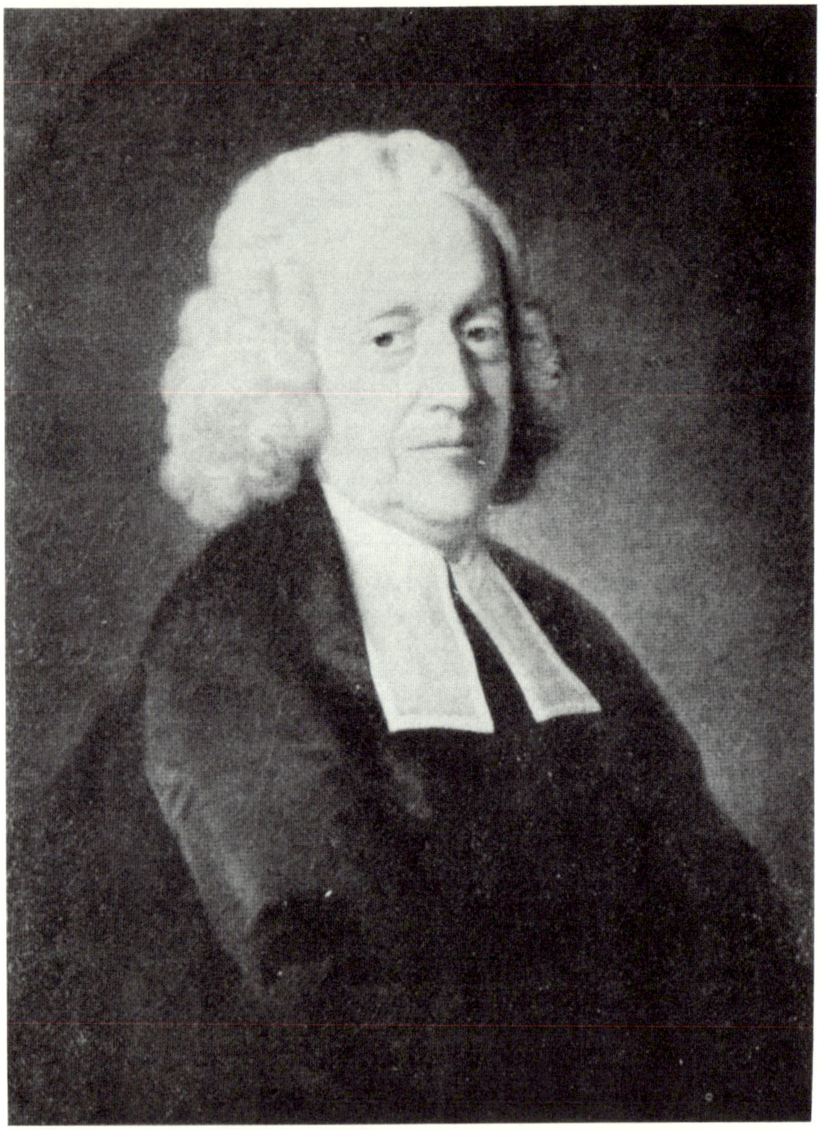

STEPHEN HALES

Portrait by Thomas Hudson

(Courtesy Charles C Thomas.)

STEPHEN HALES

(1677-1761)

ON SEPTEMBER 7, 1677, Stephen Hales was born at Beckesbourne, Kent, England. He was the sixth son of Thomas and Mary Hales. His paternal grandfather, Sir Robert Hales, was created a baronet by Charles II.

At the age of nineteen, young Hales entered the University of Cambridge as a pensioner of Corpus Christi College. He was graduated from that college with the degree of Bachelor of Arts in 1696. He then accepted a fellowship which he held for several years. In 1703 he received the degree of Master of Arts. In 1704, still at study under his fellowship, he made the acquaintance of William Stukely (1687-1765), who had come to enroll at Corpus Christi College. Stukely and Hales became friends. Both were interested in natural history, anatomy, and chemistry. They spent considerable time together, sometimes collecting fossils and sometimes in quest of butterflies. They also studied comparative anatomy and the dissection of frogs, dogs, and other animals. Among other activities they found time to repeat many of Boyle's classic experiments.

In 1710, Hales was made perpetual curate at Teddington in Middlesex. There he was ordained in the ministry and in 1711 he received the degree of Bachelor of Divinity. Hales made Teddington his home for the remainder of his long and useful life. He was a very faithful minister and his scientific interests were reflected in his curateship. Among other things, he aided his parish in obtaining a pure supply of water, helped construct the church lantern, and replaced the timber tower that held the lantern with a tower made of brick. He requested that at his decease, his remains be placed beneath this tower.

Some time after he was made curate he was married to Mary Newce, the daughter of Dr. Newce, rector of Halisham. She died in 1721, leaving him no children.

In 1718 he was elected a fellow of the Royal Society of London and in 1719 he reported before the society the results of some experiments he had made on the effects of the warmth of the sun in raising the sap in trees.

The Royal Society encouraged him to continue his researches, which Hales did with much enthusiasm. His combined efforts were published in 1727 in a volume entitled: ''Vegetable Staticks; or, an account of some statical Experiments on the Sap in Vegetables: being an Essay towards a Natural History of Vegetation; also a Specimen of an Attempt to analyse the Air by a great Variety of chemio-statical Experiments, which were read at several Meetings of the Royal Society.''

Hales published a second edition of this work in 1731. In the preface to the new edition he promised to contribute a second volume containing more of his studies. This appeared in 1733 under the title: ''Statical Essays: containing Haemostaticks; or an Account of some Hydraulick and Hydrostatical Experiments made on the Blood and Blood-Vessels of Animals; also an Account of some Experiments on Stones in the Kidney and Bladder; with an Enquiry into the Nature of these anomalous concretions. To which is added an Appendix containing Observations & Experiments relating to several Subjects in the first Volume.''

From the second volume of Hales' important work it is our privilege to reprint his classical experiments wherein blood pressure and velocity were first measured.

In his first experiments Hales placed a vertical glass tube, the first manometer, in the artery of a horse and measured the distance the blood rose to determine its pressure. He performed similar experiments upon the sheep and the dog. Much later, Jean Marie Poiseuille (1799-1869) and Karl F. W. Ludwig (1816-1895) were to measure blood pressure by the means of a mercury manometer. This in turn was to be followed by the kymograph of Ludwig and led to the present graphic methods now in use.

Hales estimated the blood pressure in man to be about 7½ feet, expressed according to his system of measurement. This is somewhat high, of course, but when we consider the crudity of his instruments and the fact that his work was done on experimental animals only, it seems to be a remarkable approximation.

Because of his ''Statical Essays,'' Hales achieved an international reputation. In 1733 he received the honorary degree of Doctor of Divinity from the University of Oxford. In 1739, in recognition of his many achievements, Hales was awarded the Copley medal. That same year he published a very instructive work which he dedicated to the Lords of the Admiralty. It was entitled: ''Philosophical experiments: containing useful and necessary instructions for such as undertake long Voyages at Sea; showing how Salt-water may be made fresh, wholesome, and how Fresh Water may be preserved sweet; how Biscuit, corn, &c., may be secured from the Weevil, Maggots and other Insects; and Flesh preserved in Hot Climates by salting Animals whole; to which is added an account of Experiments, and Observations on Chalybeate or Steel-waters, with some Attempts to convey them to distant places, preserving their virtues to a greater degree than has hitherto been done; likewise a proposal for cleansing away Mud, &c. out of Rivers, Harbours, and Reservoirs.''

In 1741 Hales, Sutton, a coffee-house keeper, and Martin Triewald, a captain of mechanics to the King of Sweden, had independently invented much-needed ventilators for the purpose of removing contaminated air from the lower decks of ships. The story of Triewald's invention was read before the Royal Society in 1742. In 1743 Hales' work on ventilators appeared. His apparatus was similar to Triewald's. It consisted of a large bellows which sucked out the foul air and could be operated either by hand or by windmill. Sutton's apparatus operated on a different principle. It drew off foul air by the means of the cook-room fire. It was of simpler design and replaced, to a large extent, the machines of Triewald and Hales. In a few years ventilators were also used for prisons and hospitals. Use of them resulted in reducing the death rate in these institutions, a rate which, hitherto, because of most unsanitary conditions, had been terrifically high.

Hales was honored with the friendship of Frederick, Prince of Wales. He also was on intimate terms with Alexander Pope, who was a neighbor.

He died on January 4, 1761, at the age of eighty-four. In accordance with his wishes his remains were placed in a vault in the vestry under the new tower he had constructed for St. Mary's Church in Teddington. A monument to his memory was erected by the mother of George II, the Princess Dowager of Wales. It stands in Westminster Abbey in London.

STATICAL ESSAYS:

CONTAINING

HÆMASTATICS;

Or, An ACCOUNT of ſome

HYDRAULIC and HYDROSTATICAL

EXPERIMENTS

MADE ON THE

Blood and Blood-Veſſels of ANIMALS.

ALSO

An ACCOUNT of ſome EXPERIMENTS on STONES in the KIDNEYS and BLADDER; with an ENQUIRY into the NATURE of thoſe ANOMALOUS CONCRETIONS.

To which is added,

AN APPENDIX,

CONTAINING

OBSERVATIONS and EXPERIMENTS relating to ſeveral SUBJECTS in the Firſt Volume. The greateſt Part of which were read at ſeveral Meetings before the ROYAL SOCIETY.

With an INDEX to both VOLUMES.

VOL. II.

Deſideratur Philoſophia Naturalis vera & activa, cui Medicinæ Scientia inædificetur. Fran. de Verul. Inſtaur. Magna.

By STEPHEN HALES, D. D. F. R. S. RECTOR of FARRINGDON, HAMPSHIRE, and Miniſter of Teddington, Middleſex.

The THIRD EDITION, Corrected.

LONDON,

Printed for WILSON and NICOL, in the Strand; T. DURHAM, near Charing Croſs; G. KEITH, in Grace-church Street; and ROBINSON and ROBERTS, N°. 25, in Pater-noſter Row. 1769.

TO THE

KING'S

Most Excellent Majesty

SIR.

Your Majesty's gracious acceptance of my former Volume of Experiments, has encouraged me, both further to pursue these natural researches, and also to lay the result of them at your feet.

The study of nature will ever yield us fresh matter of entertainment, and we have great reason to bless God for the faculties and abilities he has given us, and the strong desire he has implanted in our minds, to search into and contemplate his works, in which the farther we go, the more we see the signatures of his wisdom and power, everything pleases and instructs us, because in everything we see a wise design.

As the beautiful fabric of this world was chiefly framed for and adapted to the use of man, so the greater insight we get into the nature and properties of things, so much the more beneficial will they be to us, the more will our real riches thereby increase, the more also will man's original grant of dominion over the creatures be inlarged.

Your Majesty's subjects of Great Britain are allowed, by the candid confession of other nations, to excel in experimental philosophy, which has long been found to be most beneficial to mankind.

As the advancement of arts and sciences much depends on the protection of princes, whose patronage they are well worthy of, so we have a pleasing prospect of their flourishing under your Majesty's auspicious favour, whose care and concern for the welfare and prosperity of his people, is in every respect most extensive.

That your Majesty, after having long continued a blessing to your subjects in a prosperous reign here on earth, may hereafter enjoy a happy immortality in heaven, is the sincere prayer of,

May it please your Majesty,

Your Majesty's
Most humble and
Dutiful subject,

STEPHEN HALES

AN ACCOUNT OF SOME HYDRAULIC and HYDROSTATICAL EXPERIMENTS MADE ON THE BLOOD and BLOOD-VESSELS OF ANIMALS*

EXPERIMENT I

1. IN December I caused a *mare* to be tied down alive on her back; she was 14 hands high, and about 14 years of age, had a fistula on her withers, was neither very lean nor yet lusty: having laid open the left crural artery about 3 inches from her belly, I inserted into it a brass pipe whose bore was 1/6 of an inch in diameter; and to that, by means of another brass pipe which was fitly adapted to it, I fixed a glass tube, of nearly the same diameter, which was 9 feet in length: then untying the ligature on the artery, the blood rose in the tube 8 feet 3 inches perpendicular above the level of the left ventricle of the heart: but it did not attain to its full height at once; it rushed up about half way in an instant, and afterwards gradually at each pulse 12, 8, 6, 4, 2 and sometimes 1 inch: when it was at its full height, it would rise and fall at and after each pulse 2, 3, or 4 inches; and sometimes it would fall 12 or 14 inches, and have there for a time the same vibrations up and down, at and after each pulse, as it had, when it was at its full height; to which it would rise again, after forty or fifty pulses.

2. The pulse of a horse that is well, and not terrified, nor in any pain, is about 36 beats a minute, which is nearly half as fast as the pulse of a man in health: this *mare's* pulse beat about 55 times in a minute, and sometimes 60 or a 100, she being in pain.

3. Then I took away the glass tube, and let the blood from the artery mount up in the open air, when the greatest height of its jet was not above two feet.

4. I measured the blood as it run out of the artery, and after each quart of blood was run out, I refixed the glass tube to the artery, to see how much the force of the blood was abated; this I repeated to the eighth quart, and then its force being much abated, I applied the glass tube after each pint had flowed out: the result of each trial was as is set down in the following table, in which are noted the greatest heights it reached after every evacuation. It was usually about a minute before it rose to these several heights, and did not rise gradually, but would stand during

*This work originally appeared in 1733. We have reprinted from the edition of 1769, the title page of which appears on page 129.—F. A. W., 1940.

several pulses much lower, than what it would at length reach to; so that I often thought it had done rising, when on a sudden it would rise for sometime, 4, 8, 12, or 16 inches higher, where it would stay for sometime, and then on a sudden fall 4, 8, 12, or 16 inches.

	The several trials	The quantities of blood let out in wine measure		The several heights of the blood after these evacuations	
		Quarts	Pints	Feet	Inches
*These five ounces lost in preparing the artery	1	0	*5 ounces	8	3
	2	1	0	7	8
	3	2		7	2
	4	3		6	6½
	5	4		6	10½
	6	5		6	½
	7	6		5	5½
By this time there is a pint lost in making the several trials which is not allowed for in this table.	8	7		4	8
	9	8		3	3
	10	8	1	3	7½
	11	9	0	3	10
	12	9	1	3	6½
	13	10	0	3	9½
	14	10	1	4	3½
	15	11	0	3	8
	16	11	1	3	10½
	17	12	0	3	9
	18	12	1	3	7½
	19	13	0	3	2
	20	13	1	4	
	21	14	0	3	9
	22	14	1	3	3
	23	15	0	3	4½
	24	15	1	3	1
	25	16	0	2	4

There was about a quart lost in making the several trials; so there flowed out in all 17 quarts, and half a pint after the last trial, when she expired. This whole quantity of blood was equal to 996.18 cubick inches.

5. We may observe from this table, that the decrease of the force of the blood in the arteries, was not proportioned to the several quantities of blood which were evacuated; for at the eighth trial, when 7 quarts were drawn off, the height of the blood was four feet 8 inches, after which it decreased in the five following trials to three feet odd inches, sometimes a little lower, and then a few inches higher. But at the fourteenth trial, after ten quarts and a pint had been drawn off, it rose again up to four feet, 3 plus one-half inches, and it came nearly to the same height again at the twentieth trial, when thirteen quarts and a pint had been drawn off.

6. This disproportionate inequality in the several heights was principally owing to her violent straining to get loose, which made the blood in the fourteenth trial rise higher than it had done in several of the preceding ones.

7. About the twentieth trial she grew very faint and uneasy, and breathed quick; the violent straining to get loose, did, by the acting of

most of her muscles, especially the abdominal, impel the blood from all parts to the *vena cava,* and consequently there was a greater supply for the heart, which must therefore throw out more at each pulsation, and thereby increase the force of the blood in the arteries.

8. For the same reason, too, it would be somewhat increased in height upon deep sighing, because the lungs being then put into greater motion, and more dilated, the blood passed more freely, and in greater quantity, to the left auricle, and thence to the ventricle.

9. This plainly shows how sighing increases the force of the blood, and consequently, proportionably chears and relieves nature, when oppressed by its too slow motion, which is the case of those who are dejected and sad.

10. Hence, also we see evidently, that the blood moves fastest and most freely thro' the lungs when they are in a dilated state: for which reason animals when they are near expiring, do usually breathe quick, the lungs then laboring to heave fast, that the languid blood may thereby, have a freer course thro' them, to supply the then almost bloodless pulsations of the heart, as was, we see, the case of this mare when her blood was near exhausted.

11. When between 14 and 15 quarts of blood had been evacuated, and thereby the force of that which remained in the vessels greatly decreased, then the mare fell into cold clammy sweats, such as frequently attend dying persons; which shows to how low a state the vital force of the blood is at that time reduced. Whence we see, that these faint sweats are not occasioned by a greater protrusive force of the blood at that time, but rather by a general relaxation of the pores, as well as of all other parts of the body. And it seems hence probable, that the vigour of the blood in the arteries is much abated, when persons who are not in a dying state, have colliquative sweats, as in violent colic pains, fear, &c.

12. Upon opening the *mare's* body, I found little or no blood in the *aorta,* about an ounce in the left ventricle, but none in the right; the *vena porta* and *cava* were full; she bled two or three ounces, but very slowly, and not without pressing the jugular vein, which was opened as soon as she expired.

13. There might be about two quarts and three-quarters of blood left in the large veins, which, with what was drawn out at the artery, makes five wine gallons, which at 221 cubick inches to the gallon, amounts to 1105 cubick inches, or 42.2 pounds; which, at a low estimation, may be reckoned the quantity of current blood in a horse; there is, doubtless, considerably more, but it is not easy to determine how much.

14. As this experiment shews how much the force of the blood in the arteries is abated by different degrees of evacuation; so it may be of use to direct what quantity to let out at a time in bleeding: for whatever the real quantity of the circulating blood be, it is certain that the estimate of what can with safety be let out at once, must be taken from the propor-

tion which that bears to the whole quantity of blood, which will flow out of the vein or artery of the animal till it dies.

15. We see also from this experiment, the reasonableness of the practice of bleeding at several distant times, where it is requisite to take away a great quantity of blood; and not to do it all at once, which would too much weaken the force of the blood. For since it was found by several instances in this experiment, that when the force of the blood was much depressed by evacuations, it would be considerably raised again by the action of the muscles, out of whose very fine and long capillary vessels it moves but slowly, as also by the motion of all parts of the *mare;* so the case is doubtless the same, when the vigour of the blood is in any degree rebated in the large vessels, by blood-letting, that vigour will in some measure be in a little time restored again, not only by the action of the several parts of his body, whereby the blood would have time to flow in from all parts, to supply the most evacuated vessels, whereby there would be a just proportionate evacuation of all parts; but also because the vessels themselves would thereby have time to contract themselves in some proportion to the degree of their evacuation.

EXPERIMENT II

1. In January, I caused a *gelding* to be tied down fast on his back, in the same manner as the mare was in the foregoing experiment: he was 13 hands high, and 10 or 11 years old, but very lame, by reason of a canker in his hoof; he was lean, but somewhat lustier than the mare, and much more lively. I fixed the same brass pipe and glass tube, as above, to his left crural artery.

2. The blood rushed up the tube at once, to near two-thirds of its greatest height, and then more leisurely, as in the mare. It would rise and fall commonly, about an inch at each pulsation of the heart, but sometimes two or three inches. I let out the blood gradually, as in the mare; and after each evacuation, I refixed the glass tube to the artery, to take the several heights of the blood: the result of each trial was, as noted in the following table. [See opposite page.]

3. When I first fixed the tube to the artery, I stopped the horse's nostrils, so as to make him breathe with great difficulty, which made the blood rise five inches higher, but I could not carry this experiment almost to suffocation, as I would have done, because his plunging obliged me to take the tube from the artery. He did not bleed half a pint more after this last trial, before he expired.

4. We may observe that as this horse was more lively than the mare, so the blood mounted at the first trial 17 inches higher in the tube, than the mare's blood did; yet there flowed three pints of blood less from the horse than from the mare, one reason of this may be, that as she was 4 inches taller, than the horse, so she was probably proportionably bigger

in size every way, and should therefore have more blood; besides, bulk for bulk, the females are observed to have more blood than the males.

5. As the quantity of blood decreased, so would the projectile force of the blood in the tube proportionably decrease, so that it would not rise above a quarter of an inch at a pulse, when the horse grew very faint.

6. The great ascents or descents of the blood, *viz.* 12 or 15 inches at a time, did not seem to be owing immediately to the more vigorous or faint, faster or slower pulsations or systole of the heart; but by its continued equable beating, seemed rather to be occasioned by a more or less quantity of blood flowing in to supply the left ventricle of the heart.

The several trials	The quantity of blood let out		The several heights of the blood after those evacuations	
	Quarts	Pints	Feet	Inches
1	0	1	9	8
2	1		9	8
3	2		9	5½
4	3		8	4
5	4		8	2
6	5		7	8½
7	6		7	1
8	7		7	6½
9	8		7	4½
10	9		6	6½
11	10		6	7¾
12	11		5	11
13	12		5*	8½
	12		4†	5½
14	13		4	4
15	14		3	8
16	14	1	4‡	2
	14	1	3§	2
17	15		3	3½
18	15	1	2	10

*The highest point it would stand at for some time.
†The lowest points at which points it would continue for some time.
‡The highest point.
§The lowest point.

7. The horse's pulse beat 40 strokes in a minute, before he was disturbed or tied down; but when the glass tube was fixed to the artery, it beat 65 in a minute, and as the horse grew fainter, the pulse was more and more accelerated, so as to beat an 100 times or more in a minute; whence we see, that the pulse is weak and quick, when the heart is supplied with little blood; which is the case in the hectic fevers, etc.

8. And the diastole of the heart must necessarily be proportionably small; for if the heart dilated as much, when a small quantity of blood flowed into the ventricle, as when a large quantity entered, it must then consequently be filled partly with air each time, which would soon cause the death of the animal.

EXPERIMENT III

1. In December, I laid a common field gate on the ground, with some straw upon it, on which a white *mare* was cast on her right side, and in that

posture bound fast to the gate; she was 14 hands and 3 inches high, lean, tho' not to a great degree, and about 10 or 12 years old. This and the above mentioned horse and mare were to have been killed as being unfit for service.

2. Then laying open the left jugular vein, I fixed to that part of it which comes from the head, a glass tube, which was 4 feet and 2 inches long.

3. The blood rose in it, in 3 or 4 seconds of time about a foot, and then was stationary for 2 or 3 seconds, then in 3 or 4 seconds more, it rose sometimes gradually and sometimes with an unequally accelerated motion, 9 inches or more, on small strainings of the mare: then upon greater strainings, it rose about a yard, and would subside 5 or 6 inches: then upon a larger strain or struggle of the mare, it rose so high, as to flow a little out at the top of the tube: so that had the tube been a few inches higher, it would have risen probably to that height.

4. When the mare ceased to strain and struggle, the blood subsided about 18 or 20 inches; so the return of the blood into the vein was not hindered by the valves, which I have also observed in other parts where there are valves; tho' sometimes they absolutely hinder the return of any fluid.

5. The diameter of the brass pipe and tube which were fixed to the vein, were nearly $1/7$ of an inch: the diameter of the jugular vein about half an inch.

6. Then laying bare the left carotid artery, I fixed to it towards the heart the brass pipe, and to that the wind-pipe of a goose; to the other end of which a glass tube was fixed, which was 12 feet 9 inches long. The design of using the wind-pipe was by its pliancy to prevent the inconveniences that might happen when the mare struggled, if the tube had been immediately fixed to the artery, without the intervention of this pliant pipe.

7. There had been lost before the tube was fixed to the artery, about 70 cubick inches of blood. The blood rose in the tube in the same manner, as in the case of the two former horses, till it reached 9 feet 6 inches height. I then took away the tube from the artery, and let out by measure 60 cubick inches of blood; and then immediately replaced the tube to see how high the blood would rise in it after each evacuation; this was repeated several times till the mare expired, as follows, *viz.* [Page 137.]

8. We may observe that these three horses all expired, when the perpendicular height of the blood in the tube was about two feet.

9. These 833 cubick inches of blood weigh 31.82 pounds, and are equal to 14.4 wine quarts, the large veins in the body of the mare were full of blood, there was some also in the descending *aorta*, and in both ventricles and auricles.

	The several trials	Cubick inches let out	Perpendicular height after each evacuation	
			Feet	Inches
	1	70	9	6
	2	130	7	10
	3	190	7	6
	4	250	7	3
	5	310	6	5
	6	370	4	9
	7	430	3	9
	8	490	3	4½
*Deep sighing raised the blood.	9	550	2	9½
	10	610	3	2½
When the force of the blood was thus small, then faint sweats came on.	11	670 {	4*	5
			2	9½
	12	730	3	6
	13	790	3	5
Very faint -------------	14	820	2	0
Now expired -----------	15	833	2	5

10. In order to make an estimate with what force the heart of this mare must propel the blood, to raise it in the tube to the height of nine feet six inches, I injected the right ventricle of the heart in the following manner, *viz.*

11. I fixed a musket-barrel to the pulmonary vein, near its entrance into the left auricle, and tied the ascending and descending *aorta's* fast, at some distance from their branching off from each other: then placing the barrel in a perpendicular posture, with a funnel on the top of it, I poured in melted beeswax, till the funnel was half filled. Yet, as I had found by experience, this perpendicular height of melted wax, which was near four feet, would not have filled the auricle and ventricle, if I had not at the same time taken care to pass a small brass pipe thro' one of the ascending branches of the *aorta,* into the left ventricle; thro' which the air passed off as the wax entered into the ventricle, the brass pipe being at the same time gradually drawn up by an assistant, who, as soon as all the air was driven out, tied that branch of the *aorta,* to prevent the flowing out of the wax.

12. I chose this method of injecting from a perpendicular height rather than by a syringe, both because I was by this means assured of the force with which the injected cavity of the heart was dilated, which is more uncertain with a syringe; and also because this dilating force from the perpendicular height, continued acting uniformly till the wax was grown stiff and hard.

13. When cutting open the left ventricle, I found the thickness of its muscular coat to be 1 + ½ inch, and the thinnest part of that of the right ventricle was half an inch.

14. Then taking out the wax which was formed in the shape of the ventricle, I cut the wax of the left ventricle off, where the valves, called *mitrales,* made the separation; which valves were propelled inward by

the entering wax; and I did the same also at the orifice of the *aorta,* where the valves called *semilunares* were also propelled inward by the above-mentioned brass vent-pipe.

15. And this is the proper cavity of the left ventricle, just before its contraction; for at that instant, the blood flowing in from the auricle has opened the mitral valves inward, while at the same time the contracting arteries repel the blood forcibly against the semilunar valves; but at the instant that the ventricle contracts, the mitral valves are closed, being expelled by the blood outwards, while at the same time the semilunar are by the same action opened outwards, to make way for the compressed blood to rush into the *aorta.*

16. So that this piece of wax thus formed, may reasonably be taken to be nearly commensurate to the quantity of blood received into this ventricle at each *diastole,* and is thence propelled into the *aorta* at the subsequent *systoles.*

17. Having therefore filled a narrow-mouthed vessel brim-full of water, I immersed the wax in it; then taking it out of the water, I filled the vessel brim-full again, from another vessel, whose capacity was divided into cubick inches, which gave the bulk of the wax, and consequently the capacity of the left ventricle, equal to ten cubick inches.

18. I got the quantity of the surface of the sides of this ventricle by laying pieces of paper aptly cut to the irregular form of the several parts of the wax, and then laying those papers under another paper, which was equally divided into little squares of one-fourth inch each; by running a pin thro' both papers at every corner of each square, the under papers being thus marked too, it was easy by numbering their several squares and parts of a square, to come pretty nearly to an estimate of the whole inward surface of the ventricle; which I by this means found to be equal to 26 square inches, deducting one square inch for the area of the orifice of the *aorta,* whose diameter I measured from the injected wax.

19. The diameter of the *aorta* just before the coronary artery branches from it, was 1.15 inch, whence its area 1.036 square inch.

The diameter of the descending *aorta* 0.93, its area 0.677.

The diameter of the ascending *aorta* 0.74, its area 0.369.

20. The inward area of the sides of the left ventricle being therefore equal to 26 square inches; the sum of the whole pressure of the blood against all the sides of that ventricle, at the instant when it begins first to contract, so as to sustain the pressure of the arterial blood, will be that surface or area multiplied into the perpendicular height of the blood in the glass tube, *viz.* 26×114 inches, *viz.* 2964 cubick inches of blood.

21. And since, according to Dr. Jurin's estimate, in Motte's Abridgment of the Transactions, part 2d, page 141, a cubick inch of blood weighs 267.7 grains, these multiplied into 2964, the number of cubick inches, and then reduced into pounds, give 113.22 pounds, which is the sum of the pressure

of the blood, which this ventricle sustains, at the instant when it is going to exert a contractive force, sufficient to propel it with considerable velocity into the *aorta.*

22. The scruple avoirdupoise contains 18.25 grains, the ounce 438 grains, the pound 7008 grains.

23. The area of the greatest section of this ventricle from apex to base being 6.83 square inches, these multiplied into 114 inches, the perpendicular height of the blood, in the tube, give 778.62 cubick inches of blood, equal to 29.7 pounds, the force of the blood which the muscular fibres in that transverse section of the ventricle must resist.

24. The velocity with which the blood is thrown out of the ventricle into the orifice of the *aorta,* may be thus computed; *viz.* the capacity of this ventricle being equal to ten cubick inches, and the area of the transverse section of the *aorta* being 1.036, by which dividing the ten cubick inches, the quotient 9.65 is the length of the cylinder of blood, which is formed in passing thro' the *aorta's* orifice, at each *systole,* of the ventricle. And a horse's ventricle of his heart contracting, or his pulse beating 36 times in a minute, that is, 2160 times in an hour, then a column of blood so many times 9.65 inches, or 20,844 inches long, or 1737 feet will pass in an hour.

25. But the *systoles* of the ventricle during which that quantity of blood is propelled, being estimated to be done in one-third of the space of time between each pulse, the velocity of the blood during each *systole,* will be thrice as much, *viz.* at the rate of 5211 feet, *i.e.,* 0.98 of a mile in an hour, or 86.85 feet in a minute.

26. Now this velocity is only the velocity of the blood at its first entering into the *aorta,* in the time of the *systole,* in consequence of which the blood in the arteries, being forcibly propelled forward, with an accelerated *impetus,* thereby dilates the canal of the arteries, which begin again to contract at the instant the *systole* ceases; by which curious artifice of nature the blood is carried on in the finer capillaries, with an almost even tenor of velocity, in the same manner as the spouting water of some fire-engines is contrived to flow with a more even velocity, notwithstanding the alternate *systoles* and *diastoles* of the rising and falling *embolus* or force; and this by the means of a large inverted globe, wherein the compressed air alternately dilating or contracting, in conformity to the workings to and fro of the *embolus,* and thereby impelling the water more equably than the *embolus* alone would do, pushes it out in a more nearly equal spout.

27. And since the blood in the finest capillary arteries, presses into the veins with a much more equal velocity, than in the *aorta* and greater arteries; since also the *systole* is supposed to be nearly one-third of the time between pulse and pulse, the other two-thirds of that time must be spent in the contraction of the arteries: it may therefore reasonably be concluded, that the sum of the dilatation of all the arteries in each *systole*

is equal to about the quantity of two-thirds of the blood, which is thrown out in each *systole,* which in the case of this mare is equal to two-thirds of 10 cubick inches, *viz.* 6.66.

28. This ventricle throwing out 10 cubick inches at a time, will in the 36 pulses of a minute throw out 360 cubick inches, equal to 13.75 pounds, and in an hour 825 pounds weight of blood, nearly equal to the weight of the horse.

29. The area of the transverse section of the *aorta* being as above noted 1.036 inch; and the immediate next divisions of it being in the area of the like section of the descending *aorta* 0.677 inch; and that of the ascending *aorta* being 0.369, we find the sum of the two areas of these ascending and descending branches is greater than that of the trunk they arise from; and accordingly the velocity of the blood will be proportionably abated in them; as also on account of what passes thro' the coronary arteries, before the blood arrives at those two branches, of which the descending *aorta* is considerably the largest, thereby to furnish a greater quantity of blood, in the proportion that all the parts of the body below the heart exceed the bulk of those above the heart.

EXPERIMENT IV

1. I injected also with wax the left auricle and ventricle of an ox's *heart,* which ox was by guess supposed to weigh about 1600 pounds when alive.

The capacity of this ventricle was equal to 12.5 cubick inches.

The area of the transverse section of the *aorta* equal to 1.539 inch.

That of the descending *aorta* equal to 0.912, that of the ascending equal to 0.85.

2. The pulse of a very gentle cow, which was not terrified nor disturbed, while its pulse was counted, was at the rate of 38 in a minute, nearly the same as that of a horse.

3. The capacity of this ventricle 12.5 being divided by the area of the orifice of the *aorta* 1.539, the quotient 8.1 inches is the length of the cylinder of blood, which is formed in passing thro' the *aorta,* in each *systole* of the ventricle.

4. And an ox's pulse beating, or this ventricle contracting 38 times in a minute, that is, 2280 times in an hour, then a column so many times 8.1 inches, or 18,468 inches long, or 1539 feet, will pass in an hour.

5. But each *systole* of the ventricle being performed in one-third of that time, the velocity of the blood in each *systole* will be thrice as great, *viz.* 4617 feet, *i.e.,* 0.874 of a mile in an hour or 76.95 feet in a minute.

6. This ventricle throwing out 12.5 cubick inches at a time, will in thirty-eight *systoles,* which it performs in a minute, throw out 18.14 pounds; and in an hour, and twenty-eight minutes, it will have thrown out 1600 pounds of blood, a quantity equal to the weight of the ox. But this ox being fat,

a quantity of blood equal to his weight must be longer in passing through its heart, than in the lean horse, Exper. III. No. 27, for the fat of animals has little or no blood in it; whence, lean animals have *caeteris paribus* much more blood in them than fat ones.

EXPERIMENT V

1. I took an estimate also of the force of the blood in a fat gelt sheep or wether, by fixing glass tubes to the jugular vein and carotid artery, in the same manner as I had done to the horse in Exper. III. The sheep was three years old and weighed ninety-one pounds alive.

2. Its pulse beat 65 times in a minute.

3. The blood rose in the tube fixed to the jugular vein 5 + ½ inches, and 9 inches when the sheep struggled and strained.

4. In the tube fixed to the carotid artery it rose 6 feet 5 + ½ inches.

5. The capacity of the left ventricle of its heart, was equal to 1.85 cubick inch.

6. Its inward surface = 12.35 square inches.

7. Its greatest transverse section = 2.54.

8. The area of the transverse section of the *aorta* = 0.172 square inch, that of the descending *aorta* = 0.094, that of the left carotid artery = 0.012, and of the right = 0.07, they both rose separate immediately from the *aorta*.

9. The inward surface of this left ventricle being equal to 12.35 square inches; this, multiplied by 6 feet 5 + ½ inches, produces 957.12 cubick inches of blood = 36.56 pounds, the weight of blood which this ventricle sustains, just before its *systole* begins.

10. And the area of its greatest transverse section being = 2.54 square inches, this multiplied into 6 feet 5 + ½ inches, the height of the blood in the tube, the product is 196.85 cubick inches of blood = 7.51 pounds, the weight of blood which the fibres in this transverse section of the ventricle must sustain.

11. The capacity of the left ventricle being = 1.85 cubick inch, which divided by 0.172, the area of the transverse section of the *aorta,* the quotient 10.75 is the length of the cylinder of blood, which is formed in passing thro' the *aorta* in each *systole* of the ventricle.

12. And this sheep's pulse beating, or his left ventricle contracting 65 times in a minute, that is 3900 times in an hour, therefore a column of blood so many times 10.75 inches, or 41,925 inches long, or 3493.75 feet will pass in an hour.

13. But the *systoles* of the heart, during which that quantity of blood is propelled, being estimated to be done in one-third of the space of time between each pulse, the velocity of the blood during each *systole* will be thrice as much; *viz.* at the rate of 10,481.25 feet, *i.e.,* 1.98 mile in an hour, or 174.6 feet in a minute.

14. And the ventricle throwing out 1.85 cubick inch of blood each time, that will be 4.593 pounds in a minute, or 91 pounds, a quantity equal to the weight of the sheep in twenty minutes.

EXPERIMENT VI

1. Having fixed a tube to the left crural artery of a *fallow doe,* the blood rose 4 feet 2 inches in the tube.

2. I injected with wax both auricles and ventricles of the heart, of another doe, and found the capacity of the ventricle equal to 9 cubick inches, and the right auricle and ventricle near as big.

3. Timorous animals are observed to have larger hearts than courageous ones; as deer, asses, hares, etc. which holds true in the instance of this *doe's* heart. *Qu.* May not one reason of this be, that the fibres of the timorous are generally more lax than those of courageous animals? On which account the blood passing with less resistance through the lax fibred capillary vessels, it was requisite that the heart should at each pulse throw out a greater quantity of blood, in order to supply its more easy and plentiful flow through the lax capillary arteries into the veins. And may not this be the reason why the pulses of young animals, as of children, are found to beat faster than those of grown persons? *viz.* because the tender fibres of the coats of their blood-vessels being very lax, they give the less resistance to the flowing blood, whose globules are observed by Leewenhoeck to be all of a size both in great and small animals; whence it was needful to make provision for a proportionably greater supply of it from the heart, by increasing the velocity of the dilatations and contractions of that curious engine; in the formation of which are seen such evident marks of the consummate wisdom of the great Author of nature.

4. The area of the transverse section of the *aorta* of this *doe* = 0.476, of the descending *aorta* = 0.383, of the ascending = 0.246, and that of the pulmonary artery = 0.502. But it being not easy to obtain, in that timorous creature, the just number of pulses in a minute, I could not calculate the velocity of the blood, nor the quantity that passes in any determinate time.

EXPERIMENT VII

1. I fixed tubes also in the same manner to the jugular vein and carotid artery, of several dogs; for whatever experiment I principally intended to make on any dog, I usually began with fixing a tube first to the jugular vein, and then to the carotid artery, which was the method I used to wash the blood out of the capillary vessels, thereby the better to prepare them for my intended experiments.

2. The force of the blood in the veins and arteries is very different, not only in animals of different species, but also in animals of the same kind,

and that not only in those of different sizes and weights, but also in dogs of the same size and weight, and even in the same animal, the force of the blood in its vessels is continually varying, according to the different kinds and quantities of food, the various distances of time after taking food, the more or less plethoric state of the blood-vessels, also from exercise, rest, different states of vigour or vivacity of the animal, and many other circumstances, which may conduce to vary the force of the blood; for the healthy state of animals is not confined to the scanty limits of one determinate degree of vital vigour in the blood: but the all-wise Framer of these admirable machines has so ordered it, as that their healthy state shall not be disturbed by every little variation of this force, but has made it consistent with a very considerable latitude in the variation of it. Now since this force of the blood is so variable, it is the more requisite to be furnished with a good quantity of observations, thereby to find out, the more nearly, a medium of those forces, not only in the same animal, but also in those of different ages, sizes, and kinds, whence haply some curious observations may arise.

3. These great inequalities of the force of the blood, not only in different animals, but also in animals of the same kind, may be seen in the following table in Exper. VIII. No. 12 in which I have set down the weights of most of them, and also in different columns, the height to which the blood rose in tubes fixed to the veins and arteries.

4. I observed here, as in the above-mentioned horses, and that when the blood had subsided a little in the tubes which were fixed to the arteries of these dogs, it would, as in the horses, rise on a sudden considerably on deep sighing, as also on pressing the dogs bellies hard with the hand, the blood would immediately rise about six inches and subside as much on taking off the hand, and it was the same on several repetitions.

5. It may be objected to this method of estimating the force of the blood, that by thus fixing tubes to these large veins and arteries, the course of a considerable stream of blood was for that time stopped; and that consequently the force of the blood must be proportionably increased in all the veins or arteries; and therefore also in the veins or arteries to which the tube is fixed: and doubtless in some degree it is so. In the sheep the left carotide is nearly $\frac{1}{13}$ part of the right carotide and descending *aorta* taken together; and in the dog, Numb. 3, it is about $\frac{1}{10}$ of them.

6. To obviate therefore this inconvenience, I fixed tubes laterally to the jugular veins and arteries of the dog, Numb. 13, in the following manner: *viz.* I took two cylindrical sticks which were $\frac{1}{2}$ inch diameter, and $1 + \frac{1}{2}$ inch in length; and having bored holes through them from end to end, something larger than those veins and arteries; I then slit them in halves

length-ways, and bored another hole through the middle of one of them into its cavity, into which lateral hole the brass pipe entered; which was, at its other end, adapted to fit another pipe which was cemented to a glass tube. Then having laid the vein or artery bare, I drew a linen cloth under it, to wipe it very dry; and then placed under it one of the above-mentioned slit pieces of wood, laying the vein or artery in its cavity, which was covered with pitch, that was at that instant afresh melted with a small warm iron rod; then pouring melted pitch not very hot, over the vein or artery, I immediately put on the other half of the split wood, which had the hole bored thro' it, and tied them fast together: then entering the very slender point of a pen-knife into the above-mentioned hole, I cut an orifice in the vein or artery, and then immediately fixed the brass pipe and tube to receive the following blood, which rose from the jugular vein of the thirteenth dog, first, six inches, and on straining $9 + \frac{1}{2}$ inches, and from the artery four feet eleven inches; and would doubtless have mounted higher, if the blood had not made an outlet between the artery and the pitch, so as to prevent its rise; which inconvenience might easily be prevented by proper care; which, if done, would give us the real force of the blood against the sides of the arteries, as it did in this jugular vein.

7. I believe this would be a good method to take the force of the blood in lesser animals, where by reason of the smallness of those vessels it might be difficult to insert pipes into them, which if done, those pipes would have too small a bore for the blood freely to pass through them.

8. I have noted in the following table, Exper. VIII. Numb. 12, the several heights to which the blood rose in tubes fixed to the veins and arteries of animals, as they lay horizontally on their backs, or on one side, in the case of the mare, Exper. III. But when an animal stands on its legs, a column equal to the perpendicular height of the animal, must be added to the several heights of the blood in the glass tubes, in order to estimate the force with which the blood presses against the coats of the blood vessels, at the lower parts of the body, and so in proportion for any other part that is higher. So that these columns of blood in the arteries and veins, communicating with each other, are, on account of their equal heights, equipollent to each other: the progressive motion of them being determined by the energy of the heart. And though valves in tubes in which a fluid is propelled upwards with an equal force, would rather retard than promote its progress; yet in tubes where the fluid does not ascend equably but by reason of frequent motions of the whole machine, it is subject to many agitations; in this case valves are of great importance to check the repercussion and regurgitation of the fluid; and accordingly, the all-wise Framer of animal bodies has provided valves in the veins, to prevent this inconvenience, and that principally in the lower parts of the body, where they are most needed, especially in great motions, and in exerting the muscular force of the body.

EXPERIMENT VIII

1. The blood having risen six feet eight inches from the crural artery of the dog, Numb. 1 and to the same height from the left carotide artery of Numb. 7 in the table, Numb. 12 of this Experiment VIII, I chose to calculate the velocity, &c. of the blood of this dog.

2. The capacity of the left ventricle of the heart, being injected with wax, was found equal to 1.172 cubick inch.

3. Its inward surface equal to eleven square inches, which multiplied into the perpendicular height of the blood in the glass tube, which was fixed to the artery, *viz.* six feet eight inches, or eighty inches, gives eight hundred and eighty cubick inches of blood, which press on all sides of that ventricle, when it has contracted just so far, as to sustain and be equal to the force of the blood in the *aorta.*

4. These eight hundred and eighty cubick inches multiplied by 267.7, the number of grains in a cubick inch of blood, gives 235,567 = 33.61 pounds.

5. The area of the transverse section of the *aorta,* just before the coronary arteries branch off from it, being 0.196 square inch, by which dividing 1.172 cubick inch, the capacity of the ventricle, the quotient 5.978 inches, is the length of the cylinder of blood, which is formed in passing thro' the orifice of the *aorta,* at each *systole* of the ventricle.

6. And a dog's pulse being found to beat, or his left ventricle to contract, ninety-seven times in a minute, then a column of blood so many times 5.97 inches long, will be 34,745.4 inches, or 2,895.45 feet long; but the *systoles* of the heart during which that quantity is propelled, being estimated to be done in one third of the time between pulse and pulse, the velocity of the blood during each *systole* will be thrice as much, *viz.* 8,686.35 feet, that is at the rate of 1.64 mile in an hour, or 144.77 feet in a minute.

7. And the ventricle throwing out 1.172 cubick inch of blood in each *systole,* that is, 4.34 pounds in ninety-seven pulses, the number of pulses in one minute, hence fifty-two pounds, a quantity equal to the dog's weight, will pass thro' the heart in 11.9 minutes.

8. If, according to Dr. Keill's estimate, the left ventricle of a man's heart throw out in each *systole* an ounce or 1.638 cubick inch of blood, and the area of the orifice of the *aorta* be = 0.4187; then dividing the former by this, the quotient 3.9 is the length of the cylinder of blood, which is formed in passing thro' the *aorta* in each *systole* of the ventricle; and in the seventy-five pulses of a minute a cylinder of 292.5 inches length will pass; this is at the rate of 1462 feet in an hour. But the *systole* of the heart being performed in one-third of this time, the velocity of the blood in that instant will be thrice as much, *viz.* at the rate of 43861* feet in an hour, or 735* feet in a minute.

*The figures 43861 and 735, which appear in the 1769 edition from which we reprint, are obvious errors and should read 4,386 and 73.1.—F. A. W., 1940.

9. And if the ventricle throws out one ounce in a pulse, then in seventy-five pulses of a minute the quantity of blood will be equal to 4.4 pounds, 11 ounces, and in 34 minutes a quantity equal to a middle-sized man, *viz.* a hundred and fifty-eight pounds, will pass thro' the heart.

10. But if with Dr. Harvey and Dr. Lower we suppose two ounces of blood, that is, 3.276 cubick inches to be thrown out at each *systole* of the ventricle, then the velocity of the blood in entering the orifice of the *aorta,* will be double the former, *viz.* at the rate of 146 feet in a minute, and a quantity of blood equal to the weight of a man's body will pass in half the time, *viz.* 17 minutes.

11. If we suppose, what is probable, that the blood would rise 7 plus ½ feet high in a tube fixed to the carotide artery of a man, and that the inward area of the left ventricle of his heart, is equal to fifteen square inches, these multiplied into 7 + ½ feet gives 1350 cubick inches of blood, which presses on that ventricle, when first it begins to contract, a weight equal to 51.5 pounds.

12. That we may the more readily compare the above-mentioned several estimates together, I shall here range them in order in a table.

The several Animals		Weight of each		Height of the Blood in the Tube from Jugul		Height of the Blood in Tubes fixed to Arteries		Capacity of the left Ventricle of the Heart	Area of the Orifice of the Aorta	Velocity of the Blood in the Aorta
		Pd.	Cu.	Inches		Feet	Inch	Cubick Inches	Square Inches	Feet Inch in a Minute
Man			160			7	6	1.659	0.4187	56.55
								3.318		113. 3
Horse	1st					8	3			
	2d					9	8			
	3d		825	12 On straining	52	9	6	10	1.036	86.85
Ox			1600					12.5	1.539	76.95
Sheep			91	5½	9	6	5½	1.85	0.172	174. 5
Doe						4	2	9	0.476	
Dogs	1st		52	0	6	6	8	1.172	0.196	144.77
	2d		24	5	7	2	8	1	0.185	130. 9
	3d		18	5		4	8	0.633	0.118	130
	4	12	8	4		3	3	0.5	0.101	120
	5			4	6	at crural		1.25	0.210	144.28
	6		31			Arter.			0.196	
	7		43			6	8	1.172	0.179	156.59
	8					6	6	Tube fixed to the crural artery.		
	9			7	14	3	1			
	10		15	5	24	1	6	was very old, and died soon.		
	11		37	8½		4	9			
	12		36			6	7			
	13		24	6	9½	4	11	Tube fixed laterally to the left		
	14	37	8			5	8	carotide artery.		
	15			5	19	on sucking at the tube.				
	16			5½	8	on sucking				
	17		19	5	14	5	2			
	18		35	5		4	7			
	19		32	6	9½	3	11			
	20		23	5	7	4	10			

13. I do not see, by comparing the weights of these animals, and the several quantities of blood which pass thro' their hearts in a given time, that we can thence form any rule that is fixed, for the proportioning the quantities of flowing blood to their different sizes.

14. These quantities in larger animals are very disproportionate to the bulk of their bodies, in comparison of what they are in lesser animals, as estimated in this table.

15. But as in the bigger animals the blood had a longer course to go, and must therefore meet with a greater resistance; so we may observe in this table, by comparing the perpendicular heights of the blood in the tubes fixed to the arteries, that the force of it in the arteries is in the main greatest in the largest animals.

The several Animals	Quantities of Blood = to the Weight of the Animal in what time	How much in a Minute	Weight of the Blood sustained by the left Ventricle contracting	Number of Pulses in a Minute	Area of the transverse Section of descending Aorta	Area of the transv. Sect. of ascending Aorta	
	Minutes	Pounds	Pounds		Square Inches	Square Inches	
Man	34.18	4.38	51.5	75			
	17.6	9.36					
Horse 3d	60	13.75	113.22	36	0.677	0.369	
Ox	88	18.14		38	0.912	0.85	
						Right	Left
Sheep	20	4.593	36.56	65	0.094	0.07	0.012
					0.385	0.246	
						Right	Left
Dog 1	11.9	4.34	33.61	97	0.106	0.041	0.034
2	6.48	3.7			0.102	0.031	0.009
3	7.8	2.3	19.8		0.07	0.022	0.009
4	6.7	1.85	11.1		0.061	0.015	0.007
					0.119	0.7	0.031
					0.125	0.062	0.031
7	9.9	4.34			0.109	0.053	0.032

16. And supposing the blood-vessels in the man and horse to be equally distributed in all their homologous parts, that is, if they are proportionable to their respective weights, then the blood must move in them reciprocally as the times, in which quantities of blood equal to their respective weights, pass thro' their hearts, *viz.* as 60 to 17 minutes.

17. So that notwithstanding the arterial blood of a horse is propelled with a greater force than that of a man; yet it moves the slower in the horse, on account of a greater number of ramifications, and a greater length of vessels in the larger animal.

18. When I compared the proportion, that the area of the transverse sections of the descending *aorta* bears to the flesh and other parts which they supply with circulating blood, I found it to be as follows; *viz.* having cut the body of a dog asunder at his heart, and first weighing each part

separately, and then boiling them so as to separate the bottes [bones] from the flesh, the weight of the bones being deducted from the flesh, the flesh, etc. of the hinder part was found to weigh eleven pounds, eleven ounces; that of the forepart seven pounds and two ounces.

19. Now the areas of the transverse section of the arteries of these five animals are by measurement as follows, *viz.*

20.

	Aorta.	desc.	ascend.		
In the Mare	1.036	0.677	0.369		0.412
Ox	1.539	0.912	0.85	by Computation from the	0.556
Sheep	0.172	0.094	0.082	above found proportion of	0.057
Doe	0.476	0.383	0.246	flesh from the hinder and	0.233
1st Dog	0.196	0.106	0.075	fore parts.	0.064
6th Dog	0.196	0.125	0.093		0.076
7th Dog	0.179	0.109	0.085		0.066

21. In this table we find that the areas of the transverse section of the descending and ascending *aorta's* of the first dog are nearly proportionable to the weights of the respective parts which they supply with blood; and that in the mare and doe, the difference is not great, but greater in the ox and sheep. In estimates of this kind great accuracy in the proportions is not to be expected.

22. The velocity with which the blood is thrown out of the left ventricle, being performed in one-third of the time between *systole* and *systole,* the like quantity of blood would move with an equable motion, of one-third of that velocity, thro' the orifice of the *aorta* in the space of time between each *systole.*

23. Since in a man a cylinder of blood of the diameter of the orifice of the *aorta* and 7.92 inches long, is at each pulse impelled through a dilatable conical artery, its velocity would be greatly increased by passing thro' that narrower defile; but the arteries continually sending off innumerable branches, the sum of whose orifices are considerably larger than the main stems, hence the velocity of the blood must be proportionably rebated. So that as Dr. James Keill, in his *Tentamina Medico Physica* p. 46, has estimated it, the velocity of the blood at the heart, would be to its velocity in an evanescent artery as 5233 to 1, if it had a free unembarrassed course through those capillary arteries. And since the velocity at its passing from the heart to the *aorta* is at the rate of 146 feet in a minute, taking one-third of that, *viz.* 43.2 for its continued equable velocity, according to Dr. Keill's estimate it would move but 0.00901th part of a foot, or 0.1128 inch in a minute, in the evanescent arteries in that time.

24. This would be its velocity there, if the blood had as free and unembarrassed a course thro' the finer capillary arteries, as it has thro' their larger ramifications. But by the following experiment, it is found, that the principal obstruction to the progress of the arterial blood is in the capillary arteries.

EXPERIMENT IX

1. I slit open with a pair of scissars, from end to end, the guts of a dog, on that side which is opposite to the insertion of the mesenteric arteries and veins; and having fixed a tube 4 + ½ feet high to the descending *aorta* a little below the heart, I poured blood-warm water thro' a funnel into the tube, which descended thence into the *aorta*, with a force equal to that, with which the blood is there impelled by the heart. This water passed off thro' the orifices of innumerable small capillary vessels, which were cut asunder thro' the whole length of the slit gut. But notwithstanding it was impelled with a force equal to that of the arterial blood in a live dog, yet it did not spout out in little distinct streams, but only seem to ouze out at the very fine orifices of the arteries, in the same manner as the blood does from the capillary arteries of a muscle cut transversely.

2. Having provided a pendulum which beat seconds, and pouring in through the tube known quantities of warm water, I found that 342 cubick inches of water passed off in 400 seconds, or 6.6 minutes.

3. Then cutting all the mesenteric arteries asunder close to the guts, and taking away the guts, I found that a like quantity of water passed thro' these larger ramifications of the arteries in 140 seconds, or 2.3 minutes, that is, in one-third of the time.

4. Then cutting asunder the crural arteries, which were before tied, and cutting off the mesenteric and emulgent arteries, close to the *aorta*, a like quantity of water passed thro' this thus cut *aorta* in 0.308 minutes, that is in $\frac{1}{21}$ 4, or 0.467th part of the time, in which it passed thro' the capillary arteries of the slit guts.

5. There being 342 cubick inches which passed thro' the capillary arteries of the slit guts in 6.6 minutes, that is, thirteen pounds, if it were blood, or 1.969 pound in a minute; and it being estimated in the table [p. 147], that 4.34 pounds of blood were thrown out of the heart of the dog, Numb. 1, in a minute, the above-mentioned 0.969* pound is 1/2.2 = 0.454th part of what passes the heart in that time.

6. But on weighing all the fleshly and other membranous parts of another dog, through which the arterial blood passes, that is, exclusive of the bones and lungs, I found the whole weight to be eighteen pounds eleven ounces, of which the slit gut weighing one pound two ounces, was therefore, 1/16.6 or 0.06th part of the whole: and there going 4.34 pounds out of the heart in a minute, and 1.969 pounds passing the mesenterick artery in the same time, and the slit gut weighing but 18 ounces, and all the parts of the body weighing 299 ounces, or 18 pounds 11 ounces; therefore, 1.969 pounds pass thro' 18 ounces, whilst 2.371 pounds pass 281 ounces (for 4.34 − 1.969 = 2.371, and 299 − 18 = 281), but 1969/18 = 0.1094

*This obvious error occurs in the edition from which we reprint. It should read 1.969.—F. A. W., 1940.

and 2374/281 = 0.008474, and 0.1094 : 00.08474 :: 12.1 : 91.1.* So that bulk for bulk there passed 12.91 times more water through the arteries of these slit guts, than through the rest of the arteries of the body, and that with a force no greater than that of the heart.

7. Which may reasonably be attributed to these several causes, as to the much greater fluidity of water than of viscid blood, to the more relaxed state of these arteries in the dead than in the living animal; for tho' the arteries and veins of a dead animal being then freed from the distending force of the blood do contract, yet with equal forces, those of the dead animal will dilate more than those of a live animal: but this more plentiful flow of water is principally owing to the great difference there is in size, between these cut capillary arteries, and the succeeding series's of exceeding small ramifications, and that at right angles, thro' which the blood passes in its further progress towards the vein: as also to a want of the resistance of the venal blood, which rising six inches in the tube fixed to the jugular vein is 1/13.33 or 0.075th part of the force of the arterial blood, and must therefore proportionably retard its motion.

8. The diameters of the cut orifices of the arteries thro' which the water passed off, were at a medium, one with another, equal to twice the diameter of a hair; which Dr. Jurin, by an accurate estimation, found to be 1/324th part of an inch; hence these arteries, which are 1/162 inch diameter, as they branch off from the mesentericks, spread themselves alternately on each side of the guts; whence meeting again, their inosculating branches form *areola's* like those that are on the leaves of trees: and from these thus converging arteries and sap-vessels, there branch off nearly at right angles, without converging any more, much smaller arteries, and from these others again, both at right angles, and like the spread fingers of a hand, in successive series's in their progress towards the veins.

9. The diameters of the first series's of these unconverging branches, may in a piece of gut well injected with vermilion, be observed to be of several sizes, from ½ to ⅓ of the arteries whence they rose, and the succeeding ones finer and finer to nearly 1/3240th part of an inch, that is so fine, that only single blood globules can pass them into the veins, here therefore, so viscid a fluid as the blood must needs meet with a very great resistance.

10. These reticular converging arteries, by being thus inosculated into each other, both prevent obstructions in them, and also thereby the most plentiful supply the next series of rectangular branches with blood; for if the blood had entered the converging arteries only at one end, its velocity would thereby have been more retarded in going the whole length, than half the length of these converging arteries; by these innumerable convergencies of the arteries, the blood is more blended and mixed, as is plain to be seen in the lungs of frogs.

---

*Several obvious errors appear in this proportion which we reprint exactly as it appeared in the 1769 edition. The figure 12.91 is obtained as follows: 1.969/18 = 0.1094 and 2.371/281 = 0.008474, and 0.1094 ; 0.008474 : : 12.91 : 1.—F. A. W., 1940.

11. From this experiment we see how greatly the velocity of the water is retarded in passing thro' the several branchings of the arteries, notwithstanding the sum of the areas of their transverse section is considerably greater than that of the *aorta*. And this retardation must be still greater to the blood which is both a grosser and more viscid fluid than water, and that especially in the extreme capillary arteries which branch off at right angles, and which are about 1/1620th part of an inch in diameter, so fine that only single globules of blood can pass them.

12. And to this resistance which the blood meets with in passing the capillary arteries, is owing the great difference of the force of the blood in the arteries to that in the veins, *viz.* as 10 or 12 to 1.

13. For tho' the velocity of the blood at its first entrance into the *aorta,* depends on the proportion the area of its orifice bears to the quantity thrown into it at each *systole,* and also on the number of those *systoles* in a given time: yet the real force of the blood in the arteries, depends on the proportion, which the quantity of blood thrown out of the left ventricle, in a given time, bears to the quantity which can pass thro' the capillary arteries into the veins, in that time.

14. But the resistance which the blood meets with in those capillary passages may be greatly varied, either by the different degrees of the viscidity or fluidity of the blood, or by the several degrees of constriction or relaxation of those fine vessels; instances of which may be seen in Experiments 15, 16, 17, 18.

15. And as the state of the blood or blood-vessels is in these respects continually varying from divers causes, as motion, rest, food, evacuations, heat, cold, &c. so as probably never to be exactly the same any two minutes, during the whole life of an animal, so nature has wisely provided, that a considerable variation in these, shall not greatly disturb the healthy state of the animal.

16. We may make a pretty near estimate of the force of the blood in the capillary vessels in the following manner; *viz.* taking the diameter of a blood-globule to be as above 1/3240th part of an inch; which Leewenhoeck has observed to be of the same size both in small and great animals; and allowing these capillary vessels to be a small size larger than the globules, which swim in and are carried along by the *serum* which surrounds them on all sides, we may therefore well suppose one of these vessels to be double the diameter of such a globule, *viz.* 1/1620th part of an inch, or 0.000617; the periphery therefore of this vessel will be 0.001939, and its area 0.000000298; which multiplied by 80, the number of inches to which the blood rose in the tube when fixed to the artery of the dog, Numb. 1, gives 0.000239 parts of eighty cubick inches of blood, or of 21,416 grains, equal to 0.515 parts of a grain. But the resistance of the blood in the veins of the same dog being found equal to six inches height, or 1/13.33d, or 0.075 parts of eighty inches, this 1/33.33d part = 0.03039 being deducted

out of 0.5118 parts of a grain, the remainder 0.4734 grain is the force with which the blood would be impelled into such a capillary by a column of blood of eighty inches height, supposing it were in a stagnant state; to which also must be added the velocity which the blood has acquired at its first entrance in the capillary vessel, which can be but small, as appears by the great resistance it meets with in the capillary vessels, in this 9th Experiment, Numb. 18, whence we see, both from experiment and calculation, that the force of the blood in these fine capillaries can be but very little; and the longer such capillaries are, the slower will the motion of the blood be in them.

17. It is observable, that these parallel arteries are not as in the bowels, lungs, and other membranous parts of the body, intermixed with corresponding similar veins; but two different series's of these arteries, arising at right angles from larger arteries, one series from the upper, and the other from the lower parts of the muscles, their parallel arteries do mutually and alternately intermix; whereby the blood is conveyed in them alternately upwards and downwards, and thence flows at right angles into the veins.

18. From this very small force of the arterial blood among the muscular fibres we may with good reason conclude, how short this force is of producing so great an effect, as that of muscular motion; which wonderful and hitherto inexplicable mystery of nature, must therefore be owing to some more vigorous and active energy, whose force is regulated by the nerves: but whether it be confined in canals within the nerves, or acts along their surfaces like electrical powers, is not easy to determine.

19. That a vibrating electrical virtue can be conveyed and freely act with considerable energy along the surface of animal fibres, and therefore on the nerves, is evident from curious experiments, made by that skillful and indefatigable experimenter, Mr. Stephen Gray, of which he has given an account in the *Philosophical Transactions,* Numb. 417, 422; where he shews that electrical virtues from a glass heated by rubbing, will not only be conveyed along the surface of lines to very great lengths, but will also be freely conveyed from the foot to the extended hand of a human body suspended by ropes in a horizontal posture in the air; and also from that hand to a long fishing-rod held in it, and thence to a string and a ball suspended by it: and also that an electrical virtue may be carried along a surface of water.

20. And it has been frequently observed, that when some part of the body has upon itching been gently scratched by the nails, there has at the same time been felt in a distant part, a very pungent *stimulus* or sensation answering exactly stroke for stroke to the action of the scratching nails. Thus particularly, on scratching a small pimple, a little below the right knee on the outside, a like pungent sensation has been felt on the left

shoulder-blade, and sometimes on that arm some inches below the shoulder: and *vice versa* the right shoulder or arm has in like manner been affected, when the scratching has been made near the left knee, but this effect does not always follow: there are many instances of the sympathy of the nerves.

21. That the animal spirits, whether they act within or on the outsides of the nerves, are elastick, seems probable not only from their great activity and energy; but also from the sudden and strong effects that sulphureous vapours, which are known to destroy elasticity, are found by experience to have on them. Thus the fumes of burning brimstone will instantly deprive all animals whatever of life: thus also the subtile and most penetrating fumes of fermenting spirituous liquors, are known either to strike those instantly dead who smell to them, or to infatuate or render paralytic for life, those who smell to them in lesser degrees. Thus also the sulphureous foetid fumes of burnt feathers, etc. have an effect on the disordered spirits of those who are in fits. Thus also *assa foetida, castor,* &c. which abound with a subtile sulphur, are found to be friendly to the spirits of the hysteric; as on the contrary are many fumes most offensive to the spirits of others.

22. If the skin be flead off the belly of a live frog, and the abdomen opened on each side, so as that its strait muscles may, by drawing a little on one side, have a strong focal light cast on the inside of them; if in this posture those muscles be viewed thro' a good microscope, the parallel fibres of the muscles are plain to be seen, with the blood running alternately up and down between each fibre, in capillary arteries so fine that only a single globule can pass them. If the muscle happens to act while thus viewed, then the scene is instantly changed from parallel fibres, to series's of *rhomboidal pinnulae,* which immediately disappear as soon as the muscle ceases to act. It is not easy to get a sight of this most agreeable scene, because that on the action of the muscle, the object is apt to get out of the focus of the microscope; but those who are expert in the use of those glasses may readily move them accordingly. I have found small frogs best for this purpose, *viz.* such as are not above ⅓ or ¼ of their full growth. Stimulating the foot of a frog, will sometimes make it contract these muscles. The frog must be fixed in a proper frame. If repeated observations were made on the muscles thus in action, it might perhaps give some farther insight into the nature of muscular motion.

23. It may not be improper here to take notice, that having about twenty-seven years since, read the unsatisfactory conjectures of several, about the cause of muscular motion, it occurred to me, that by fixing tubes to the arteries of live animals, I might find pretty nearly, whether the blood, by its mere hydraulic energy, could have a sufficient force, by dilating the fibres of the acting muscles, and thereby shortening their lengths, to produce the great effects of muscular motion. And hence it was, as I mentioned in the preface to Vol. I, that I was insensibly led on from time to

time, into this large field of statical and other experiments, whence we see what great encouragement we have to spur us on in these pursuits; since the wonderful works of the great Author of nature are so fruitful in furnishing us, from its inexhaustible fund, with fresh matter for our researches, and thence with the inexpressible delight, of new and farther motives to adore and praise our all-glorious Maker in his works.

*EXPERIMENT XI**

1. As to the force with which the blood is impelled from the right ventricle of the heart into the pulmonary artery, it seems impracticable to attempt the finding of it, by fixing a tube to that artery, in the same manner as to the carotid and crural arteries of living animals, because the animal must needs die while it is doing.

2. The area of the transverse section of the pulmonary artery being in one part, before it divaricates into branches, of the same dimension with the orifice of the *aorta,* the velocity of the blood in that part may be accounted the same as in the orifice of the *aorta.* But tho' the quantities and velocities of the blood, in passing out of both ventricles, be the same, yet it does not thence follow, that their expulsive forces must be both the same: for if the blood in passing into the pulmonary artery, finds less resistance from the preceding blood, than the blood does in entering into the *aorta,* then a less force will expel it out of the right ventricle with equal velocity; and accordingly, as there is not so much force required to drive the blood thro' the lungs, as thro' the rest of the whole body, so we may observe, that the substance of the muscle of the right ventricle has not near the thickness of that of the left. The following experiments and observations may give us some light into this matter, *viz.*

3. I fixed a glass tube to the pulmonary artery of a calf's lungs, and then thro' a tunnel† poured warm water into it; then with a large pair of bellows fixed to the wind-pipe, I alternately dilated the lungs, to try if by that means the water would pass into the pulmonary vein: but I soon found myself disappointed; for the water flowed so freely from the capillary arteries thro' the tunicles of the vesicles, into the vesicles themselves, and thence into the *bronchiae,* as to flow plentifully thro' the wind-pipe, when it hung down in a depending posture. At first I suspected that the force of the water, which was four feet high, in the tube affixed to the artery, might have burst the thin blood-vessels; but I found it the same in several trials, on the fresh warm lungs of sheep, oxen, and calves, even when the perpendicular height of the water of the tube was less than a foot; and doubtless the force with which the blood is thrown into the lungs by the right ventricle of the heart, is greater than this.

4. And that so small a force of water could not burst the blood-vessels, I was assured by the following experiment, *viz.* I dissolved 4 ounces of nitre

*Experiment X has been omitted from the present printing.—F. A. W., 1940.
†Funnel.—F. A. W., 1940.

in a pint of hot water, into which water there flowed from the cut throat of a calf, a quart and a quarter of a pint of blood, which was kept in a diluted state by the nitrated water. Having then fixed a tube which was 2 feet long, to the pulmonary artery of the above-mentioned calf's lungs, I poured gradually into the tube, of the nitrated blood, as much as the artery and its ramifications would contain, which was near a quart, none passing, that I could perceive, into the pulmonary vein. The lungs were much dilated, and looked very red: but notwithstanding the perpendicular height of the blood in the tube was 2 feet, yet no blood passed through the tunicles of the vesicles, into the vesicles and *bronchiae;* for when the wind-pipe was held downwards, nothing flowed out but a white froth; a plain proof that when the water was less than a foot perpendicular in height, in the foregoing experiments, it did not forcibly break through the blood-vessels, but must pass through pores which were too fine for the globules of nitrated blood to pass: those pores being perhaps something larger in the lungs of a dead animal, than when alive; for upon death all the fibres of the body are relaxed. When I cut a slash into the substance of the lungs, the nitrated blood freely flowed out.

5. And that the capillary arteries were not burst by the force of the water, seems farther probable from hence; *viz.* I fixed a tube 5 feet long to the pulmonary vein of a hog's lung's and poured in warm water, which neither flowed into the pulmonary arteries, nor among the *bronchiae;* an argument that this force did not burst the veins, which some anatomists say, have no valves in them.

6. When I fixed the same tube to the wind-pipe of those lungs, and poured in water, it passed through the *bronchiae,* and ran out of the orifice of the pulmonary artery, but not above one-fifth so fast, as when its course was the reverse, *viz.* from the pulmonary artery to the *bronchiae,* in which case it run at the rate of a pint in a minute. Yet when air was blown into the cavity of the lungs, thro' the wind-pipe, none passed thence, either into the pulmonary artery or vein.

7. Another time I tried also whether the thin serum of a hog's blood would pass from the pulmonary arteries, thro' the corresponding veins of the lungs, of the same hog, which lungs were kept warm in water; the serum passed most freely thro' into the *bronchiae,* but not into the veins.

1749

JEAN-BAPTISTE DE SÉNAC

TREATMENT OF "REBELLIOUS PALPITATION" WITH QUININE

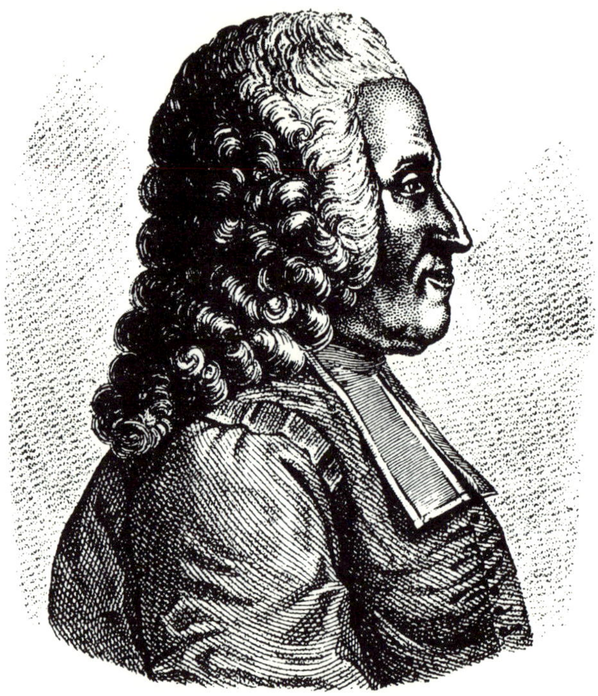

JEAN-BAPTISTE DE SÉNAC

(Courtesy American Heart Association.)

JEAN-BAPTISTE DE SÉNAC

(1693-1770)

"Theory reduced to consequences drawn from facts alone, is the light of practice."

—Sénac, in preface to *Le Traité de la Structure du Cœur* (1749), quoted by Renouard.

JEAN-BAPTISTE DE SÉNAC was born in 1693 in the district of Lombez in Gascony, France. From his birth to the date of publication of his first work in 1724 nothing definite about him is known, but it is said that at first, encouraged by his parents, he decided to study for the ministry. Later he changed his studies to medicine.

There is no definite knowledge as to where or when Sénac studied medicine. Degris wrote that Eloy, in his "Biographical Dictionary," said that Sénac received his Bachelor's degree from the Faculté de Paris but Degris thought that this was an error, since Hahn could not find Sénac's name in the "Commentaries of the Faculty" or in Baron's list of recipients of the Bachelor's or Doctor's degree of the Faculty.

Sénac, it is known, accepted the appointment of consulting physician to the King in 1738 and on his first publication he signed himself as a member of the faculty of the University of Montpellier, which Noé Legrand called the oldest university in Europe.

According to Degris, it is believed that Sénac came to Paris when he was about thirty years of age. In Paris he published his first work in 1724, a translation of Heister's "Anatomy."[1] In 1724 and 1725 he communicated before the Royal Academy of Sciences two memoirs: "On the Organs of Respiration" and "On Drowning." In 1724 he became an associate member of this academy.

In 1727 he published an appreciative account showing the different methods of the lithotomists entitled: "Discours sur la méthode de France et sur celle de Rau Touchant l'Opération de la Taille." Sénac published many more interesting contributions, but none is as famous as his "Traité de la Structure du Coeur" (1749), which we shall later discuss in more detail.

Sénac moved to Versailles in 1733 where he became physician to the Royal House of Saint-Cyr and to the Royal Hospital of Versailles.

In 1745, Sénac cured the great French general, Maurice, Count de Saxe (1693-1750), of a serious disease and later accompanied him on his campaigns. In 1751, after the death of Maurice, who was given Turenne's title of "Marshal general of the King's armies and camps," Sénac became chief physician to the Duke of Orleans and in 1752, after the death of Chicoyneau, he became chief physician to Louis XV. He treated the dauphin during his illness from smallpox in 1752, and again during the young man's fatal illness from tuberculosis in 1765. In addition to the members of the court, he numbered among his patients Madame de Pompadour.

---

[1]Sénac, J. B.: *L'Anatomie d'Heister avec des essais de physique sur l'usage des parties du corps humain,* Paris, 1724.

In 1760 and again in 1761, Voltaire addressed two letters to Sénac. The first supported Sénac's memoir on a certain contagious disease which had devastated the country around Ferney, and the second was a missive of thanks to the ''chief physician'' for his good work in aiding some people who lived close to a contaminated marsh.

Louis XV appointed Sénac counsellor of state and superintendent of the mineral waters and medicinals of the kingdom.

Sénac died on December 20, 1770, at the age of seventy-seven years. He was survived by two sons, one of whom, Gabriel Sénac de Meilhon (1736-1803), was a writer and was invited to Russia in 1792 by the Empress Catherine II, and the other of whom was a superintendent of agricultural revenues.

Sénac's fame in cardiology rests, of course, on his important work first published in 1749 in two volumes, ''Traité de la Structure du Coeur, de son Action et de ses Maladies.'' A second edition of this valuable work appeared in 1777, seven years after the author's death.

In his original work, which greatly surpassed studies of the heart made by his predecessors, Sénac made many noteworthy observations. Among these are his descriptions in detail of the structure of the heart and the direction in placement of its fibers. He discussed the transfusion of blood. He noted the increase in incidence of cardiac disease with the increase in age and considered dilatation to be the most common of all cardiac conditions. Sénac related pericarditis to inflammation of the lungs and mediastinum. He acknowledged that hydrothorax played a conspicuous part in failure of circulation. He was the first physician to use quinine for palpitation, and it is this classic description which we are republishing herein in translation. According to Long, the germ of the modern idea of septicemia is seen in Sénac's conception of the condition as caused by pus which flowed back into the blood from the loci of external ulcers.

Sénac regarded with skepticism the remarks of early writers on ''hairy'' hearts, and on stones and worms in the heart. He believed that polyp of the heart was a formation occurring at the time of death. Sénac entertained a curious idea about the remote cause of movements of the heart. He thought these motions were transmitted by an animal spirit situated in the brain and spinal marrow. He thought of this spirit as an extremely elastic fluid, which the impression of the blood on the delicate tissue of the parietes of the heart and the columns of the ventricles put into action.

TRAITÉ
DE
LA STRUCTURE DU CŒUR,
DE SON ACTION,
ET
DE SES MALADIES

Par M. SENAC, Médecin Consultant du Roy.

Multùm egerunt qui ante nos fuerunt, multùm etiam adhuc restat operis, multùmque restabit; nec ulli nato post mille sæcula præcludetur occasio aliquid adjiciendi. Ann. Seneca.

TOME PREMIER.

A PARIS,
Chez JACQUES VINCENT, rue & vis-à-vis l'Eglise de S. Severin, à l'Ange.

MDCCXLIX.
AVEC APPROBATION ET PRIVILEGE DU ROY.

OPERATION OF STOMACHIC REMEDIES IN PALPITATION*

[Including the use of quinine in rebellious palpitations]

THE above are not the sole resources of Medicine against palpitation; aid has been found in various remedies of which the properties are very different. These remedies are the stomachics, the cordials and the sedatives. The stomachic remedies have appeared to various physicians as a resource against palpitations, for it is often in the stomach that their cause resides; if they do not arise from this as an immediate cause, there is in many cases an occasional cause which sets the other in motion. The ancients, attentive to sensible effects, have accused *flatulence.* Pisanus, Higmer and Bartholin have had the same idea. It is true that if the first instrument of digestion is inflated by the action of the air that it contains, it will produce the same effects as if it were full of aliment, and when it cannot empty itself it will agitate its viscera and its nerves and may excite palpitation, as Widelius has judiciously remarked. The majority, he says, of those who are subject to palpitations are *hypochondriacs,* the functions of their stomachs are deranged, and this derangement troubles the action of the heart.

The derangements of the viscera are thus an object that one must not lose sight of in the treatment of palpitations; it excites them often when it is overloaded; thus regularity is one of the necessary conditions to avoid the agitation of the heart or to calm it. If it comes from a vice of that organ, sobriety is not less essential; excess adds to this vice a new irritation, the viscera of the lower abdomen being overloaded, are too much pressed on by the mass of the full stomach, and these push the blood with more force and give stimuli to the nerves which may trouble the movements of the heart.

When patients are put on a regime one must facilitate digestion if this is possible; such a resource will be the more necessary if the palpitations are excited by the viscera, or if they are occasioned by the derangement of its functions; when one must first of all attempt to prevent food from staying too long in the stomach, and see that food of poor quality be not taken.

Bitter extracts and other similar remedies aid the stomach to empty itself, they act on the membranes to stimulate and urge them; they have

*Sénac, J. B.: *Traité de la structure du coeur, de son action et de ses maladies,* Paris, Chez Jacques Vincent, 1749, Tome Second, XVIII, p. 524. Translated by Maurice N. Walsh, M.D., Mayo Clinic.

some of the qualities of the bile, which they replace when it does not flow easily or has lost its qualities; but their operation carries with it some disadvantages, they are warming and thus it is necessary to avoid or to moderate their usage in bodies which are too sensitive and susceptible to impressions of heat. The usage of carminatives necessitates the same management, these are not remedies that one can neglect as they have produced happy results according to Widelius and other physicians.

If aliments degenerate in the stomach the bad qualities that they produce reduce to two: they become acid or rancid. It is to absorb the bitter and to correct rancid oils that physicians have resource to earthy absorbents as remedies that may calm palpitations. The efficacy of these remedies is recognized by all observers in the malady called *Soda,* that is to say in that derangement of the stomach which sends into the esophagus a burning heat, or a kind of caustic liquor which appears to leave impressions of fire in its passage.

In general, remedies which facilitate digestion have been regarded as remedies for palpitation of the heart. Widelius has prescribed the elixir de propriété (simple elixir?) ; Marcatus recommends Rhapontic as a proven remedy, he gives an infusion of it in wine with Panax, round Aristolochus, Greek Fennel. Rivièrè has given his approval to this remedy which in truth acts at the same time as a purgative and appropriate to hysterical affections.

Of all the stomachic remedies the one whose effects have appeared to me the most constant and the most prompt in many cases, is Quinine mixed with a little rhubarb. Long and rebellious palpitations have ceded to this febrifuge, seconded with a light purgative.

One must place among the stomachic remedies the cordials which have been regarded as effective remedies against palpitation. . . .

1755

ALBRECHT VON HALLER

DESCRIPTION OF CALCIFICATION OF THE HEART AND PERICARDIUM

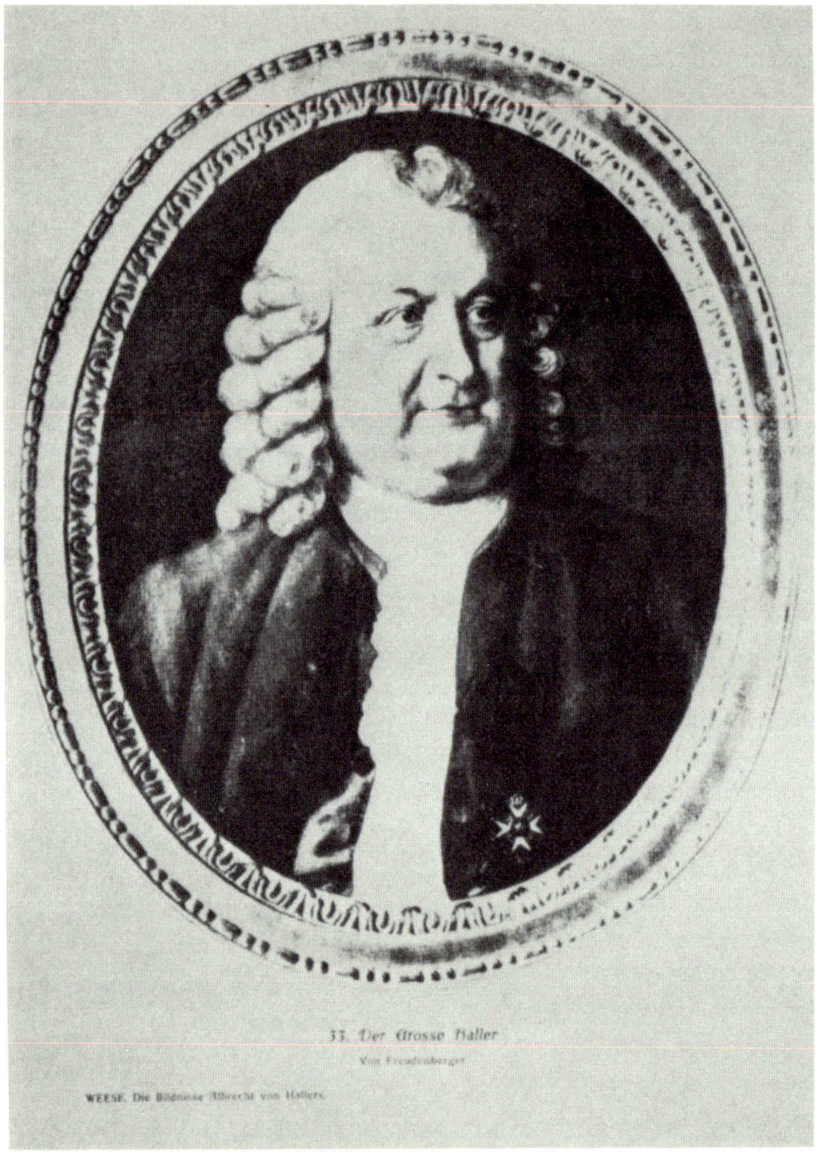
33. Der Grosse Haller
WEESE, Die Bildnisse Albrecht von Hallers.

ALBRECHT VON HALLER

Portrait by Sigmund Freudenberger

(Courtesy Charles C Thomas.)

ALBRECHT VON HALLER

(1708-1777)

"The Prince of Physiologists."

—Pettigrew.

ALBRECHT VON HALLER was born in October, 1708, at Bern, Switzerland. His father was a prominent lawyer and Albrecht was his fourth and youngest son. Young Haller showed a large capacity for knowledge in early childhood. At the age of four he expounded the Scriptures to the servants; at eight years of age, he had written 2,000 brief biographies, and by the time he was ten years old he had written a brief lexicon of Greek, Hebrew, and Chaldean.

Haller continued to astound his family with his intellectual achievements, for at the age of twelve he began to write verse. When he was either fourteen or fifteen, we are told, he wrote an epic poem of 4,000 stanzas on the "Origin of the Swiss Union of States." At this time he also translated Ovid, Horace, and Virgil.

In 1723 Haller matriculated at the University of Tübingen. Two years later he traveled to Holland, where he studied under the renowned Boerhaave. He later wrote a commentary on the works of his great teacher. At the age of eighteen, Haller received his medical degree from the University of Leyden. In his dissertation he disproved Coschwitz' supposed discovery of a new salivary duct. Haller proved this anatomic structure to be a blood vessel.

After receiving his degree, Haller traveled to France and England where he studied for a time before returning to Switzerland. Then he went to his native country, studied mathematics under Bernouilli in Basel and later returned to Bern to practice medicine. In 1734, when the Republic of Bern established an amphitheater, Haller was invited to give demonstrations in anatomy.

With the founding of the University of Göttingen in 1736, Haller was asked by George II, King of England, who was also Elector of Hanover and Brunswick, to fill the chair of anatomy, surgery, and botany. Haller accepted and remained in Göttingen for seventeen years. At Göttingen he founded the Anatomical Museum and Laboratory, the Botanical School and Garden and the Department of Obstetrics. He also founded there a journal entitled: "Göttinger gelehrten Anzeiger," to which he contributed more than 12,000 book reviews. During this time, also, he received attractive offers from Oxford, Leyden, and Berlin, but refused them all. In 1752 the Emperor Joseph conferred a baronetcy on Haller. This he did not accept.

Haller returned to Bern in 1753, where he remained until his death in 1777. In his last days he suffered from an inflammatory condition of the bladder so painful that he could be relieved only by large doses of opium.

The most productive period of Haller's literary career began in Göttingen. He was perhaps, the most prodigious and versatile writer of all times. According to Garrison, while Haller was in Göttingen he wrote some 13,000 scientific papers. We have mentioned his 12,000 book reviews contributed to the journal he had founded. At Göttingen, also, Haller began his classic experiments on nerve sensibility and muscular irritability which were to be published in 1757. And at Göttingen he laid the foundation for his huge and most authoritative work in physiology, ''Elementa Physiologiae corporis humani.'' This was published in nine volumes at Lausanne from 1759 to 1769.

It is impossible in this brief account even to mention all of Haller's contributions to medicine. As far as we know, he was the first to describe calcification of the pericardium. This description we are including herein.

Before Haller published his great work on physiology, he contributed several monographs on physiology and its relationship to embryology, circulation, reproduction, formation of bone and irritability.

According to Hemmeter, the principal contributions of Haller to anatomy were: (1) a demonstration that the so-called salivary duct was a vein, (2) an investigation of the respiratory muscles and an exhaustive description of the diaphragm, with an interpretation of the intercostal muscles as elevators of the ribs, (3) a demonstration of the uterine musculature, (4) a demonstration of the coni vasculosi, (5) a correct description of the musculature of the heart and an accurate description of the pericardium and the valves in the veins, (6) a description of a number of hitherto unknown arteries, (7) recognition of the higher situation of the bladder above the pubes in children, (8) description of the omentum and (9) demonstration of the tela cellulosa as a connective tissue substance.

To cardiac physiology Haller made many contributions. He stressed the changes of the heart occurring during contraction and he was familiar with the influence of gravity and respiratory aspiration of the thorax on the circulation of the veins. He also succeeded in demonstrating the automatism of the heart.

Haller gained universal admiration for his several works on botanical subjects and in his ''Historia stirpium indigenarum Helvetiae'' he described 2486 species of plants. He holds an important place in the history of German literature, his poetry having been regarded as outstanding. His well-known poem, ''The Alps,'' was published in English in 1729. Twenty-two editions of it were published in German and it was also translated into French, Italian, and Latin. He also contributed to history his splendid biography, ''Life of Alfred the Great.''

By all means, mention should be made of his numerous bibliographic undertakings. Haller had made it a custom to write a concise summary of the books he read. His ''Bibliothecae,'' comprising his bibliographies on anatomy, botany, surgery, and medicine, compiled from his lifetime of reading, include 52,000 works! According to Fulton, next to the ''Index Catalogue of the Surgeon General's Office'' of the United States Army, this collection represents the greatest compilation of medical titles ever assembled. Not only is it an index to the world's medical literature up to and including Haller's era, it is also a compendium in which each author's biographic data are given, a summary of the work is presented, critical comments on the author's views are offered, and other considerations that Haller thought of interest are included.

Haller was married three times. His first two wives died and by his third wife he had eleven children. Of these, four sons and four daughters survived him. Among the few honors that he chose to accept were membership in the Academy of Sciences of Paris and fellowship in the Royal Society of London. Gustavus III, King of Sweden, also made him a knight of the Polar Star.

ALBERTI HALLERI

PRÆSIDIS S. REG. SC. GOTTING.

OPUSCULA PATHOLOGICA

Partim recusa partim inedita:

QUIBUS

SECTIONES CADAVERUM

MORBOSORUM

Potissimum continentur.

ACCEDUNT EXPERIMENTA

DE RESPIRATIONE,

QUARTA PARTE AUCTA.

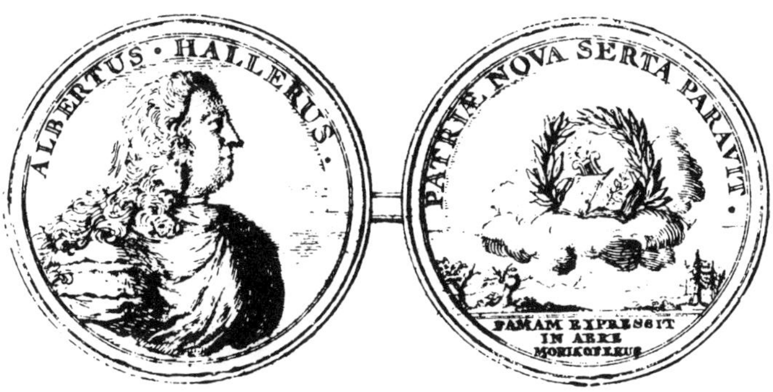

LAUSANNÆ,

Sumpt. MARCI-MICH. BOUSQUET & Soc.

MDCCLV.

DESCRIPTION OF CALCIFICATION OF THE HEART*

. . . .

But the following unusual disease is worthy to be remembered, from it a most admirable young person died not long since. The mother of the boy I perceived on medical examination eight years previously to be subject to palpitation of the heart, the youth now fell into the same illness. He himself, on the day of his death, was without the pulse which you feel in the wrist; however I found the carotids to be violently throbbing. [The patient] chilling, then drenched with sweat, I reluctantly gave a bad prognosis.

Shortly after death we opened the body. The pericardium of the heart and the pleura of the lungs were everywhere attached, and all over the surface of the pericardium were white hard masses, some firm and some filled with white material like pus. These hard swellings were totally and indissolubly united to the pericardium by bands. The semi-stone-like inferior part of the right ventricle was strongly adherent to the pericardium by a mass of tophaceous calculi like fine sand. The sinus between the two membranes of the aortic valves was hard and in part stony. In the aortic valves between the membranes there was a strange material, in fact the tendons which held back these valves were even found to be fleshy, and with variable bony scales.

But a special disorder was concealed in the valves of the pulmonary vein. These were all excessively hard and solid; they were completely filled with stony material, to the extent that the fibres grated whenever they were cut. Even the tissue of the pulmonary sinus was formed of stony material. Neither the heart nor the great vessels exceeded the usual size.

The patient's age, twenty years, increases the rarity of the disease. The heart of this youth was not stopped up, neither was it satisfactorily open; it lacked alternate rest, without which no heart can live. Now the left ventricle received blood with great difficulty from its sinus and by its contraction sent it through the rigid opening of the osseous mitral valves to its sinus. Thus from the aorta in like manner the blood could return between the inexplicably rigid aortic valves into the heart. Whence, with the heart perpetually stimulated, it palpitated uninterruptedly, and since it could not send enough blood to the brain, in this manner a stupor was produced, like that which befalls with loss of blood from venesection or from wounds.

---

*Von Haller, Albrecht: *Opuscula Pathologica,* Lausannae, Bousquet et soc., 1755, p. 135. Translated by Maurice N. Walsh, M.D., Mayo Clinic.

1761

JOHN BAPTIST MORGAGNI

DESCRIPTIONS OF MITRAL STENOSIS, HEART BLOCK, CALCAREOUS STENOSIS OF THE AORTIC VALVE WITH REGURGITATION, CORONARY SCLEROSIS, AND ANEURYSM OF THE AORTA

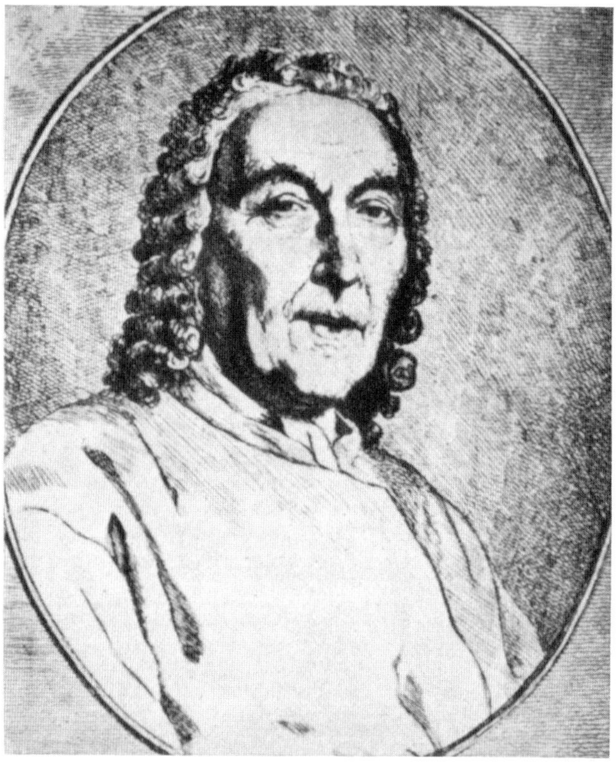

JOHN BAPTIST MORGAGNI

(Courtesy Charles C Thomas.)

JOHN BAPTIST MORGAGNI

(1682-1771)

"Those who have dissected or inspected many (bodies), have at least learned to doubt; when others, who are ignorant of anatomy and do not take the trouble to attend to it, are in no doubt at all."

—Morgagni, letter 16, article 25, of *De sedibus et causis morborum,* after Adams.

MORGAGNI was born on February 25 near Bologna at Forli, at that time an important Italian town. He matriculated at the University of Bologna, where he studied under the faculties of philosophy and medicine. He was graduated from Bologna in 1701, with high honors from both faculties.

Soon after graduation Morgagni accepted at Bologna the position of prosector in anatomy under the famous teacher, Antonio Maria Valsalva, a pupil of Malpighi. Morgagni assisted Valsalva in the preparation of the latter's famous work on the anatomy and diseases of the ear.[1] This work was published in 1704.

Morgagni esteemed Valsalva and later edited the anatomic writings of his former teacher. Morgagni's editing of Valsalva's work was supplemented by some of his own observations, and he later added a memoir to the life of Valsalva (1740).

When Valsalva resigned his position to accept an offer at Parma, Morgagni succeeded him at Bologna as demonstrator in anatomy. In 1706 Morgagni became president of the Academia Inquietorum of Bologna. At this time he published in six parts his first notable work, "Adversaria anatomica," comprising the substance of his communications to the Academia. Therein are contained some of his independent discoveries, more especially, as Nicholls points out, "in connection with the muscles of the hyoid bone, the uvula and the larynx."

After some time, Morgagni resigned his position at Bologna and went to Padua and Venice, at which universities he continued his anatomic studies for the space of two to three years. He then moved to his native town, Forli, and began the practice of medicine. Although Morgagni was successful at the physician's art he did not enjoy the practical aspects of medical practice, and, therefore, on the death of Domenicho Guglielmini, he accepted a chair of theoretical medicine in the University of Padua made vacant when Antonio Vallisnisei succeeded to Guglielmini's post.

Thus began Morgagni's long and uninterrupted academic career, for he taught at Padua until his death fifty-one years later. After three years he was appointed by the Venetian Senate to the chair of anatomy at Padua made vacant by the death of Michel Angelo Molinetti. This was the most distinguished position on the faculty, and among the renowned anatomists he succeeded were Vesalius, Fallopius, Gasserius and Spigelius.

Shortly after coming to Padua, Morgagni married a noble lady, Paola Vergieri, of Forli. Fifteen children were born of the union, eight of whom were living when Morgagni died.

[1]*De aure humana.*

Morgagni was popular with his students, and his distinguished friends, according to Pettigrew, included King Charles Emanuel III of Sardinia, and Popes Clement XI, XII, and XIII and Benedict XIV. In his own profession he enjoyed an international reputation and was esteemed by Valsalva, Albertini, Lancisi, Verheyen, Heister, Ruysch, Boerhaave, Mead, Sénac, Haller, Meckel, Le Clerc, Fantoni, Nigrisoli, Michelotti, Molinetti, and numerous others.

Morgagni was the recipient of scientific honors from all Europe. He was elected a member of the Academia Naturae Curiosorum in 1708, the Royal Society of London in 1724, the Academy of Sciences of Paris in 1731, the Imperial Academy of St. Petersburg in 1735, and the Academy of Berlin in 1754.

Apart from his scientific studies, Morgagni was a man of unusual attainments. He wrote on philology, archaeology, literature and history. Nicholls mentioned these works as typical: Morgagni's letters to Lancisi on the ''Manner of Cleopatra's death,'' ''Commentaries'' on Celsus and Sammonicus, and notes on Varro, Alpinus, Vegetius, Columella, and Vitruvius, as well as archaeologic papers on the districts around Ravenna and Forli.

It was not until 1761, when Morgagni was seventy-nine years old that his monumental work, ''De sedibus et causis morborum per anatomen indagatis libri quinque,'' was published. This work has immortalized Morgagni as the father of pathologic anatomy, chiefly because the records of post-mortem descriptions are correlated with clinical observations on a grand scale in addition to the fact that he was the first to describe many diseases. Before Morgagni's work was published, the standard printed work on the subject was the ''Sepulchretum'' of Theophilus Bonetus, published at Geneva three years before Morgagni himself was born. This work contained what was known about morbid anatomy up to the date of the publication. The more Morgagni studied the ''Sepulchretum,'' the less satisfied with it he became and finally he concluded to supplement it with his own observations.

As was the custom of the time, Morgagni wrote his observations in the form of letters to a friend, a procedure that resulted in the production of seventy letters. The letters were then returned to Morgagni, were revised and published in a huge work of five books.

The five books of ''De sedibus et causis morborum'' deal with: (1) diseases of the head, (2) diseases of the thorax, (3) diseases of the abdomen, (4) diseases of a general nature, and diseases requiring surgical treatment and (5) such things as were added to the other four books.

The work is based on the results of 640 post-mortem examinations, generally occurring in his own experience but occasionally taken from the unpublished notes of Valsalva and Albertini.

Morgagni devoted several letters of ''De sedibus'' to a study of the diseased heart, in which he accurately described the principal cardiac lesions which he found after the death of his patients. We have chosen to reproduce his classic descriptions of (1) mitral stenosis, (2) heart block, (3) calcareous stenosis of the aortic valve with regurgitation, (4) coronary sclerosis, and (5) aneurysm of the aorta.

As we have noted in our study of Heberden, Morgagni also included an early description of angina pectoris, which he noted in 1707, and published in his ''De sedibus'' in 1761 (vol. 1, p. 282). Morgagni observed that certain disorders, such as asthma and dyspnea, formerly considered to be the result of pulmonary disease, also might be caused by diseases of the heart. He suggested the possible relationship, as did many of his predecessors, of syphilis to aneurysm. He also described rupture of the heart, but did not mention the cause of this condition. He also described vegetative endocarditis.

Nicholls called attention to the fact that Morgagni ''came far short of establishing a complete system of Morbid Anatomy.'' Morgagni could not entirely shake himself free from the erroneous conceptions of disease prevalent in his day. Although the microscope was in use before his time, as we have shown, he does not appear to have used it in his investigations. However, by basing his views on personal observation and making an effort to harmonize clinical manifestations of disease with the morbid appearances of diseases, Morgagni established a firm basis for those great principles that underlie modern methods of scientific research.

Morgagni's death occurred on December 5, 1771, when he was at the advanced age of ninety. The citizens of Forli erected a bust to him in the principal palace of the town in 1763. In Dryden's ''Oedipus,'' the play he wrote with Nathaniel Lee, are found the lines which provide an excellent strophe on the last years of Morgagni:

> ''Of no distemper, of no blast he died,
> But fell like autumn-fruit that mellowed long,
> Ev'n wondered at because he dropp'd no sooner.
> Fate seemed to wind him up for fourscore years
> Yet freely ran he on ten winter's more;
> 'Till, like a clock worn out with eating time,
> The wheels of weary life at last stood still.''

(Quoted by Pettigrew)

THE SEATS and CAUSES OF DISEASES INVESTIGATED BY ANATOMY;

IN FIVE BOOKS,

CONTAINING

A Great Variety of DISSECTIONS, with REMARKS.

TO WHICH ARE ADDED

Very ACCURATE and COPIOUS INDEXES of the PRINCIPAL THINGS and NAMES therein contained.

TRANSLATED from the LATIN of

JOHN BAPTIST MORGAGNI,
Chief Professor of Anatomy, and President of the University at PADUA,

By BENJAMIN ALEXANDER, M. D.

IN THREE VOLUMES.

VOL. I.

LONDON,
Printed for A. MILLAR; and T. CADELL, his Successor, in the Strand;
and JOHNSON and PAYNE, in Pater-noster Row.
MDCCLXIX.

LETTER THE THIRD*

WHICH CONCLUDES THE OBSERVATIONS ON THE SANGUINEOUS APOPLEXY

[Description of Mitral Stenosis]

. . . .

26. Peter Fasolati, an engraver, at Padua, in the sixty-second year of his age, yet still of a full habit, and liable to no indisposition, died at the very same season as Tita (*m*), and even the very day after him, in the following manner. He had gone through no labour, had not been troubled with care and anxiety, as he had been us'd at other times, and made no complaint of any thing. He had even supp'd heartily, for he always us'd to eat freely; and desir'd to go to bed more early than usual, which he did: but two hours afterwards, his wife happening to wake, found him not only dead, but even cold, and stretch'd out in the same manner he had lay'd himself when he went to bed.

The day following, when the integuments of the cranium were cut into, and while the upper part of the skull was saw'd through, and taken off, much blood was discharg'd. Yet there was none at all extravasated within the skull; none in the substance of the cerebrum, or cerebellum: and both these parts seem'd, to the touch, to be perfectly natural: there was, I say, nothing ruptur'd, nothing injur'd in any part. There was some water in the lateral ventricles almost limpid, but in small quantity; and some also seem'd to flow from the sides of the cerebellum, which was found, as I have said; or might it not come from the tube of the vertebrae? But such a quantity of fluid blood distended all the vessels in and about the brain, that I do not remember to have seen the like before: even some small vessels, which us'd to be scarcely perceptible, were extremely large and turgid (†). I order'd, however, that the thorax should be open'd also. The left lobe of the lungs was strongly connected to the ribs, but both of them were sound. The colour of the fat, in the mediastinum, was brown; which I attributed to the blood remaining in the smallest vessels. In the pericardium was some bloody water, but not much. The heart was large, and its proper vessels and auricles turgid with blood, which came forth very black and grumous while the heart was cut off from its larger vessels, that I might examine it the more

*Morgagni, John Baptist: *De sedibus et causis morborum per anatomen indagatis libri quinque,* 1761. We are reprinting from the English translation of 1769.—F. A. W., 1940.

(*m*) Vide supra n. 11.

†Vid. etiam. Epist. 60. n. 12.

closely, out of the body. The blood was also black and grumous in the ventricles of the heart, yet not in very great quantity. The right valvula mitralis was white; and in like manner some of the semilunar valves: the former were much harder than usual, and the latter a little so: but in both mitral and semilunar, the membranous nature had degenerated almost into the nature of a ligament. In the middle and posterior surface of the heart, a kind of little membrane protruded, of a white colour, and look'd like the remains of an hydatid. On the right auricle externally, also, were some white spots. But the aorta and other vessels, as far as I could see, were according to their natural appearances.

27. It does not escape me, that you may think this man's death is rather to be imputed to a syncope, than to an apoplexy; as well when you consider the celerity of it, as the sudden coldness of the body at that hot season, and in bed; or even the appearances observ'd in the heart. But, to begin with these last, and to compare them with the quantity of blood found within the cranium; we certainly find greater marks of disorder in the hearts of those, who had not the slightest appearance of fainting, and much less the most violent syncope. And Galen has taught us, that an apoplexy may be form'd from such an abundance of blood within the cranium, though I have never seen any other case of the kind that I remember: Galen's (*n*) words are, "By this means apoplexies are brought on, to wit, by much blood rushing tumultuously into the principle of animation." Nor did Petrus Salius (*o*), who first wrote a separate chapter on the sanguineous apoplexy, as I have mention'd in the former letter (*p*), imagine, that the disorder was, in general, brought about by other means, in the cerebrum, than from "too great a repletion of the veins, arteries, and sinusses, with blood; for which reason a very great stricture is brought upon the brain, whereby, not only the free passage of the spirits is prevented, but they are even choak'd up, and suffocated thereby; so that sense and motion are suddenly lost, and the intelligent faculties are suspended: that is, a true and exact apoplexy succeeds." And, indeed, such a quantity of blood could not be collected in all the vessels within the cranium, but that the soft substance of the cerebrum and cerebellum must be violently compressed, both from within and from without; the small vessels also, which escape the senses, being streighten'd, the circulation of the blood is intercepted; and consequently the secretion of spirits, which cannot happen without it, is prevented: for as there is no vacuity in the cranium, and the bones of it are incapable of giving way, the whole force of the pressure must be expended on the brain. These things cannot happen to the cerebellum, as it seems, and as I have already said (*q*), without a sudden suffocation of respiration and the motion of the heart, being the consequences thereof; that is, with-

(*n*) Vid. apud Salium, de Affect. partic. c.2.
(*o*) Ibid.
(*p*) n. 1.
(*q*) Epist. 2. n. 24.

out sudden death: and this death, if you would rather have it so, from a syncope; but a syncope that would proceed from the head, and not from the heart; or if from the heart also, on account of the appearances spoken of, yet, at least, certainly more from the head, than from the heart. But wherever there is a syncope, from whencesoever it proceeds, there is no reason to wonder at the sudden coldness of the body: though I should rather suppose, that it was only a diminution of warmth, which seemed to a woman who was herself warm, to be cold. And, as far as I can judge, you would not err much, if you should call that kind of syncope, which Herophilus (*r*) seems to have particularly pointed out, an apoplexy from the cerebellum: for he says, "When sudden death happens without any manifest cause, then it is owing to a palsy of the heart:" for what an apoplexy from the cerebrum does in other parts of the body, the same an apoplexy from the cerebellum does in the heart: but in an apoplexy which proceeds both from cerebrum and cerebellum at the same time, motion is destroy'd in all parts of the body at once. And such, I think, was the case under consideration, since there was evidently a material cause of compression upon them both; nor did I find that any of those symptoms had preceded, which are generally antecedent to a syncope from the heart, or any of its nearest vessels.

. . . .

LETTER THE NINTH

WHICH TREATS OF THE EPILEPSY

[Description of Heart Block]

. . . .

7. To which, therefore, that I may return, I will just skim over, in as few words as I shall be able, those many things which I have observ'd, for a long time, in my fellow-citizen Anastasio Poggi, a grave and worthy priest. He was in his sixty-eighth year, of a habit moderately fat, and of a florid complexion, when he was first seiz'd with the epilepsy, which left behind it the greatest slowness of pulse, and in like manner a coldness of the body. But this coldness of the body was overcome within seven hours, nor did it return any more, though the disorder often return'd; but the slowness of the pulse still remain'd. The first epilepsy had succeeded to a pain of the right hypochondrium, which was resolv'd by bilious dejections: the other paroxysms, which were slighter, generally succeeded to the sensation of a kind of smoke, ascending up to the head from the hypochondria, the fullness of which parts was continually troublesome to the patient, and was certainly encreas'd from the ingesta, but especially from liquids. And this being the state of the case, and as the pain of the head, and all the marks of its being affected of itself, were absent, the senior physicians, who

(*r*) Apud Cael. Aurelian. Chronic. L. 2. c.I.

had not wish'd for me to be their companion, in the cure of this refractory disorder, less than the patient himself, made no scruple to pronounce, that it arose from the irritation of the hypochondria. And indeed, as you have it also in this section of the Sepulchretum (*m*), there is extant in Galen a history of a certain grammarian, "who, having abstain'd too long from food, became epileptic, from no other cause than bile." And examples are very common of adults (*n*), not only of children (*o*), who have been troubl'd with epilepsies, from worms harbour'd in the intestines. And to this purpose also is that observation of Spigellius (*p*), on a whelp thus kill'd by worms; not very unlike to which, is that formerly written by me to Vallisneri, and by him publish'd (*q*). And you know that this disorder often arises, also, from other viscera of the belly being diseas'd, which the section, that I have already quoted, confirms (*r*).

But although that kind of cure was applied to my fellow-citizen Poggi, with my assent, which was proper to open, cleanse, and relax, the hypochondria, yet, nevertheless, the accessions still return'd frequently; so that we now began to fear, lest the head itself had also contracted the injury, especially as, upon a very quick turn of the head, the epileptic insults recurr'd, and left a sense of weight with stupidness in the head; and frequently some blood came, together with the mucus, from the nose. Wherefore, as in the beginning, they had already drawn blood once and again from the arm, nor had omitted to give such things as are generally of use to the head, I persuaded them to let blood be taken away from those veins, which lie about the anus also; and that several things should be given internally, which are recommended as extremely proper against this disease, by the most excellent physicians. These remedies, however, were of no advantage; but the bleeding, whether it reliev'd the head, or rather those viscera which are serv'd with blood by the vena portarum, was so far of advantage, that for a short time the paroxysms were quiet. When, therefore, they return'd again more frequently, it was of use to make the patient sit up, sometimes to rub the lower limbs, and sometimes to tie them alternately with bandages thrown round about, and sometimes to fix cupping-glasses without scarification, and presently to vex the patient by taking them off; for thus he seemed to have a longer intermission from his paroxysms. And I was even assur'd, that when they sometimes attack'd him much more often, the spirit of salt ammoniac, applied to the nostrils, had driven them away as they were coming on; or, even when they were already, in a manner begun, had suppress'd them, although the patient was entirely without the power of smelling. They were, for the most part, very short, but by no means slight. For distortions of the eyes, agitations of the limbs, and a suspension of all the senses, always accompanied the

(*m*) Sect. 12. in schol. ad. obs. 19.
(*n*) Ibid. schol. ad obs. 41. (*o*) Obs. ead. § 2. & schol. ad obs. 15. in additam.
(*p*) Ibid. obs. 41. § 1. (*q*) Consideraz. in. a la gener. de'Vermi.
(*r*) Obs. 39. cum schol.

attack: oftentimes there was a strangulation, and that sometimes join'd together with a stertor; and even, now and then, an involuntary efflux of urine attended. But he was exceedingly bad that day on which the solstice happen'd, and in like manner, that on which the eclipse of the sun happen'd.

And though you may suppose this might be by chance, yet you cannot suppose it merely accidental, that when the quantity of urine was either naturally or artificially encreas'd (*s*), the epileptic paroxysms not only became not slighter, but were even very frequently exasperated. For we were oblig'd to have regard to this excretion sometimes, when a sudden difficulty of breathing rous'd the patient, as he was beginning to sleep, and compell'd him to sit up; which symptom, doubtless, gave us some suspicion of a dropsy of the thorax; and the more so, because the patient told us, that his right leg had, for a long time past, been accustom'd to swell a little with water, and that even then, which, when he told us, we examin'd into, the swelling was ascending up the thigh. But it was easy to encrease the quantity of urine, by obvious and innocent remedies, and therefore to diminish the tumour, and that suspicion, which was afterwards entirely remov'd; but not so the force of the attacks, which, from the encreas'd afflux of urine, and that of itself, sometimes opaque, and blackish, was so far from being weaken'd, or diminish'd, that even on the contrary, as I said above, they grew stronger and stronger. When these things, and others, which for the sake of my promis'd brevity I pass over, were of no effect against the inroads of this disease, and even such as had been sometimes useful to retard or suppress them, as I said above, were now of no advantage, as they did not continue to afford these effects; there was one thing, however, which was constantly of service; I mean opium, given at the beginning of the night, in quantity of half a grain. For the frequency and force of the insults, and added to these also, obstinate watchings, so weaken'd the patient in other respects, that we were under a necessity of gaining a truce by some means or other. And by this means, good nights, and easy sleeps, were procur'd to the patient: and so far was his head from being made heavy, or dull, by the use of this medicine, that even the heaviness and dullness, left behind by the daily attacks, were by this means taken away; which otherwise, that is, when the use of the opium was intermitted, continu'd, while the former restlessness and watchings also oppressed him. And, indeed, after he had pass'd a night of that kind, which was far more troublesome than the rest, when to the greatest rarity of the pulse, which I mention'd in the beginning, an inequality had suddenly been added, so that very often they were perceiv'd to be even much more rare, then not more so, than usual, and presently much rarer again; which symptom made us the more uneasy, because the disease, at that time, was wont, first of all, entirely to obscure the pulse, and then immediately to begin its attack; and when we had tried all the remedies, recom-

(*s*) Vid. infra. n. 11.

mended to dissolve, and promote, the circulation of the blood, in vain; upon giving the opium again, the quiet nights again return'd, and diminish'd that inequality of the pulse: and, by the continu'd use of opium every night, it was entirely remov'd, and even the former rarity was diminish'd.

But, perhaps, you will suspect, whether the rarity of the pulse be, in fact, a very uncommon symptom, to remain after an epilepsy, in hypochondriac patients, when you shall have compar'd this observation of mine with that of the celebrated Gerbezius (*t*) which describes the pulse of a strong hypochondriac man, "who was now and then subject to slight epileptic paroxysms," even when he was in health, "as being so very slow, that before the subsequent pulsation follow'd that which went before, three pulsations would certainly have pass'd in another healthy person." But to return to my subject; after that no fit had now returned for thirteen days, and the use of opium was intermitted, the first night indeed was not bad; but the following ones, by reason of the continual watching, and restlessness, and at length by reason of that difficulty of breathing, which I spoke of above, were exceedingly troublesome; so that we were oblig'd to have recourse again to opium, in order to procure quiet nights, which nothing but opium would procure. And, to comprehend all in a few words; that the attacks of the disease, from being very frequent, as they had happen'd every day, in the month of June, had been so far reduc'd in their number, that but one happen'd in July, one in August, nor more in September, and after that none in the two next months at least, and upwards, till I departed to teach medicine publicly, we judg'd was owing to the use of opium, given opportunely, sometimes every night, sometimes every other night, and at length at the intervals of many nights. For by that medicine we were able to appease the tumultuary motions, which arose, and frequently by a very manifest sensation, from the hypochondria, to the thorax, and head; and by this means procure a truce, both for nature and art; and this gave us sufficient time to cleanse and confirm the hypochondriac viscera, which we had determined to do, in the beginning, but in vain attempted, among those first continual tumults, with which the patient was harrass'd: and from these viscera alone, and not from water being redundant in the brain, that these sudden commotions arose, this history, or I am much deceiv'd, indeed, evidently shews.

. . . .

(*t*) Eph. N. C. Cent. 7. in Append.

LETTER THE TWENTY-THIRD

TREATS OF PALPITATION AND PAIN OF THE HEART

[Description of Calcareous Stenosis of the Aortic Valve with Regurgitation]

. . . .

8. A woman, a little younger than that last describ'd, complain'd, in the same hospital, of a palpitation of the heart sometimes, but always of a difficulty in her breath, which she could not draw but with her neck erect; and still more of so great a streightness and anxiety at her heart, that very often she seem'd just at the point of death. Some suppos'd her to labour under a dropsy of the pericardium. Her pulse never was intermitting; but her veins were large. She died at the time that the genital parts of a woman were wanted to finish the public demonstrations of the year 1731, a little before the middle of March.

The thorax and belly being open'd, some quantity of water was found in both cavities; but there was no dropsy of the pericardium. The valves of the aorta were indurated, and one of them even bony. The trunk of the artery itself shew'd, up and down on its internal surface, either something bony, or something verging to the nature of a bone; so that the part of the artery which went through the belly, and which I dissected after demonstration of the genital parts, was in the same state. Nor did I find it bony only at the side of the inferior mesenteric artery, and in other places, but even at the very division of it into the iliacs: and in several places it was unequal, and here and there of a whitish colour, as it generally is when it begins to become bony.

9. It certainly cannot be denied, that the aorta, in the state I have describ'd it, must resist the blood, as it is driven by the heart, and, for that reason, be able to create a palpitation, a difficulty of breathing, and that sense of streightness with which the woman was tormented. But at the same time it is necessary to declare, why, out of so great a number of persons in whom there was an aorta of this kind, as I have already written to you, and shall write hereafter, many of them, certainly, did not labour under these disorders at all, or, at least, not so vehemently. And in order to do this, other circumstances, without doubt, must be added to the disorder of the aorta, which did exist in this woman, and did not exist in the others; as, for instance, a different fault in the organs, or a different constitution of the blood, different quantity, and other things of a similar kind besides, that we may not seem to be always bringing in the more exquisite sense of the nerves, and convulsions. So in an observation of Verdriesius, already pointed out (*m*), after a violent palpitation of the heart, and a very great asthma, the aorta was found to be internally bony near the heart; but the heart itself was found to be of a stupendous magnitude, hard, and tumid. So in another person, who having been long afflicted with various

(*m*) Epist. 18. n. 4.

disorders, had been, in the beginning of them, very much subject to a palpitation of the heart, the celebrated Plancus (*n*) not only found the aorta in many places become bony, but also both the coronaries of the heart, and the heart itself very large, particularly its right auricle, which was the largest and strongest of all: and from hence you may easily perceive, that, in consequence of this one disorder, the heart might be more vehemently irritated by the blood being more strongly impell'd into the subjected ventricle; and may the less wonder, if in the observation of Grassius the younger, spoken of already in this work (*o*), it shall perhaps appear, that nothing else could be the cause of the palpitation, but the right auricle being enlarg'd to the double of its usual capacity. Finally, not to detain you too long, in a woman of an illustrious family, whose palpitation of the heart was so great, and so constant, as to be heard by those who stood near her, and be discern'd by those who were at some distance, the celebrated Cohausen (*p*) not only saw the aorta entirely callous; but he even saw in the heart itself, not to mention the lungs, scirrhi, and the blood viscid and mucous.

Wherefore, in the woman, also, spoken of by me, besides the aorta being here and there bony, or inclining to a bony state, the valves of it are also to be attended to. For as one of these was bony, and the others indurated, so being, of consequence, less yielding to the blood, they might encrease the obstacles to its exit, and, on the other hand, not sufficiently prevent its return, when, soon after, repuls'd by the contraction of the great artery; so that, as some portion of it return'd into the left ventricle of the heart, when this ventricle ought to receive the blood that was coming in from the lungs, it would necessarily happen, that the returning portion, as well as the portion which had not been extruded just before, must occupy some part of that space, which, from the design of nature, was entirely due to the blood that was coming in from the lungs. Which circumstance, finally, could not but overload both the lungs and the heart, and compel the latter to throw out, every now and then, with a great impetus, the blood that stagnated in it.

And these things, which reason seems to lead us to, are confirm'd by more than one observation of the anatomists. Thus Vieussens (*q*), in a man and a matron, both of whom had been long troubl'd with a palpitation of the heart, and incapacity of lying down with the head low, join'd with an inequality of the pulse, relates, that the aorta and its valves were found to be bony in the matron; and in the man, that the aorta was very hard, and in a manner cartilaginous; and the valves not only bony, but also with their edges cloven asunder, and the same really become stony; I say really, lest you should, perhaps, imagine, that what was bony should have been taken for being stony in the heart, as it has happen'd sometimes in other

(*n*) Epist. de Monstr. (*o*) Epist. 18. n. 4. (*p*) Commerc. Litter. A. 1743. Hebd. 21. n. 4.

(*q*) Traité du Coeur, ch. 16.

places. For besides those which will be mention'd below, you will read of similar cases, here, in the Sepulchretum, in observations which are pretty ancient; as that of Gregorius Horstius the elder (*r*), who found "a calculus concreted from tartar adhering to the membranous substance of the valves" of the right ventricle of the heart; and that of Jo. Georgius Greiselius (*s*), who saw one of those valves of the aorta which we are speaking of "half-consum'd, and lost, and that part where it adher'd to the artery even friable into a kind of sand"; and there was "a kind of white particle, like the nail of a little finger," which was the part of the valve that the blood had lately torn away; the heart being in both of them, who died after a palpitation, very much enlarg'd, in the same manner as the left ventricle had been in that man of Vieussens.

. . . .

LETTER THE TWENTY-FOURTH

TREATS OF PRETERNATURAL PULSES

[Description of Coronary Sclerosis]

. . . .

16. In an old man, who was of a lean habit, and whom I dissected in the month of December of the year 1743, the pulse had been weak and small, but not intermitting, when, on account of an *incarcerated* hernia, as it is call'd, he was brought into the hospital at Padua. And notwithstanding it was out of my power certainly to inform myself, whether the pulse had been in that state before this disorder came on, or whether it was rather brought on by this disease, join'd with an inflammation of the intestines, to such a degree, that a speedy death prevented any method of cure being attempted; yet the appearances which I observ'd in many parts of the body, and particularly in the heart itself, and demonstrated to a very crowded circle of students, are of such a nature, that I cannot judge them to be unworthy of being communicated to you.

As I examin'd the external surface of the heart, the left coronary artery appear'd to have been chang'd into a bony canal, from its very origin to the extent of many fingers breadth, where it embraces the greater part of the basis. And part of that very long branch, also, which it sends down upon the anterior surface of the heart, was already become bony to so great a space, as could be cover'd by three fingers plac'd transversely. For which reasons, a passage was open'd on both sides, not through a membranous canal, or one which was made somewhat hard, here and there, by disjoin'd bony lamellae, but through a continued bony tube, which for hardness might with justice have been compar'd with any other hard bone, except that in some places it was less hard; though those were very small, and inconsiderable, and resembl'd the transverse lines form'd by the

(*r*) Obs. 35. (*s*) Obs. 13.

knots of a slender reed. The heart then being open'd, and some polypous concretions being taken away, although I saw the tubercles of the valves of the great artery much harder than usual, and almost bony; yet I found nothing bony either in them, or in any other valves, or in that artery near the heart. But at some interval from the heart, and at the origins of the upper arteries, and from thence downwards quite to the divisions into the iliacs, the internal surface of the aorta was frequently unequal on account of very hard bony laminae, many of which equall'd in bigness the nail of a man's thumb: yet I found the thin internal membrane, by which all these ossifications were cover'd, to be hurt only in one place, a thickish kind of humour showing itself there: in regard to which, and the seat itself of these laminae, I shall have a more convenient opportunity of speaking hereafter (*x*), and telling you what I observ'd in this man, and in others. And bony scales were not wanting, either at the division into the subclavian and carotid arteries, on the right side, or in the iliacs, nor yet in the splenic in particular, in which they were found very thick, quite to the spleen. Nevertheless, within the cranium, and in like manner, both in the upper limbs, and in the lower limbs, I observ'd nothing bony in the arteries; although this class of vessels was, in the limbs, more firm and hard than usual, and perhaps even somewhat wider than they generally are: and while I was cutting into these arteries, I saw that the blood which remain'd in the crural vessels was not fluid indeed, yet not polypous.

. . . .

LETTER THE TWENTY-SIXTH

TREATS OF SUDDEN DEATH, FROM A DISORDER OF THE SANGUIFEROUS VESSELS, ESPECIALLY THOSE THAT LIE IN THE THORAX

[Description of Aneurysm of the Aorta]

. . . .

9. A man who had been too much given to the exercise of tennis and the abuse of wine, was, in consequence of both these irregularities, seiz'd with a pain of the right arm, and soon after of the left, join'd with a fever. After these there appear'd a tumour on the upper part of the sternum, like a large boil: by which appearance some vulgar surgeons being deceiv'd, and either not having at all observ'd, or having neglected, the pulsation, applied such things as are generally us'd to bring these tumours to suppuration; and these applications were of the most violent kind. As the tumour still encreas'd, others applied emollient medicines, from which it seem'd to them to be diminish'd; that is, from the fibres being rubb'd with ointments and relax'd; whereas they had been before greatly irritated by the applications. But as this circumstance related rather

(*x*) Epist. 27. n. 22.

to the common integuments, than to the tumour itself, or to the coats that were proper thereto, it not only soon recover'd its former magnitude, but even was, plainly, seen to encrease every day. Wherefore, when the patient came into the Hospital of Incurables, at Bologna, which was, I suppose, in the year 1704, it was equal in size to a quince; and what was much worse, it began to exsude blood in one place; so that the man himself was very near having broken through the skin (this being reduc'd to the utmost thinness in that part, and he being quite ignorant of the danger which was at hand) when he began to pull off the bandages, for the sake of showing his disorder. But this circumstance being observ'd, he was prevented going on, and order'd to keep himself still, and to think seriously and piously of his departure from this mortal life, which was very near at hand, and inevitable. And this really happen'd on the day following, from the vast profusion of blood that had been foretold, though not so soon expected by the patient. Nevertheless, he had the presence of mind, immediately as he felt the blood gushing forth, not only to commend himself to God, but to take up with his own hands a bason that lay at his bed-side; and, as if he had been receiving the blood of another person, put it beneath the gaping tumour, while the attendants immediately ran to him as fast as possible, in whose arms he soon after expired.

In examining the body before I dissected it, I saw that there was no longer any tumour, inasmuch as it had subsided after the blood, by which it had been rais'd up externally, had been discharg'd. The skin was there broken through, and the parts that lie beneath it with an aperture, which admitted two fingers at once. The membrana adioposa of the thorax discharged a water during the time of dissection, with which some vessels were also turgid, that were prominent, here and there, upon the surface of the skin in the feet and the legs. In both the cavities of the thorax, also, was a great quantity of water, of a yellowish colour. And there was a large aneurism, into which the anterior part of the curvature of the aorta itself being expanded, had partly consum'd the upper part of the sternum, the extremities of the clavicles, which lie upon it and the neighboring ribs, and partly had made them diseas'd, by bringing on a caries. And where the bones had been consum'd or affected with the caries, there not the least traces of the coats of the artery remain'd: to which, in other places, a thick substance everywhere adher'd internally, resembling a dry and lurid kind of flesh, distinguish'd with some whitish points; and this substance you might easily divide into many membranes, as it were, one lying upon another, quite different in their nature from those coats to which they adher'd, as they were evidently polypous. And these things being accurately attended to, nothing occur'd besides that was worthy of remark.

1761

LEOPOLD AUENBRUGGER

ON PERCUSSION

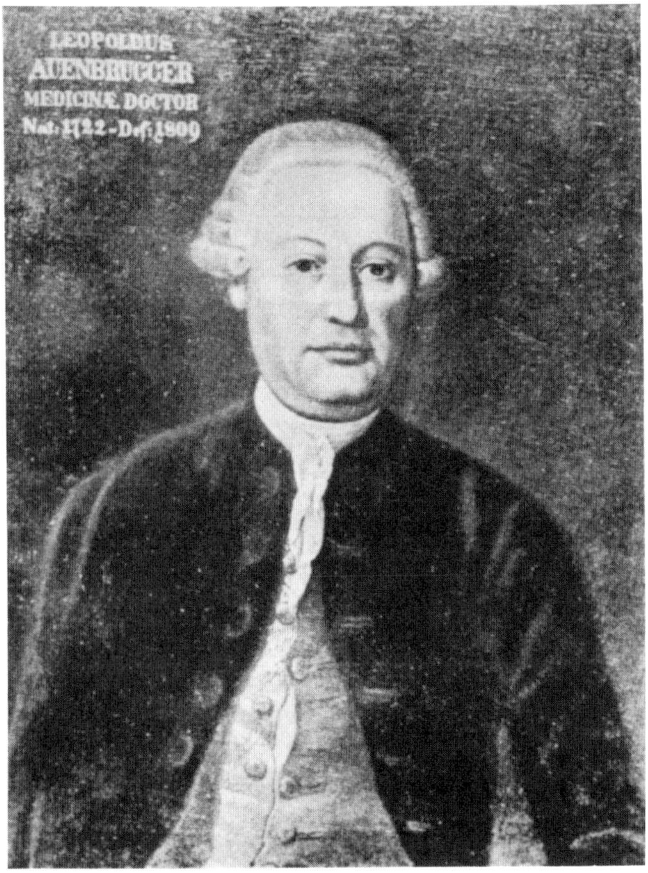

LEOPOLD AUENBRUGGER

Painted in 1770 by an unknown artist; restored by Kurz von Goldenstein

(Courtesy Annals of Medical History.)

JOSEPH LEOPOLD AUENBRUGGER

(1722-1809)

[*Durdles:*] *'Now, lookee here. You pitch your note, don't you, Mr. Jasper?'*

[*Mr. Jasper:*] *'Yes.'*

[*Durdles:*] *'So I sound for mine. I take my hammer, and I tap . . . I tap, tap, tap. Solid! I go on tapping. Solid still! Tap again. Holloa! Hollow! Tap again, persevering. Solid in hollow! Tap, tap, tap, to try it better. Solid in hollow; and inside solid, hollow again! There you are! Old 'un crumbled away in stone coffin, in vault!'*

—From *The Mystery of Edwin Drood,* by Charles Dickens.

PERCUSSION as a means of testing whether walls were solid or whether they covered hiding places, whether barrels were empty or full and for many other purposes, must have been in use since the beginnings of civilization. It is surprising, therefore, that no one before Auenbrugger seems to have thought of using percussion of the human body as a means of diagnosis.

Joseph Leopold Auenbrugger was born at Gratz in Stryria, Austria. His father was an innkeeper, and the younger Auenbrugger himself was an accomplished musician.[1] These two facts had no little significance in his development of percussion. The technic he probably learned from tapping wine barrels in his father's inn and his good musical ear helped him greatly in the interpretation of sounds.

In due course Auenbrugger studied medicine at the University of Vienna, where he was the pupil of van Swieten who at an earlier date had been a student of Boerhaave at Leyden. Van Swieten had been called from Holland to the Austrian capital by the Empress Maria Theresa. He became court physician and because of his royal backing he was able to found the great medical school at Vienna.

From 1751 to 1762 Auenbrugger was connected with the Spanish Hospital at Vienna, first as assistant, later as physician. In 1754 he first noted the difference in sounds produced by striking the wall of the chest in various places. Not until he had pursued the line of clinical research this opened up to him for seven years did he publish his results and observations. The 95-page book, ''Inventum novum ex percussione thoracis humani ut signo abstrusos interni pectoris morbos detegendi,'' was published in Vienna in 1761, the same year that brought forth Morgagni's ''De sedibus et causis morborum per anatomen indagatis libri quinque.''

After describing the sound produced by striking the chest of a healthy person in different regions, Auenbrugger gave a detailed account of his method of practicing percussion. Had he but applied his ear as well as his hand he would have anticipated Laënnec. But he came near to the discovery of auscultation when, under part three of his Eleventh Observation in ''On percussion of the chest,'' he wrote: ''If at this time, while the patient is coughing and spitting, the palm of the

[1]He wrote the libretto for Antonio Salieri's *Der Rauchfangkehrer, oder die unentbehrlichen Verrater ihrer Herrschaften aus Eigennutz,* which was presented at Vienna in 1781. This libretto attracted the attention of the Empress Maria Theresa. She asked him to write another, but Auenbrugger replied that he had something better to do than to write operas.

hand be placed over the site of the vomica, i.e., over the place where its existence had been detected by percussion—the noise of fluid within the chest will be sufficiently manifest.''

It is of interest to notice, especially, the diseases which he was able to detect merely by means of the preternatural sounds heard through percussion, diseases whose existence he was later able to confirm by studies at necropsy. These diseases included ''scirrhus'' of the lungs, vomica, empyema, pleural effusion, dropsy of the pericardium, extravasation of blood into the cavity of the pleura or pericardium, and aneurysm of the heart.

Auenbrugger's discovery was ignored by those occupying the high places of medicine of his day. Even his own teacher, Baron van Swieten, for whom Auenbrugger had the highest respect, was not impressed by the remarkable new aid to diagnosis. The only well-known physicians in good standing who appreciated Auenbrugger's work at that time were Dr. Stoll of Vienna, who both used and taught percussion from 1776 to 1784, and Charles G. Ludwig of Leipzig. The ''Inventum novum'' was translated into French by Rozière of Montpellier in 1770. And although the book went through two French editions it seems to have been practically unknown until the clinician Jean-Nicholas Corvisart, noted teacher[2] and physician to Napoleon Bonaparte, revived the discovery.

It is said that Corvisart had never heard of Auenbrugger and his ''Inventum novum'' until he read of it in the works of Stoll. From that time on he practiced percussion with perseverance on living subjects as well as cadavers. After twenty years of experience he translated Auenbrugger's work and added his own voluminous commentaries to it in 1808, only a year before Auenbrugger's death. Corvisart, in his 440-page translation, gave full credit to Auenbrugger as the discoverer of percussion, but Corvisart's renown at home and abroad quickly placed the discovery of Auenbrugger on a high pinnacle. In his preface, Corvisart said: ''I declare from experience, that this sign of which I treat is one of the greatest importance, not only in detecting disease, but also in curing it, and therefore merits first place after exploration of the pulse and respiration.'' (Quoted from Otis.)

Notwithstanding the neglect of Auenbrugger's sign during his own lifetime, it cannot be said that he was not appreciated. He had a large practice, was noted for his philanthropy, had a genuine devotion to the science and the art of medicine, and had a high regard for the poor as well as the rich.

His life at home was happy. He had fallen in love with Marianna von Priestersberg when he was a student, and he married her in 1754. They had two children, both daughters, one of whom was a remarkable pianist, and the other of whom was noted for her beauty and wit.

As has been mentioned, Auenbrugger had early found favor with the Empress Maria Theresa, and the Emperor Joseph raised him to noble rank in 1784, probably not because of his discovery but in recognition of his skill as a physician and his services to the public.

In the latter part of his life Auenbrugger lost the sight of one eye, but the other was so good that he could tell time by the town clock, which was a considerable distance from his window. Two years before his own death his beloved wife, Marianna, died. (They had celebrated their golden wedding anniversary in 1804.) From that time onward Auenbrugger took little interest in life, remained most of the time in his study and enjoyed only the company of his granddaughters. His death, the result of a cold, occurred in 1809. He was in his eighty-seventh year.

---

[2]Laënnec was one of his pupils.

LEOPOLDI AUENBRUGGER

MEDICINÆ DOCTORIS
IN CÆSAREO REGIO NOSOCOMIO NATIONUM
HISPANICO MEDICI ORDINARII.

INVENTUM NOVUM

EX

PERCUSSIONE THORACIS HUMANI
UT SIGNO

ABSTRUSOS INTERNI
PECTORIS MORBOS
DETEGENDI.

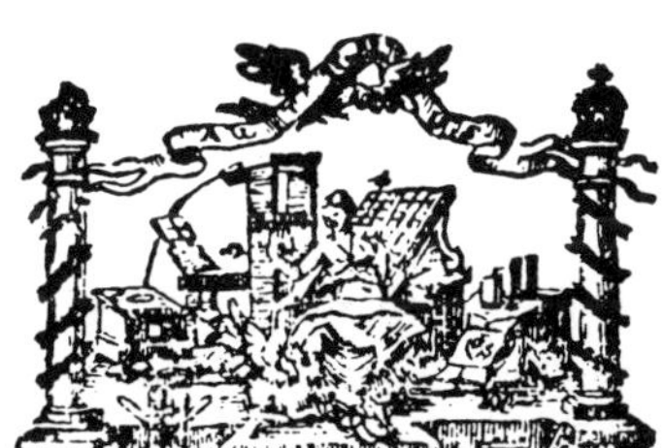

VINDOBONÆ,

TYPIS JOANNIS THOMÆ TRATTNER, CÆS. REG. MAJEST. AULÆ TYPOGRAPHI.

MDCCLXI.

ON PERCUSSION OF THE CHEST*

By

LEOPOLD AUENBRUGGER

PREFACE

I HERE present the Reader with a new sign which I have discovered for detecting diseases of the chest. This consists in the Percussion of the human thorax, whereby, according to the character of the particular sounds thence elicited, an opinion is formed of the internal state of that cavity. In making public my discoveries respecting this matter, I have been actuated neither by an itch for writing, nor a fondness for speculation, but by the desire of submitting to my brethren the fruits of seven years' observation and reflexion. In doing so, I have not been unconscious of the dangers I must encounter; since it has always been the fate of those who have illustrated or improved the arts and sciences by their discoveries, to be beset by envy, malice, hatred, detraction and calumny.

This the common lot, I have chosen to undergo; but with the determination of refusing to every one who is actuated by such motives as these, all explanation of my doctrines. What I have written I have proved again and again, by the testimony of my own senses, and amid laborious and tedious exertions—still guarding, on all occasions, against the seductive influence of self-love.

And here, lest any one should imagine that this new sign has been thoroughly investigated, even as far as regards the diseases noticed in my Treatise, I think it necessary candidly to confess, that there still remain many defects to be remedied—and which I expect will be remedied—by careful observation and experience. Perhaps, also, the same observation and experience may lead to the discovery of other truths, in these or other diseases, of like value in the diagnosis, prognosis and cure of thoracic affections. Owing to this acknowledged imperfection, it will be seen, that, in my difficulties, I have had recourse to the Commentaries of the most illustrious Baron Van Swieten, as containing every thing which can be desired by the faithful observer of the nature; by which means I have not only avoided the vice of tedious and prolix writing, but have, at the same time possessed myself of the firmest basis whereon to raise, most securely

Inventum novum ex percussione thoracis humani, ut signo abstrusos interni pectoris morbos detegendi, Vienna, 1761. Translated by John Forbes, M.D., London, 1824. Reprinted from Sigerist, H. E.: Bull. Inst. Hist. Med. **4**: 379-403, 1936.

and creditably, the rudiments of my discovery. In submitting this to the public, I doubt not that I shall be considered, by all those who can justly appreciate medical science, as having thereby rendered a grateful service to our art, inasmuch as it must be allowed to throw no small degree of light upon the obscurer diseases of the chest, of which a more perfect knowledge has hitherto been much wanted.

In drawing up my little work I have omitted many things that were doubtful, and not sufficiently digested; to the due perfection of which it will be my endeavour henceforth to apply myself. To conclude, I have not been ambitious of ornament in my mode or style of writing, being contented if I shall be understood.

December 31, 1760.

FIRST OBSERVATION

OF THE NATURAL SOUND OF THE CHEST, AND ITS CHARACTER IN DIFFERENT PARTS

I

The thorax of a healthy person sounds, when struck.

Scholium. I deem it unnecessary to give in this place, any description of the thorax. I think it sufficient to say, that by this term I mean that cavity bounded above by the neck and clavicles, and below by the diaphragm: in the sound state, the viscera it contains are fitted for their respective uses.

II

The sound thus elicited (I) from the healthy chest, resembles the stifled sound of a drum covered with a thick woollen cloth or other envelope.

III

This sound is perceptible on different parts of the chest in the following manner:

1. On the right side anteriorly it is observed from the clavicle to the sixth true rib; laterally, from the axilla to the seventh rib; and posteriorly, from the scapula to the second and third false ribs.

2. The left side yields this sound from the clavicle to the fourth true rib, anteriorly; and on the back and laterally, in the same extent as the other side: over the space occupied by the heart the sound loses part of its usual clearness, and becomes dull.

3. The whole sternum yields as distinct a sound as the sides of the chest, except in the cardiac region where it is somewhat duller.

4. The same sound is perceptible over that part of the spinal column which contributes to form the chest.

Scholium. The sound is more distinct in the lean, and proportionably duller in the robust; in very fat persons it is almost lost. The most sonorous region is from the clavicle to the fourth rib anteriorly; lower down, the mammae and pectoral muscles deaden the sound. Sometimes, owing to the presence of muscle, the sound is dull beneath the axilla. In the scapular regions on the back, owing to the obstacle afforded by the bones and thick muscles there, it is also less distinct. Sometimes, but rarely, it exists over the third false rib—owing, I conceive, to a very unwanted length of the thoracic cavity.

SECOND OBSERVATION
OF THE METHOD OF PERCUSSION

IV

The thorax ought to be struck, slowly and gently, with the points of the fingers, brought close together and at the same time extended.

Scholium. Robust and fat subjects require a stronger percussion; such, indeed, as to elicit a degree of sound equal to that produced, by a slight percussion, in a lean subject.

V

During percussion the shirt is to be drawn tight over the chest, or the hand of the operator covered with a glove made of unpolished leather.

Scholium. If the naked chest is struck by the naked hand, the contact of the polished surfaces produces a kind of noise which alters or obscures the natural character of the sound.

VI

During the application of percussion the patient is first to go on breathing in the natural manner, and then is to hold the breath after a full inspiration. The difference of sound during inspiration, expiration, and the retention of the breath, is important in fixing our diagnosis.

VII

While undergoing percussion on the fore parts of the chest, the patient is to hold his head erect, and the shoulders are to be thrown back; in order that the chest may protrude, and the skin and muscles be drawn tight over it: a clear sound is thus obtained.

VIII

While we are striking the lateral parts of the chest, the patient is to hold his arms across his head; as, thereby, the thoracic parietes are made more tense, and a clearer sound obtained.

IX

When operating on the back, you are to cause the patient to bend forwards, and draw his shoulders towards the anterior parts of the chest, so as to render the dorsal region rounded; and for the same reasons, as stated in VIII.

Scholium. Any healthy person may make experience of percussion in his own person or that of other sound subjects; and will thus be convinced from the variety of the sounds obtained, that this sign is not to be dispised in forming a diagnosis.

THIRD OBSERVATION
OF THE PRETERNATURAL OR MORBID SOUND OF THE CHEST, AND ITS GENERAL IMPORT

X and Scholium

To be able justly to appreciate the value of the various sounds elicited from the chest in cases of disease, it is necessary to have learned by experience on many subjects, the modification of sound, general or partial, produced by the habit of body, natural conformation as to the scapulae, mammae, the heart, the capacity of the thorax, the degree of fleshiness, fatness, etc., etc.; inasmuch, as these various circumstances modify the sound very considerably.

XI

If, then, a distinct sound, equal on both sides, and commensurate to the degree of percussion, is not obtained from the sonorous regions above mentioned, a morbid condition of some of the parts within the chest is indicated.

Scholium. On this truth a general rule is founded, and from this certain predictions can be deduced, as will be shown in order. For I have learned from much experience that diseases of the worst description may exist within the chest, unmarked by any symptoms, and undiscoverable by any other means than percussion alone.

A clear and equal sound elicited from both sides of the chest indicates that the air cells of the lungs are free, and uncompressed either by a solid or liquid body. (Exceptions to this rule will be mentioned in their place.)

XII and XIII

If a sonorous part of the chest, struck with the same intensity, yields a sound duller than natural, disease exists in that part.

XIV

If a sonorous region of the chest appears, on percussion, entirely destitute of the natural sound—that is, if it yields only a sound like that of a fleshy limb when struck,—disease exists in that region.

Scholium. The nature of the indications above pointed out, will be understood by any one who attends to the difference of sound elicited by percussion of the chest, and of the thigh, in his own person

XV

The superficial extent of this unnatural sound (XIV) in a sonorous region, is commensurate with the extent of the morbid affection.

XVI

If a place, naturally sonorous, and now sounding only as a piece of flesh when struck, still retains the same sound (on percussion) when the breath is held after a deep inspiration,—we are to conclude that the disease extends deep into the cavity of the chest.

XVII

If the same results (XVI) are obtained both before and behind, on points precisely opposite, we are to conclude that the disease occupies the whole diameter of the chest.

Scholium. These varying results depend on the greater or less diminution of the volume of air usually contained in the thorax (lungs); and the cause which occasions this diminution, whether solid or liquid, produces analogous results to those obtained by striking a cask, for example, in different degrees of emptiness or fulness: the diminution of sound being proportioned to the diminution of the volume of air contained in it.

FOURTH OBSERVATION
OF THE DISEASES IN GENERAL IN WHICH THE MORBID SOUND OF THE CHEST IS OBSERVED

XVIII

The preternatural or morbid sound occurs in acute and chronic diseases; it always accompanies a copious effusion of fluid in the thoracic cavity.

Scholium. It must be admitted that whatever diminishes the volume of air within the chest, diminishes the natural sound of that cavity; but we know from the nature, the causes, and the effects, of acute and chronic diseases of the chest, that such a result is possible in these cases; and the fact is finally demonstrated by examinations after death. The effect of effused fluids in producing the morbid sound, is at once proved by the injection of water into the thorax of a dead body; in which case it will be found that the sound elicited by percussion, will be obscure over the portion of the cavity occupied by the injected liquid.

FIFTH OBSERVATION
OF ACUTE DISEASES IN WHICH THE CHEST YIELDS THE MORBID SOUND

XIX

The morbid sound which is observed in acute diseases, occurs during their progress, or at their termination.

Scholium. This consideration ought to lead all medical men to use percussion in acute diseases; as they will thereby be enabled to form a more correct judgment, which in such cases is always a matter of difficulty. It has often occurred to me to see cases of acute diseases, apparently over, and imposing on the physician under the mask of intermittent or remittent fevers, and which have eventually ended in a fatal vomica or fatal schirrus of the lungs.

XX

The preternatural sound which is perceived during the course of acute diseases of the chest, occurs most frequently in inflammatory affections.

Scholium. The reason of this observation (XX) will be obvious to any one acquainted with the nature of inflammation. The preternatural sound may also be observed sometimes in epidemic exanthematous diseases, previously to the eruption;—as was the case in the petechial epidemic of 1757, 1758, 1759, and in the miliary epidemic of the present year (1760). In the latter instance, I observed that the preternatural sound, when once present, continued to the termination of the eruption.

XXI

The morbid sound which occurs towards the termination of acute diseases, is observed, when the excretion of morbid matter is not adequate to the severity of the affection.

XXII

The morbid sound occurring in inflammatory diseases is commonly observable on the fourth day; it rarely precedes, but often follows this period.

Scholium. This sign occurs rarely on the third, and very often on the fourth, fifth, and seventh day—but never later. It is observed in those inflammatory affections of the pleura or lungs, or both, which are accompanied by a humid cough; but not in those attended by a dry cough,—such (e.g.) as the dry pleurisy, and inflammation of the mediastinum, pericardium, and heart. At least in these latter affections, the sound is not observed, until such time as they verge towards a fatal termination, or have degenerated into obvious abscesses or vomicae.

XXIII

The morbid sound increases, from the time of its appearance, according to the nature, severity, and duration of the disease; it diminishes proportionably to the nature, duration, and copiousness of the excretions.

Scholium. The progressive augmentation of the preternatural sound depends on the gradual deposition of the morbific matter, which I have often found in such quantity as to occupy the inferior two-thirds of the affected side.

XXIV

The disease in which the preternatural sound is once present, either proves fatal [on a decretory day, reckoning from its origin]; passes off with due excretion; or terminates in other affections.

XXV

The following corollaries are the result of my observation of inflammatory diseases of the chest, studied under the sign of morbid resonance:

1. The duller the sound, and the more nearly approaching that of a fleshy limb stricken, the more severe is the disease.

2. The more extensive the space over which the morbid sound is perceived, the more certain is the danger from the disease.

3. The disease is more dangerous on the left than on the right side.

4. The existence of the morbid sound on the superior and anterior part of the chest (i.e. from clavicle to the fourth rib) indicates less danger, than on the inferior parts of the chest.

5. The want of the natural sound behind, indicates more danger than it does on the anterior and superior part of the chest.

6. The total destitution of sound over one whole side, is generally (passim) a fatal sign.

7. The absence of sound along the course of the sternum is a fatal sign.

8. The entire absence of the natural sound over a large space in the region of the heart, is a fatal sign.

Scholium. I have sometimes observed that the fatal prognostics given in the corollaries 6 and 7, were not verified when the matter made its way outwards, or abscesses formed in parts less essential to life. And this natural process has been often happily imitaded by the ancients, by cauterising or otherwise incising, the affected parts.

SIXTH OBSERVATION

OF CHRONIC DISEASES IN WHICH THE PRETERNATURAL SOUND IS OBSERVED

XXVI

The preternatural sound observed in chronic diseases is owing either to (1) some hidden condition of the organs, which disorders them with a slow progress and finally destroys them; or exists (2) when certain obvious causes have induced a slow disorganisation of the same.

Scholium. These are the general sources of chronic diseases of the chest; and from whichever of the two classes of causes these arise; the morbid sound will equally and always be present.

XXVII

The diseases of the first class are, (1) those which depend on hereditary predisposition; (2) those which arise from affections of the mind, particularly ungratified desires, the principal of which is Nostalgia; (3) those which affect certain artisans, naturally possessing weak lungs.

Scholium. 1. The influence of an hereditary taint in producing diseases we know by experience, though we cannot explain it.—See Van Swieten.

2. Mental affections, we find, produce quite opposite effects, while acting as causes of pectoral diseases. Of these affections of the mind I have observed none more powerful in rendering obscure the natural resonance of the chest, than the destruction of cherished hopes. And as among this class of diseases, Nostalgia (commonly called *heimwehe*—home ail) occupies the first place, I shall here give a short history of it.

When young men, not yet arrived at their full growth, are forcibly impressed into the military service, and thereby at once lose all hope of returning safe and sound to their beloved home and country, they become sad, silent, listless, solitary, musing and full of sighs and moans, and finally quite regardless of, and indifferent to, all the cares and duties of life. From this state of mental disorder nothing can rouse them,—neither argument, nor promises, nor the dread of punishment; and the body gradually pines and wastes away, under the pressure of ungratified desires, and with the preternatural sound of one side of the chest. This is the disease Nostalgia. I have examined the bodies of many youths who have fallen victims to it, and have uniformly found the lungs firmly united to the pleura, and the lobes on that side where the obscure sound had existed, callous, indurated, and more or less purulent. Some years ago, this disease was very common, but is now rarely met with, since the wise arrangement has been adopted of limiting the period to military service to a certain number of years only.

3. The various arts and occupations of life have their peculiar diseases, in like manner as the ages, temperaments, and sexes have theirs. This truth is exemplified in the case of the man of letters, the husbandman, the workers in metals, painters, etc., etc. Our particular business, however, at present, is with those arts which dispose to diseases of the chest indicated by the sound so often described. Thus I have remarked that Tailors, Millers, etc. who are forced to inhale, during their labours, a fine dust, become phthisical; while shoemakers, weavers, etc. from the forced position or application of their weak chests, during their various occupations, become asthmatical, with scirrhous lungs, etc.

I may here state a fact which I have frequently proved by dissection, but which I cannot well account for—it is this: in the above mentioned class of cases it is extremely rare to find both lungs affected at the same time; and, when this happens, one lung is always more diseased than the other.

XXVIII

The diseases mentioned (in XXVI, 2) arise either from (1) a vitiated condition of the fluids, gradually produced; or (2) from acute affections imperfectly cured.

Scholium. 1. The vitiation of the humours arises from ingesta which cannot be assimilated, the effect of which in producing chronic diseases is well known.

2. An acute disease is said to be imperfectly cured when some morbid affection still remains after it, in some part of the body. This morbid condition will be observed either in the site of the primary disease, or, at least, in that portion of the chest, which yields the morbid sound;—namely, the pleura, or lungs, or both these together, or the mediastinum or pericardium. When the primary inflammatory disease is succeeded by a collection of pus in the chest, the affection is readily recognized; but if the secondary affection is a scirrhus of the lung, how often and how grievously are medical men thereby deceived! Often have I met with cases of fancied convalescence from acute fevers, in which there was hardly any cough or dyspnoea, or indeed any other sign of disease (as appeared to the attendants) but a trifling degree of irregular fever. In these cases, however, on percussion the preternatural sound was found over one whole side of the chest, and the final result was death, preceded either by dropsy or extreme emaciation; the real seat of the disease remaining, perhaps, unknown to the very last!

XXIX

For the above reasons, it may be received as a general rule in chronic diseases, that when, together with the indication stated XXVI, there are emaciation and debility,—the case is desperate.

Scholium. This result is inevitable whensoever the disease does not yield to medicine. In such cases we may always conclude, that the lung of the side which yields the preternatural sound, is either compressed by some foreign body; is indurated by disease, or destroyed by some morbid acrimony developed within its own structure.

SEVENTH OBSERVATION

OF THE PRETERNATURAL SOUND OF THE CHEST WHICH RESULTS FROM COPIOUS EXTRAVASATION OF THE FLUIDS CONTAINED IN THE VESSELS OF THAT CAVITY

XXX

The fluids contained in the vessel of the chest are: 1. Chyle; 2. Blood; 3. Serum and Lymph.

Scholium. I must candidly admit that I have never seen a case of extravasated chyle. I however believe the thing possible, although I am well aware that the thoracic duct runs outside the pleura: the same causes that produce erosion and perforation of the thoracic parietes, may produce this.

XXXI

The extravasation of these fluids (XXX) may arise from the following causes: (1) rupture of the containing vessels; (2) too great tenuity of the contained fluids; (3) nonabsorption of the same, etc., etc.

Scholium. 1. Under this head come wounds, contusions, etc.

2. Extravasations from internal causes arise from rupture of relaxed and debilitated vessels, during a state of plethora and overactivity of the circulation.

3. A third class of causes are obstructions originating in a bad habit of body.

XXXII

When from these causes the fluids mentioned are poured out in considerable quantity, the preternatural sound will exist over the space occupied by them.

Scholium. The correctness of this statement is evinced by the experiment mentioned at the end of the scholium of XVII.

According to the plan formerly proposed (XI), I shall now proceed to notice those affections of the chest which are not indicated by percussion.

EIGHTH OBSERVATION

OF THOSE AFFECTIONS OF THE CHEST WHICH ARE NOT INDICATED BY PERCUSSION

XXXIII

Certain diseases attended by a violent cough, and thereby creating a suspicion that the lungs are certainly implicated, are nevertheless truly diseases of the abdomen, and affect the pulmonary organs merely sympathetically.

Scholium. Under this head are ranged the gastric and convulsive coughs of infants, pregnant women, and such other persons as have their abdominal viscera oppressed by the lentor of autumnal agues, or a superfluity of phlegm.

XXXIV

Violent coughs, dyspnoeas, asthmas and consumptions, are also occasionally observed which originate in some incomprehensible irritability of the nerves of the chest.

Affections of this sort rarely give rise to the preternatural sound: from the absence of this, however, and the presence of a copious watery urine, their existence may be pretty confidently presumed.

Scholium. Under this head are ranged the coughs, dyspnoeas, and asthmas so common in hysterical and hypochondriacal affections; the nervous consumption and asthma of old persons; and, perhaps we may add the polypous concretions found near the heart in young subjects.

XXXV

A slight engorgement of the lung, a scirrhus of small extent, a small vomica, and a trifling extravasation, are not detected by percussion,—unless, sometimes, by the decreased resonance of the affected part.

Scholium. These affections are not dangerous until they reach a size when they become more readily discoverable by means of percussion.

XXXVI

There is another class of diseases of the lungs [undiscoverable by percussion] in which the distinguishing symptoms are a very severe cough, with expectoration of fatty, chalky, gypseous and stony matters.

Scholium. The cases are known by the nature of the expectoration. I have frequently observed a cough of this kind (but without the peculiar expectoration) succeeding miliary fevers improperly treated.

NINTH OBSERVATION
OF THE APPEARANCES ON DISSECTION, IN CASES WHERE THE PRETERNATURAL SOUND OF THE CHEST HAD BEEN OBSERVED

XXXVII

These are the following:

1. Scirrhus of the lungs;
2. The conversion of this into an ichorous vomica;
3. A purulent vomica (simple or ruptured) in the pleura, lungs, mediastinum or pericardium.
4. Empyema;
5. Dropsy of the chest, in one or both cavities;

6. Dropsy of the pericardium;

7. Extensive extravasation of blood in the cavity of the pleura or pericardium;

8. Aneurism of the heart.

Scholium. I will now proceed to notice these diseases in order, premising, occasionally, some account of the general symptoms.

TENTH OBSERVATION

OF SCIRRHUS OF THE LUNGS, AND ITS SYMPTOMS

XXXVIII

By scirrhus of the lungs I mean the degeneration of the natural spongy substance of the organ into an indolent fleshy mass.

Scholium. A portion of sound lung swims in water, but this carniform degeneration sinks. There is often observed a vast difference in the character of these scirrhi, in respect of hardness, colour, and component parts. Thus, in inflammatory diseases of the chest proving fatal on the fifth, seventh, or ninth day, the lung is very often found so completely gorged with blood, as to resemble liver in every respect, both as to colour and consistence. One appearance deserves to be noticed: the lung is frequently invested with a purulent adventitious membrane, in those instances wherein the fatal peripneumony has succeeded an acute pleurisy. In chronic diseases of the lungs the appearances are extremely various. Frequently they are interspersed and as it were marbled with a fatty kind of matter; frequently along with the fleshy appearance, they have the consistence of cartilage; and very often they are found indurated by means of a thickened and black blood. These varieties, doubtless, depend on varieties of the morbific matter.

XXXIX

The presence of scirrhus of the lungs, in its primary unsoftened condition, may be suspected from the following signs:

Together with the diminution or entire loss of the natural sound over the affected part, there is an infrequent cough without any expectoration, or with only a scanty excretion of viscid and crude sputa. During a state of quiescence there is nothing to be observed much amiss, either in the condition of the pulse or respiration; but upon any considerable bodily motion, or after speaking for some time, these persons become speedily exhausted, anxious, and breathless, and complain of a sense of dryness and roughness in the throat. At the same time the pulse, which had previously been of moderate frequency, becomes quick and unequal; the respiration and speech are broken and interrupted by sighs; the temporal, sublingual, and jugular veins of the affected side, are more than usually distended; while it will be observed that this side of the chest is less moveable than the other, during inspiration. Meanwhile the natural and animal functions continue to be well performed; and the patient can lie on either side indifferently.

All the above symptoms are more severe in proportion as the scirrhus is more extensive.

ELEVENTH OBSERVATION

OF VOMICAE IN GENERAL

XL

When an humour, sound or morbid, is deposited from the circulating mass in a solid form, and (together with the extreme vessels) is afterwards, by means of the vital powers softened and converted into matter, and contained in a sort of capsule, I term this collection of matter a Vomica.

Scholium. This notion applies to every vomica, whether produced by a vice of the solids or fluids, as is clear from the history of obstruction and inflammation.

XLI

I have observed two kinds of Vomica—the Ichorous and Purulent. The former occupies the lungs only; the latter, both the lungs and other thoracic viscera. They are both either close, or communicating with the Trachaea.

Scholium. By the term Ichorous Vomica, I mean a sac containing a thin fluid frequently of a reddish yellow colour, frequently of a reddish brown, often of a colour between these, different from pus, and arising from the destruction of a scirrhus lung. By Purulent Vomica, I understand an encysted abscess of the chest, resulting from the conversion of an inflamed spot into a white, thick, glutinous, fatty matter. When these communicate with the Bronchia and discharge any of their contents by expectoration, they are called open; otherwise, close or shut.

XLII

1. Ichorous Vomica.—If a scirrhus of the lung, recognized by its proper signs (XXXIX) is converted into matter, it presents the following symptoms: The patient begins to languish and waste away insensibly (although the usual quantity of food is taken), with a quick, contracted, and unequal pulse. The respiration, even during a state of quietude, is unnaturally anxious and frequent; and is remarkably interrupted by sighing. The forehead, during the more severe attacks, is sometimes covered with a cold sweat. The eyes are dim; the veins of the cheeks and lips are livid, and the tongue, especially on the affected side, is of a leaden hue. At the same time there is neither pain nor thirst. The diseased side, however, is observed to be less mobile than natural, and the degree of immobility is proportioned to the bulk of the vomica into which the scirrhus has been

resolved. The cough is infrequent, interrupted, and dry; or the expectoration, if any, is dirty or blackish (coenosum aut fuscum).

When things have got to this height, the appetite begins to fail, and at length is entirely lost; and whatever is eaten only produces an increase of anxiety during the process of digestion: this process however, takes place without any hectic flushing, which always accompanies the purulent vomica.

In some cases, when there is a dissolution of the central parts of the scirrhus, the abdomen and hypochondres sink in; in a very few instances, the same parts are slightly swollen, and with an indistinct feeling of fluctuation. The urine rarely presents any deviation from the natural state; sometimes, however, it is red, and with a sediment (if any exists) of a cinnabar colour. The stools are of natural character, except under the influence of medicine. The extremities, even when of a livid colour, are never hotter than natural, until a few days before death; the affected side is, moreover, observed to swell, and the hand and foot in the first place. The patient now suffers from frequent sinkings and faintings; and from having hitherto been able to lie easily on either side, he is able to remain on the affected side only.

2. Close Purulent Vomica.—The following are the symptoms of this affection: While the abdominal organs still continue to perform their functions well, there is often present a very troublesome, frequent, dry cough, so severe as to irritate the fauces, to render the voice hoarse, and often to excite vomiting. At this time are observed frequent irregular chills, followed by heat, and strong flushing of the cheeks and lips, particularly of the affected side. A degree of lassitude is experienced, more remarkable after a full meal; and at the same time there is perceived a degree of quickness and straitness of the respiration, sufficient to excite suspicion of some morbid affection of the chest. The pulse is also found to be contracted, frequent somewhat hard and unequal during the period of digestion; and even at other times it is never in a perfectly natural state,—more especially under the influence of bodily motions, laughing, or speaking.

If at this time the Vomica has reached a size to be detected by percussion, the following additional signs exist: The patient is not nourished by the food taken, partly because it is, in a greater or less degree, rejected by vomiting, and partly on account of the imperfect assimilation of what is retained. As the disease increases, the whole process of respiration is at length carried on by one lung; an incessant state of anxiety prevails, and the patient remains fixed on the diseased side, through dread of impending suffocation if he turn on the other. The face, hands, feet, and the affected side are oedematous; while the opposite side of the body, from deficient assimilation, hectic heat, and nocturnal perspirations, is extenuated. The urine now becomes scanty, red, turbid, with a copious branny sediment, and soon putrefies; and the scene is finally closed, with short and asthmatic breathlessness, lividity of the cheeks, lips, and nails, etc.

3. Purulent Vomica communicating with the Trachea.—When a Vomica of considerable size, discoverable by percussion, bursts into the Trachea, or rather Bronchia, by a large opening, it produces instant suffocation; if by a small aperture, it is recognized by the following marks: By means of a violent cough, pus is expectorated, which is, in different cases, white, yellow, saffron, green, brown, bloody; which sinks in water, and, when thrown on hot coals, emits a stinking nidorous smell. If at this time, while the patient is coughing and spitting, the palm of the hand be placed over the site of the vomica, i.e. over the place where its existence had been detected by percussion,—the noise of fluid within the chest will be sufficiently manifest. This kind of expectoration will cease for some days, with relief to the patient; but it speedily returns, and is always preceded, for four and twenty hours, by an increase of the febrile state. During this state of things, and before the return of the expectoration, if percussion is applied over the site of the vomica a sound exactly like that from a fleshy limb is obtained; but if this is delayed until the evacuation of the accumulated pus, then there is perceived a distinct, though obtuse sound. The slow fever which invariably accompanies this condition, is encreased after eating, and is still higher during the night; and at these times, the forehead, neck, and chest, are covered with perspiration. With the increase of these symptoms, and the continuation of the purulent expectoration, the breath becomes tainted, insomuch as to be extremely disagreeable both to the patient and the attendants. The thirst continues great, but the appetite is lost, even for the greatest delicacies, which, however sparingly taken, produce, in place of refreshment, langour and anxiety. (The case is very different with them whose sputa are inodorous, the appetite in many being even great.) The urine is uniformly frothy, grows speedily putrid, and deposits a viscid, tenacious, white sediment. The patient now daily grows more emaciated: the bones almost pierce the skin, the hair falls off, the nails become curved, the legs swell; at length a colliquative diarrhaea supervening first lessens, and then suppresses the expectoration, and the sufferer finally dies suddenly, on the third day after that on which he began to remain obstinately fixed on his back, with his legs drawn under him.

XLIII

Empyema.—When a vomica (XXXVII), ascertained by percussion, discharges its contents into the cavity of the pleura, and upon the diaphragm, Empyema is produced.

Scholium. I premise this definition to prevent the affection now in question from being confounded with a vomica that has discharged its contents into the trachaea.

XLIV

If a large vomica, whose superficial and central extent is supposed to have been recognized by the marks pointed out (Obs. Third: XV, XVI, XVII), shall have burst as above mentioned (XLIII), it may be recognized by the following signs:

The patient who had usually lain on the affected side, starts up with a sudden pain (as if nearly suffocated), and begs to be held in the erect posture.

If percussion is now applied, it will be found that the natural sound, which had been nearly lost in the site of the vomica, has in some degree been restored in that place; while it is more or less destroyed (according to the quantity of pus effused) over the posterior and inferior parts of the chest.

There is now a very frequent cough, which is either dry, or with a scanty, frothy and noisy expectoration. The respiration becomes very laborious, with frequent faintings, and a cold sweat bedews the forehead and throat; the cheeks and lips are of an ominous red, while the nails grow livid, the pupils dilate, and death (which follows in a few hours the rupture of a large vomica) is finally preceded by dimness of sight, etc.

A small vomica, ruptured in the same manner, produces the same symptoms, and is equally fatal. This issue, however, is of later occurrence, and is preceded by the marks of pleuro-peripneumony.

TWELFTH OBSERVATION

OF DROPSY OF THE CHEST

XLV

When water is collected in the cavity of the chest, between the pleura (costalis) and the lungs, the disease is called dropsy of the chest; and this is said to be of two kinds, namely, according as the fluid occupies one, or both sides.

Scholium. This is ascertained by percussion in the living subject; and is demonstrated by anatomical examination after death. The general symptoms of this disease are chiefly the following:

1. Difficult and laborious respiration;

2. A cough at intervals, which is dry, or only attended by sputa of a thin watery nature, or occasionally somewhat viscid;

3. A pulse contracted, somewhat hard, frequent, unequal and often intermitting;

4. A sense of breathlessness and suffocation on the slightest motion;

5. An incipient dislike of warm food;

6. Perpetual anxiety about the scrobiculus cordis;

7. Great pressure on the chest, and distention of the stomach during the period of digestion;

8. A murmuring noise about the hypochondres, and frequent eructation of flatus, with momentary relief;

9. Scarcely any thirst;

10. Urine very scanty, and rarely made, red, with a lateritious sediment;

11. Swelling of the abdomen, more especially in the Epigastrium, and particularly in that point on which the incumbent water gravitates;

12. A sublivid swelling of the extremities, especially of the feet, which are moreover cold to touch;

13. Oedematous tumescence of the inferior palpebrae;

14. A pallid, or, according to the nature of the affection, a sublivid discoloration of the cheeks, lips, and tongue;

15. Inability to lie down; anxious distressing nights, with heaviness, yet frequently sleepless.

All these symptoms vary in a wonderful manner according to the disease.

First Kind.—Dropsy of one side of the Chest. Beside the general signs of this disease above enumerated, the affected side, if completely filled with water, is enfeebled (effoeminatum), and appears less moveable during inspiration. In this case, also, the affected side yields no where the natural sound on percussion. If the chest is only half-filled, a louder sound will be obtained, over the parts to which the fluid does not extend; and, in this case, the resonance will be found to vary according to the position of the patient, and the consequent level which the liquid attains. The Hypochondre of the affected side is also unusually tumid, and more resisting to pressure than the rest of the abdomen. The palpebra, hand, and foot of the affected side are slightly oedematous. It is a remarkable fact, that the reclining posture (decubitus declivis) is easily borne when the chest is entirely full; while the contrary is the case, when there remains space for the fluctuation of the water.

Second Kind.—Dropsy of both sides of the Chest. If fluid is contained in both sides of the chest, the following specific signs, in addition to the general symptoms, exist: The natural sound is destroyed over the space occupied by the water in either side. The patients uniformly become asthmatic; and resemble, in many respects, those labouring under Ascites, only that the former have their inferior palpebrae and hands swollen. They cannot lie in an horizontal posture, and are equally threatened with suffocation on whichever side they turn; on which account, they are forced to remain sitting, day and night, to prevent the pressure of the fluid from being felt on the upper parts of the chest (which would be the case on lying down), in the same degree on which it now gravitates on the abdomen. The effect of this state of things might lead to the suspicion of Ascites, only that we find, on examining the patient in the erect position, that the hypochondriac regions are more swollen than the inferior parts, which is not the case in Ascites.

All these subjects die as if from peripneumony, that is to say,—the pulse fails, the whole body, except the chest and head, grows cold, the cheeks and extremities become livid, the respiration is at first laborious, then interrupted, and finally ceases altogether.

XLVI

Dropsy of the Pericardium.—When the liquor pericardii is morbidly increased, so as to be capable of disturbing the natural action of the heart, the disease is called Dropsy of the Pericardium: of this there are two species, as the fluid is purulent or serous.

Scholium. The fluid naturally present in the pericardium accumulates in still greater quantity in those who suffer a long protracted mortal agony, as we find on examination after their death. But it is not to this accumulation, originating in the relaxation of death, but to that produced by obstruction during life, that I apply the term dropsy. I have ventured to divide the affection into two species, because I have often witnessed both of them. In the first variety, the heart is rough, and as it were shagged, with a coating of the purulent matter; while in the latter, the organ is only of a paler colour than natural. Many may be of the opinion that the purulent dropsy would be better classed under the head of Empyema; but I shall never quarrel about words, when there are appearances to instruct us.

Signs of Hydropericardium.—Almost all the symptoms which have already been enumerated as accompanying dropsy of the chest generally, accompany this species also: in addition to these, however, I have observed the following specific signs of the dropsy of the pericardium:—

The sound in the cardiac region, which I have already stated (III: 2, 3) to be naturally more obscure than in the other parts of the chest; is now as completely deadened as if the percussion were applied to a fleshy limb. A swelling is perceived in the praecordia, which can readily be distinguished, by its superior resistance, from the stomach distended by flatus.

The patients fall asleep, while sitting, the body being inclined forwards; but they soon are roused by the unconscious dropping of the head. On this account, they complain to all around them of the distressing propensity to sleep which they experience. At the same time they suffer from faintings (accompanied by a pulse frequently unequal in respect both of its rythm and volume), and, indeed continue to undergo to the end of their wretched life, and in every position of body, the greatest distress. A few days before death, in many cases, the neck is swollen, and the eyes become extremely red, as if from crying. This state of things is sometimes terminated suddenly by a stroke of apoplexy, or more slowly by leipothymia.

The same signs are furnished by percussion in the purulent, as in the proper dropsy of the pericardium; but in the former, the other symptoms are precisely the same as those which exist in the close purulent vomica. In the purulent dropsy, the fluid commonly resembles turbid whey,—the thicker portions of it (quod purulentum est) being found adhering to the heart like fringes.

THIRTEENTH OBSERVATION

OF THE SYMPTOMS OF A COPIOUS EXTRAVASATION OF BLOOD

XLVII

The causes of a large extravasation of blood into the cavity of the chest have been noticed in the Scholium of XXXI. The following are the symptoms of this affection.

Scholium. There is incessant and indescribable anxiety and oppression at the praecordia and on the chest, while there is constant jactitation of the body, and complete intolerance of the horizontal posture. Percussion elicits none of the natural sound over the space occupied by the extravasated blood. In all cases the pulse is extremely contracted, frequent, and irregular in every way. The respiration is extremely laborious, with a frequent cough, and broken by profound sighing. All the veins become flaccid, and the eyes are at first red but ultimately pale. Cold sweats etc. follow, and the patient dies stertorous.

These are the symptoms when the blood flows into the cavity of the pleura without any accompanying lesion of the lungs: when these are wounded, there is also bloody expectoration, and a passage of air to and from the wound in the parietes of the chest.

FOURTEENTH OBSERVATION

OF ANEURISM OF THE HEART

XLVIII

When the heart becomes so much distended by blood, accumulated in its auricles and ventricles, as to be unequal to propel forward its contents, it frequently becomes thereby enormously dilated. This dilatation has been called Aneurism of the Heart.

Scholium. We frequently observe this state of the heart on dissection, (1) in sudden and extensive peripneumonies of both lobes at the same time, and (2) in those fatal inflammatory diseases which are noticed towards the end of the Scholium on XXII.

The pathognomonic sign of this affection is the complete fleshy sound on percussion existing over a considerable space in the region of the heart. Whenever this sound is perceptible in the acute peripneumony it is a sign that the patient will not survive twenty-four hours: in fact, he is already at the last gasp, and is speedily carried off as in apoplexy, unconscious of his fate.

In the second class of inflammations, the sign is equally fatal, but is attended by different symptoms. In this case, the patients suffer dread-full anxiety and by the constant jactitation of their limbs, are perpetually uncovering themselves. Older persons, indeed bear more tranquilly their sufferings; but the younger are pertinaciously restless and violent, struggling and talking, attempting to get out of bed, demanding their clothes, and endeavouring to walk or go about their usual occupations. Meanwhile the eyes become dull, the cheeks livid, and the nails and extremities are tinged with a leaden hue, and death is ushered in by cold sweats, and the gradual extinction of the pulse and respiration.

Cedant haec miseris in solatium, veris autem medicinae cultoribus in incrementum artis: Quod opto!

1772

WILLIAM HEBERDEN

ON ANGINA PECTORIS

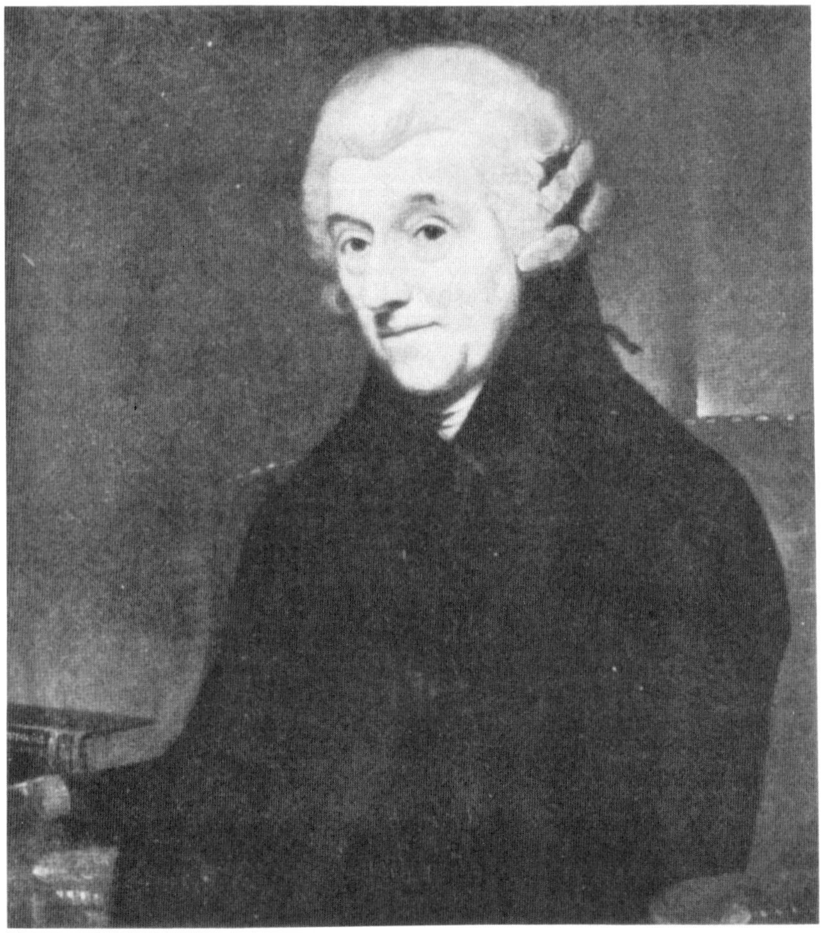

WILLIAM HEBERDEN

Portrait by Sir William Beechey, R.A., in the Royal College of Physicians, London

(Courtesy Charles C Thomas.)

WILLIAM HEBERDEN

(1710-1801)

"Good readers are almost as rare as good authors."

—William Heberden.

DURING the Eighteenth Century, which was characterized in medical history as an age of theories and individual systems, few medical men were outstanding. Except for the original contributions of such men as Morgagni, Hales, John and William Hunter, Kaspar Friedrich Wolff, and Jenner, as Garrison has shown (p. 310), the century represented a period of retrogression. Too few physicians were practicing bedside medicine, and the ideas which Harvey, Bacon, and Newton had put forth during the preceding century had not fired the general practitioners with enthusiasm. One of the reasons, other than his singular accomplishments, why William Heberden is given a conspicuous place in medical history is that he made it a point to battle the dogma and tyrannic ideologies of many of his contemporaries who were still wrangling over the medical interpretations of the ancient writers. Moreover, in his medical practice, which was very extensive, Heberden had the modern attitude of first studying the patient as an individual and later relegating his illness or disease to its proper place in the classification of disease.

William Heberden was born in London. He was next to the youngest son of Richard and Elizabeth Cooper Heberden. His preliminary education was obtained at the Grammar School of St. Saviour, Southwark. He entered St. John's College, Cambridge, in 1724. In 1728 he was granted the degree of Bachelor of Arts. Two years later he obtained a fellowship in the same college. In 1732 he received the degree of Master of Arts. From that year on, he seems to have directed his attention to medical studies, and he received his degree of Doctor of Medicine in 1739.

During his stay in medical school and while he was studying materia medica, Heberden was engaged in writing "An Essay on Mithridatium and Theriaca." In that work he exposed the use of mithridatics as antidotes for poisons, so that these glamorous drugs thereby lost their importance. The work was not published until 1745. It is of interest in the present account to note Heberden's broad acquaintance with the classics. Not only did he call on Hippocrates to elucidate some points, but he also quoted from Homer, Plautus, Virgil, Juvenal, and others.

In 1746 Heberden was elected a fellow of the Royal College of Physicians, and in 1748 he began the practice of medicine in London. Heberden was further honored in 1749 when he was elected a fellow of the Royal Society. Some of his most valuable contributions to medicine subsequently were published in the "Philosophical Transactions" of the Royal Society.

In 1752 Heberden married Elizabeth Martin, daughter of John Martin, a prominent citizen and a member of Parliament. His wife died in 1754, leaving him with two sons: John, who died in infancy, and Thomas, father of the well-known physician, Thomas Heberden. In 1760 William Heberden married again, this time to Mary Wollaston. By his second marriage he had eight children, only two of whom survived their father. These were Mary and William, the latter of whom later became physician to the King.

Heberden, in his practice of medicine, stressed the importance of experience in the study and treatment of disease. He makes this interesting comment, ". . . the practice of physic has been more improved by the casual experiments of illiterate nations, and the rash ones of vagabond quacks, than by the reasonings of all the once celebrated professors of it, and theoretic teachers in the several schools of Europe: very few of whom have furnished us with one new medicine, or have taught us better to use our old ones, or have in any one instance at all improved the art of curing diseases."[1]

From all published accounts it seems that both Heberden's professional and social contacts were pleasant. He treated William Cowper and Bishop Warburton, but perhaps his most famous patient was Samuel Johnson, whom he attended in his final illness. Johnson, in the codicil to his will, left Heberden one of his books. According to a note by Nichols in Boswell's "Life of Samuel Johnson,"[2] Dr. Johnson once called Heberden, "Dr. Heberden, ultimum Romanorum, the last of our learned physicians." Among Heberden's friends and colleagues were John and William Hunter, Fothergill, Jenner, Sir George Baker, Withering, Pitcairn, and Robert Gooch. He also was acquainted with Benjamin Franklin, who induced him to publish for the American colonies a most interesting pamphlet,[3] giving instructions for inoculation for the prevention of the smallpox (1759). According to Pettigrew, Heberden was also on intimate terms with the chief literary men of his day, among them Gray, Jacob Bryant, Mason, Cavendish, Bishop Hurd, Bishop Lowth, Dr. Kennicott, Dr. Jortin, Tyrwhitt, and Stuart. Heberden himself translated the plays of Euripides.

George III thought well of Heberden and, upon Queen Charlotte's arrival in England in 1761, he was named physician to her, an honor which he declined because he felt it might interfere with life as he wished to live it.

In 1778 Heberden was elected an honorary member of the Royal Society of Medicine of Paris. He retired from the practice of medicine in 1782. His last paper, "Of the Measles," was read at the College of Physicians in 1785. In 1787, being still rather active, he was elected vice-president of the Royal Humane Society. He had retired years ago, of course, from active practice and, as he declares in his preface to the "Commentaries," a preface which because of its beautiful sentiment and sage advice we have chosen to reprint in this book, he spent his last years in teaching what he knew to his sons. Dr. Heberden died in Pall Mall on May 17, 1801, in his ninety-first year. Included in LeRoy Crummer's prefatory essay to the publication of the Heberden manuscript, "An Introduction to the Study of Physic," is a list of Heberden's published writings as well as a check list of Heberden's manuscripts.

Heberden's major opus was, of course, his "Commentaries on the History and Cure of Diseases," published posthumously by his son, William. The Royal College of Physicians owns the original two volumes of manuscript which Heberden had carefully written in Latin. According to Crummer (p. 11-12), each volume contains about the same material. William Heberden, Jr., in 1802 chose to have published one of these volumes, which had been completed by the senior Heberden in 1782. The younger Heberden also translated the English edition of the "Commentaries," published the same year (1802). There were many subsequent editions of the work in both languages, for it was one of the most popular books on medicine of the first part of the Nineteenth Century. For those who are interested in the evolution of medical

---

[1]Pettigrew, Thomas J.: "William Heberden," in *Medical portrait gallery*, London, 1840, Whittaker and Co., vol. 3, pp. 11-12.

[2]Boswell, James: *The Life of Samuel Johnson*, Bath, England, George Bayntun, 1925, vol. 2, p. 1013.

[3]Heberden, William: *Plain instructions for inoculation in the small-pox; by which any person may be enabled to perform the operation, and conduct the patient through the distemper.* Printed at the expense of the author, to be given away in America, London, 1759, 12 pp.

thought, this book holds many fascinations. In Heberden's description of disease the keen, trained logical power of observation not surpassed by Hippocrates or Sydenham is noticed. The book represents a careful analysis of the professional experience of more than forty years of active practice of a physician possessed of a high mental endowment. In it are contained his original portrayals of varicella which he originally published in 1768,[4] of angina pectoris, a condition which he named and which was first described by him in 1772[5] which we are reproducing, and his notation of the nodules in the fingers which occur in arthritis deformans. An actual case of angina pectoris was described in the memoirs of the Earl of Clarendon (1632)[6] and Morgagni[7] presented a description of this disease (1707). It is also of interest to note that at the same time Heberden reported his cases, Dr. Rougnon[8] of Besançon wrote a letter about it concerning a captain of cavalry who had d unexpectedly during an attack of pain situated in the retrosternal region. The pain appeared after effort, similar attacks having occurred before. Several other accounts of angina pectoris were then reported, including Home's account of John Hunter's angina pectoris, which we are also reproducing. But none was so clear and concise as the classic of Heberden, who not only gave the disease its name but also gave it a masterful description.

---

[4]Heberden, William: On the Chicken-Pox, Med. Tr. Roy. Coll. Phys., London **1**: 427-436, 1768.

[5]Heberden, William: Some account of a disorder of the breast, Med. Tr. Roy. Coll. Phys., London **2**: 59-67, 1772.

[6]Case of Henry Hyde, 1632. In his: *Life.* Oxford, 1759, p. 9.

[7]Morgagni, J. B.: *De sedibus et causis morborum per anatomen indagatis libri quinque. Dissectiones, et aminadversiones, nunc primum editas complectuntur propemodum innumeras, medicis, chirurgis, anatomics profuturas.* vol. **1**: p. 282, Venice, 1761.

[8]Rougnon de Magny, N. F.: *Lettre à M. Lorry, touchant les causes de la mort de feu Monsieur Charles, ancien capitaine de cavalerie, arrivée à Besançon le 23 février,* 1768, 55 pp.

COMMENTARIES

ON

THE HISTORY AND CURE

OF

DISEASES

BY

WILLIAM HEBERDEN, M.D.

Γέρων, καὶ κάμνειν οὐκέτι δυνάμενος, τοῦτο τὸ βιβλίον ἔγραψα, συντάξας τὰς μετὰ πολλῆς τριβῆς ἐν ταῖς τῶν ἀνθρώπων νόσοις καταληφθείσας μοι πείρας.

ALEX. TRALL. Lib. XII.

LONDON:

PRINTED FOR T. PAYNE, MEWS-GATE;

By S. Hamilton, Falcon-Court, Fleet-Street.

1802.

COMMENTARIES ON THE HISTORY AND CURE OF DISEASES*

PREFACE

PLUTARCH says,† that the life of a vestal virgin was divided into three portions; in the first of which she learned the duties of her profession, in the second she practised them, and in the third she taught them to others. This is no bad model for the life of a physician: and as I have now passed through the two first of these times, I am willing to employ the remainder of my days in teaching what I know to any of my sons who may choose the profession of physic; and to him I desire that these papers may be given.

The notes from which the following observations were collected, were taken in the chambers of the sick themselves, or from their attendants, where several things might occasion the omission of some material circumstances. These notes were read over every month, and such facts, as tended to throw any light upon the history of a distemper, or the effects of a remedy, were entered under the title of the distemper in another book, from which were extracted all the particulars here given relating to the nature and cure of diseases. It appeared more advisable to give such facts only, as were justified by the original papers, however imperfect, than either to supply their defects from memory, except in a very few instances, or than to borrow any thing from other writers.

The collections from the notes, as well as the notes themselves, were written in Latin, the distempers being ranged alphabetically; and this is the reason that the titles are here in that language. In making the extracts it was not only more easy to follow the order in which the observations had been ranged, but there was likewise less danger of any confusion or omission; and little or no inconvenience can arise from preserving the Latin names of the distempers.

An useful addition might have been made to these papers by comparing them with the current doctrine of diseases and remedies, as also with what is laid down in practical writers, and with the accounts of those who treat of the dissections of morbid bodies; but at my advanced age it would be to no purpose to think of such an undertaking.

*Heberden, William: *Commentaries on the History and Cure of Diseases,* London, 1802.

†Plutarch. in Numâ, et.

CHAPTER 70

PECTORIS DOLOR*

Beside the asthma, hysteric oppressions, the acute darting pains in pleurisies, and the chronical ones in consumptions, the breast is often the seat of pains, which are distressing, sometimes even from their vehemence, oftener from their duration, as they have continued to tease the patient for six, for eight, for nine, and for fourteen years. There have been several examples of their returning periodically every night, or alternately with a head-ach. They have been called gouty, and rheumatic, and spasmodic. There has appeared no reason to judge that they proceed from any cause of much importance to health (being attended with no fever), or that they lead to any dangerous consequences; and if the patient were not uneasy with what he feels, he needs never to be so on account of any thing which he has to fear.

If these pains should return at night, and disturb the sleep, small doses of opium have been found serviceable, and may be used alone, or joined with an opening medicine, with a preparation of antimony, or with the fetid gums. Externally, a small perpetual blister applied to the breast has been successful, and so has an issue made in the thigh. A large cumin plaster has been worn over the seat of the pain with advantage. The volatile, or saponaceous liniment, may be rubbed in over the part affected. Bathing in the sea, or in any cold water, may be used at the same time.

But there is a disorder of the breast marked with strong and peculiar symptoms, considerable for the kind of danger belonging to it, and not extremely rare, which deserves to be mentioned more at length. The seat of it, and sense of strangling, and anxiety with which it is attended, may make it not improperly be called angina pectoris.

They who are afflicted with it, are seized while they are walking, (more especially if it be up hill, and soon after eating) with a painful and most disagreeable sensation in the breast, which seems as if it would extinguish life, if it were to increase or to continue; but the moment they stand still, all this uneasiness vanishes.

In all other respects, the patients are, at the beginning of this disorder, perfectly well, and in particular have no shortness of breath, from which it is totally different. The pain is sometimes situated in the upper part, sometimes in the middle, sometimes at the bottom of the os sterni, and often more inclined to the left than to the right side. It likewise very frequently extends from the breast to the middle of the left arm. The pulse is, at least sometimes, not disturbed by this pain, as I have had opportunities of observing by feeling the pulse during the paroxysm. Males are most liable to this disease, especially such as have past their fiftieth year.

*Heberden's original publication appeared in 1772. We are reprinting from the *Commentaries* published in 1802.—F. A. W., 1940.

After it has continued a year or more, it will not cease so instantaneously upon standing still; and it will come on not only when the persons are walking, but when they are lying down, especially if they lie on the left side, and oblige them to rise up out of their beds. In some inveterate cases it has been brought on by the motion of a horse, or a carriage, and even by swallowing, coughing, going to stool, or speaking, or any disturbance of mind.

Such is the most usual appearance of this disease; but some varieties may be met with. Some have been seized while they were standing still, or sitting, also upon first waking out of sleep: and the pain sometimes reaches to the right arm, as well as to the left, and even down to the hands, but this is uncommon: in a very few instances the arm has at the same time been numbed and swelled. In one or two persons, the pain has lasted some hours, or even days; but this has happened when the complaint has been of long standing, and thoroughly rooted in the constitution: once only the very first attack continued the whole night.

I have seen nearly a hundred people under this disorder, of which number there have been three women, and one boy twelve years old. All the rest were men near, or past the fiftieth year of their age.

Persons who have persevered in walking till the pain has returned four or five times, have then sometimes vomited.

A man in the sixtieth year of his life began to feel, while he was walking, an uneasy sensation in his left arm. He never perceived it while he was travelling in a carriage. After it continued ten years, it would come upon him two or three times a week at night, while he was in bed, and then he was obliged to sit up for an hour or two before it would abate so much as to suffer him to lie down. In all other respects he was very healthy, and had always been a remarkably strong man. The breast was never affected. This disorder, its seat excepted, perfectly resembled the angina pectoris, gradually increasing in the same manner, and being both excited and relieved by all the same causes. He died suddenly without a groan at the age of seventy-five.

The termination of the angina pectoris is remarkable. For if no accident intervene, but the disease go on to its height, the patients all suddenly fall down, and perish almost immediately. Of which indeed their frequent faintness, and sensations as if all the powers of life were failing, afford no obscure intimation.

The angina pectoris, as far as I have been able to investigate, belongs to the class of spasmodic, not of inflammatory complaints. For,

In the 1st place, the access and the recess of the fit is sudden.

2dly, There are long intervals of perfect health.

3dly, Wine, and spiritous liquors, and opium, afford considerable relief.

4thly, It is increased by disturbance of the mind.

5thly, It continues many years without any other injury to the health.

6thly, In the beginning it is not brought on by riding on horseback, or in a carriage, as is usual in diseases arising from scirrhus, or inflammation.

7thly, During the fit the pulse is not quickened.

Lastly, Its attacks are often after the first sleep; which is a circumstance common to many spasmodic disorders.

Yet it is not to be denied that I have met with one or two patients, who have told me they now and then spit up matter and blood, and that it seemed to them to come from the seat of the disease. In another, who fell down dead without any notice, there immediately arose such an offensive smell, as made all who were present judge that some foul abscess had just been broken.

On opening the body of one, who died suddenly of this disease, a very skilful anatomist could discover no fault in the heart, in the valves, in the arteries, or neighbouring veins, excepting small rudiments of ossification in the aorta. The brain was likewise every where sound. In this person, as it has happened to others who have died by the same disease, the blood continued fluid two or three days after death, not dividing itself into crassamentum and serum, but thick, like cream. Hence when a vein has been opened a little before death, or perhaps soon after, the blood has continued to ooze out as long as the body remained unburied.

With respect to the treatment of this complaint, I have little or nothing to advance: nor indeed is it to be expected we should have made much progress in the cure of a disease, which has hitherto hardly had a place, or a name in medical books.* Quiet, and warmth, and spiritous liquors help to restore patients who are nearly exhausted, and to dispel the effects of a fit when it does not soon go off. Opium taken at bed-time will prevent the attacks at night. I know one who set himself a task of sawing wood for half an hour every day, and was nearly cured. In one also, the disorder ceased of itself. Bleeding, vomiting and purging, appear to me to be improper.

*Cœlius Aurelianus, as far as I know, is the only ancient writer who has noticed this complaint, and he but slightly: "Erasistratus memorat paralyseos genus, et *paradoxon* appellat, quo ambulantes repente sistuntur, ut ambulare non possint, et tum rursum ambulare sinuntur."—*Chron.* lib. ii. c. 1.—M. Saussure in his *Voyage dans les Alpes* says, that at the height of 13 or 1,400 toises above the sea, a peculiar tiredness often comes upon those who are ascending such high hills, so that it is impossible to proceed four steps further; and if it were attempted, such strong universal palpitations would come on, as could not fail to end in swooning. Upon resting three minutes, even without sitting down, this tiredness passes, and the power of going on is perfectly restored. The climbing of steep hills, which are not so high above the sea, does not occasion this peculiar fatigue.—Vol. i. p. 482.

1785

WILLIAM WITHERING

AN ACCOUNT OF THE FOXGLOVE

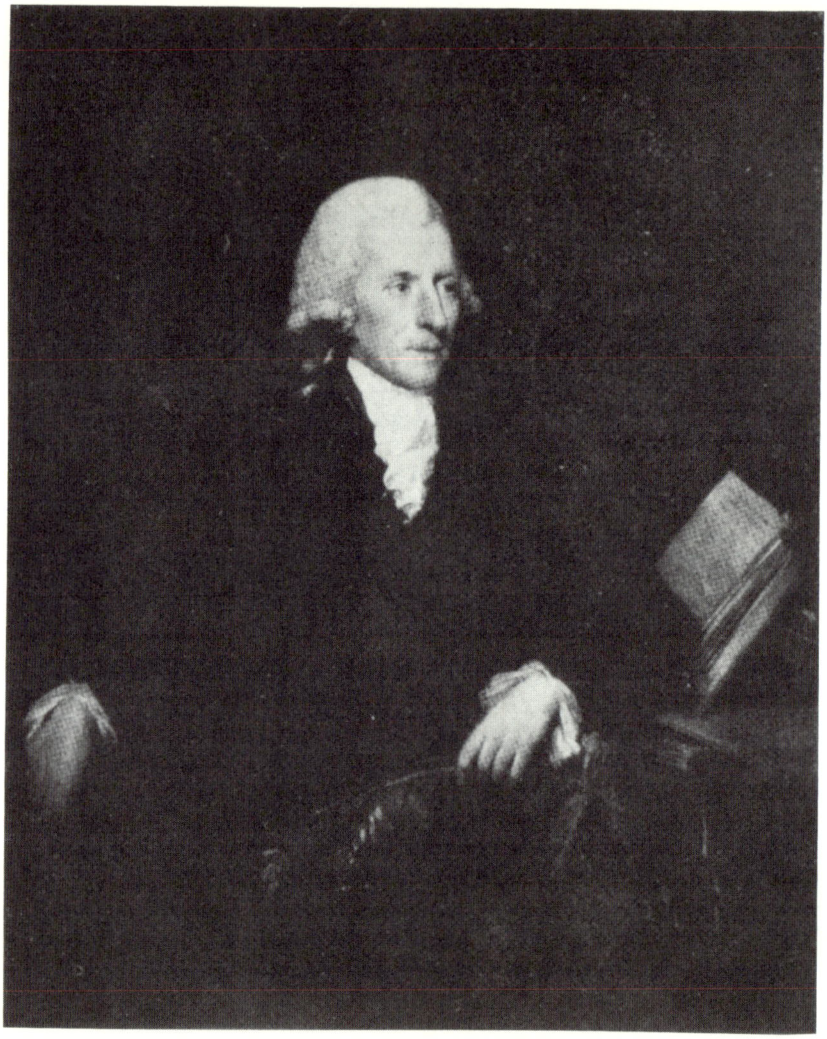

WILLIAM WITHERING

Painting by Carl Fredrik von Breda in the National Museum, Stockholm

(Courtesy Dr. Drew Luten.)

WILLIAM WITHERING

(1741-1799)

"The Flower of Physicians."

ALTHOUGH he was only fifty-eight years of age at the time of his death, William Withering lived an abundant life, and the period in which he lived was a most interesting one. He saw the development of the steam engine, the use of gas lighting in Birmingham, the invention of the spinning jenny and the cotton gin. It was his destiny to live through both the American and French Revolutions and to have been sympathetic with the citizen classes who fought for their freedom. Moreover, he was a contemporary of such men as the elder Pitt, Burke, Samuel Johnson, Goldsmith, Robert Burns, Voltaire, Washington, Haydn, Beethoven, Mozart, Franklin, and Linnaeus.

William Withering was born at Wellington in Shropshire in 1741. According to Cushny, Withering's father, Edmund Withering, was an apothecary, but it is apparent that the father practiced medicine.[1] Withering's maternal uncle was a physician in Lichfield. His mother's father, Dr. George Hector, had delivered Samuel Johnson. Thus, early in life, William Withering made contact with the profession which was his eventual choice.

Withering was tutored privately at home by the Rev. Henry Wood of Ercall. Such a method of preliminary education was a common practice in the eighteenth century. In 1762 he matriculated at the University of Edinburgh where he studied medicine. Edinburgh was the residence of David Hume (1711-1776), the famous Scotch philosopher and political economist, who during Withering's stay in this city was at the height of his brilliant career. Among Withering's professors were Hope in botany, Whytt (an authority on hysteria) in medicine, Alexander Monro "Secundus" (who in 1769 discovered the foramen of Monro) in anatomy, and Cullen in chemistry and medicine. Withering seems to have been on intimate terms with the last-named professor. William Cullen (1712-1790) held the chairs of medicine and chemistry at both Glasgow and Edinburgh. He was one of the first to give clinical lectures in Great Britain, and these lectures established a precedent in that they were delivered in English instead of in Latin. Cullen was a source of great admiration and inspiration to his pupils and it is of interest to know that he supported Withering in his therapeutic use of foxglove. Cullen was the teacher of Benjamin Rush (1745-1813), and it was Rush who introduced into America the complicated system of "fevers" as the basis for most diseases which Cullen had formulated and preached at Edinburgh. According to Shryock, the influence of Cullen, as transmitted through the teachings of his pupil, Rush, had an effect on American clinical medicine that endured for a generation. Withering received the degree of Doctor of Physic in 1766; his thesis was "De Angina Gangraenosa" (malignant putrid sore throat).

From 1767 until 1775 Withering practiced medicine at Stafford. It was here that he began studying the local flora and soon he became an expert in botany. During this time he was compiling notes for his first book, "A Botanical Arrangement of

[1]Roddis and other biographers say that he was a physician with a highly successful practice at Wellington.

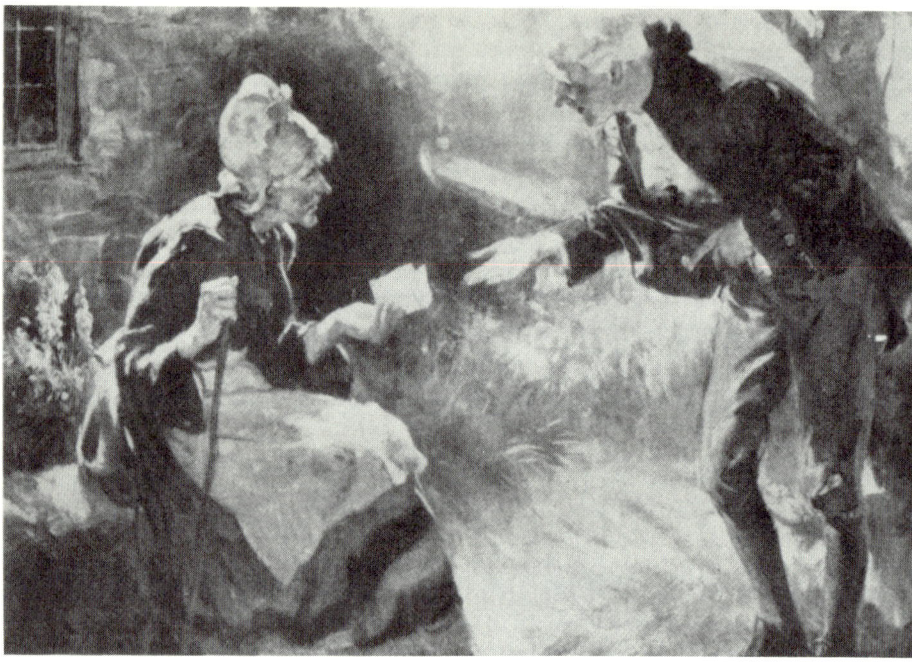

WILLIAM WITHERING RECEIVING FROM OLD MOTHER HUTTON OF SHROPSHIRE THE RECIPE FOR HER HERB TEA WHICH HAD "RELIEVED AN OXFORD DEAN OF HIS DROPSY"

(Courtesy Parke, Davis and Co.)

(It will be noted, on p. 238 of this work, that Withering himself does not say that he actually visited or met this old lady, although he does mention Shropshire, and also Dr. Cawley, of Oxford, who "had been cured of a Hydrops Pectoris" by foxglove root.)

all the Vegetables Naturally Growing in Great Britain'' (London, 1776, v. 2). This was a masterful work and went through several editions. The author not only gave a description of the plants but also indicated uses to which they might be put and often cited references made to them by the poets.

Withering was very popular in Stafford, and it seems that his latent interest in botany had been revived not because of his course in the subject under Hope, a course which had been disagreeable to him, but because of his labors in supplying suitable flowers for a young lady to paint. The young lady was his patient, Helena Cook, whom he married in 1772.

Although he enjoyed his practice in Stafford and was the only physician at the county infirmary, the practice was a poor one, and counseled by Erasmus Darwin, Withering began the practice of medicine in Birmingham in 1775. At Birmingham, Withering found a congenial circle in the Lunar Society, of which the most eminent members were Joseph Priestley, the great chemist, and James Watt, who perfected the steam engine. Withering was very successful in the practice of medicine and soon he was reputed to have the best practice outside of London. He aided in the completion of the general hospital at Birmingham and at his own house on stated days he gave the poor free medical advice.

Withering's extensive practice caused him to travel day and night. While he traveled, he read and wrote. On winter nights, to aid him in his studying, he had a light installed in his carriage. In this manner he prepared his work, ''An Account of the Scarlet Fever and Sore Throat, or Scarlatina Anginosa'' (London, 1779). Withering also interested himself in chemistry and in mineralogy. In 1783 he translated a treatise by Bergman on mineralogy. To Withering's discovery of ''Terra Ponderosa'' (the natural barium carbonate), Werner, the German geologist, gave the name ''Witherite.'' In 1784 the Royal Society elected Withering a fellow and in 1791 the Linnaean Society similarly honored him (Cushny, p. 88).

In 1785, Withering published the little book, ''An Account of the Foxglove,'' which still has the greatest of interest to his profession and which, more than either his botanical or chemical work, entitles him to immortality. In this superb monograph on the foxglove (from which we reprint the more important parts) Withering states that his attention was drawn to digitalis in 1775 by the discovery that it was important in the cure of dropsy. This remedy was a decoction of herbs which an old woman in his native town, Shropshire, had compounded and used to cure the dropsy in instances in which qualified physicians had failed. After carefully analyzing the remedy, Withering found the important ingredient to be foxglove. After experimenting with foxglove at great length and satisfying himself as to his results, he prescribed it in his personal dispensary. Apparently, his interest was further stimulated by hearing that the drug had been employed successfully in the case of the principal of Brasenose College, Oxford. At first he made the leaves of the plant into a decoction, later into an infusion, and sometimes he used the powdered form. The use of digitalis quickly spread among Withering's friends in the profession at Birmingham and Edinburgh. In 1783 the drug made its appearance in the ''Edinburgh Pharmacopoeia.'' Erasmus Darwin, among others, used it (1785) and his son, Charles Darwin, the uncle of the great naturalist, also prescribed it at an early date.

On the basis of Withering's description of the patients he treated, it has been assumed that some of his patients suffered from auricular fibrillation. But Withering recommended the use of digitalis in dropsy and anasarca only, and was careful to state that it was valueless in the treatment of ovarian cysts and similar conditions. His book was a curb on the unqualified uses of digitalis which grew out of the tremendous popularity of the drug. Withering did not understand how this drug acted in dropsy nor did he differentiate its action on cardiac dropsy from its action on other forms of dropsy. At the same time he was aware that it exerted some action on the heart and that it retarded the pulse, for he wrote, ''That it has a power over the motion of the heart, to a degree yet unobserved in any other medicine, and that this power may be converted to salutary ends.''

Besides enjoying a large circle of friends in Birmingham, Withering maintained connections with many of his profession in London. His botanical work (ed. 2, 1787-1792) served to introduce him to many continental scientists; and the French botanist, L'Heritier de Brutelle, named a genus of plants Witheringia in his honor.

In politics Withering was a moderate progressive and held the viewpoint that the constitution under George III required some modifications. In spite of this viewpoint and probably because he was sympathetic to the French revolutionists, Withering's house was attacked and he was forced to leave when the home of Priestley was burned in 1791 by a mob. He succeeded, however, in carrying off his most precious books and herbariums in wagons camouflaged with straw.

Withering suffered from tuberculosis of the lungs which finally undermined his health in 1780. Because of this, he chose to retire from active practice in 1783. From 1790 to 1791 he had repeated attacks of pleurisy and from this time onward his strength declined. In 1792 he spent the winter in Lisbon, Portugal, to try the effect of a warmer climate on his health. At Lisbon he continued his botanical studies and also made an analysis of the waters of the springs at Caldas da Rainha. Withering was not favorably impressed by the climate at Lisbon as a cure for phthisis and felt he had obtained little benefit from his stay. He returned there, however, for the winter of 1793.

In 1794 his health grew worse; he had inflammatory pulmonary attacks, dyspnea, and repeated hemoptysis. His health seemed to improve in 1795, so that he was able to publish in 1796 the third edition of his ''Arrangement of British Plants,'' this time expanded to four volumes. From 1797 to 1798 his illness grew worse and he was so dyspneic that even writing was difficult for him. He died on October 6, 1799, after twenty-five years of illness. He was buried in the old church at Edgbaston. In this church is a monument inscribed in his name and encircled with the Witheringia and the purple foxglove of which he wrote.

AN

ACCOUNT

OF THE

FOXGLOVE,

AND

Some of its Medical Ufes:

WITH

PRACTICAL REMARKS ON DROPSY, AND OTHER DISEASES.

BY

WILLIAM WITHERING, M. D.
Phyfician to the General Hofpital at Birmingham.

——*nonumque prematur in annum.*
HORACE.

BIRMINGHAM: PRINTED BY M. SWINNEY;
FOR
G. G. J. AND J. ROBINSON, PATERNOSTER-ROW, LONDON.
M,DCC,LXXXV.

AN ACCOUNT OF THE FOXGLOVE*

PREFACE

AFTER being frequently urged to write upon this subject, and as often declining to do it, from apprehension of my own inability, I am at length compelled to take up the pen, however unqualified I may still feel myself for the task.

The use of the Foxglove is getting abroad, and it is better the world should derive some instruction, however imperfect, from my experience, than that the lives of men should be hazarded by its unguarded exhibition, or that a medicine of so much efficacy should be condemned and rejected as dangerous and unmanageable.

It is now ten years since I first began to use this medicine. Experience and cautious attention gradually taught me how to use it. For the last two years I have not had occasion to alter the modes of management; but I am still far from thinking them perfect.

It would have been an easy task to have given select cases, whose successful treatment would have spoken strongly in favour of the medicine, and perhaps been flattering to my own reputation. But Truth and Science would condemn the procedure. I have therefore mentioned every case in which I have prescribed the Foxglove, proper or improper, successful or otherwise. Such a conduct will lay me open to the censure of those who are disposed to censure, but it will meet the approbation of others, who are the best qualified to be the judges.

To the Surgeons and Apothecaries, with whom I am connected in practice, both in this town and at a distance, I beg leave to make this public acknowledgement, for the assistance they so readily afforded me, in perfecting some of the cases, and in communicating the events of others.

The ages of the patients are not always exact, nor would the labour of making them so have been repaid by any useful consequences. In a few instances accuracy in that respect was necessary, and there it has been attempted; but in general, an approximation towards the truth, was supposed to be sufficient.

The cases related from my own experience, are generally written in the shortest form I could contrive, in order to save time and labour. Some of them are given more in detail, when particular circumstances made such detail necessary; but the cases communicated by other practitioners, are given in their own words.

*Withering, William: *An Account of the Foxglove,* London, 1785.

I must caution the reader, who is not a practitioner in physic, that no general deductions, decisive upon the failure or success of the medicine, can be drawn from the cases I now present to him. These cases must be considered as the most hopeless and deplorable that exist; for physicians are seldom consulted in chronic diseases, till the usual remedies have failed: and, indeed, for some years, whilst I was less expert in the management of the Digitalis, I seldom prescribed it, but when the failure of every other method compelled me to do it; so that upon the whole, the instances I am going to adduce, may truly be considered as cases lost to the common run of practice, and only snatched from destruction, by the efficacy of the Digitalis; and this in so remarkable a manner, that, if the properties of that plant had not been discovered, by far the greatest part of these patients must have died.

There are men who will hardly admit of anything which an author advances in support of a favorite medicine, and I allow they may have some cause for their hesitation; nor do I expect they will wave their usual modes of judging upon the present occasion. I could wish therefore that such readers would pass over what I have said, and attend only to the communications from correspondents, because they cannot be supposed to possess any unjust predilection in favor of the medicine: but I cannot advise them to this step, for I am certain they would then close the book, with much higher notions of the efficacy of the plant than they would have learnt from me. Not that I want faith in the discernment or in the veracity of my correspondents, for they are men of established reputation; but the cases they have sent me are, with some exceptions, too much selected. They are not upon this account less valuable in themselves, but they are not the proper premises from which to draw permanent conclusions.

I wish the reader to keep in view, that it is not my intention merely to introduce a new diuretic to his acquaintance, but one which, though not infallible, I believe to be much more certain than any other in present use.

After all, in spite of opinion, prejudice, or error, *Time* will fix the real value upon this discovery, and determine whether I have imposed upon myself and others, or contributed to the benefit of science and mankind.

Birmingham, 1st July, 1785.

INTRODUCTION

The Foxglove is a plant sufficiently common in this island, and as we have but one species, and that so generally known, I should have thought it superfluous either to figure or describe it; had I not more than once seen the leaves of Mullein* gathered for those of the Foxglove. On the continent of Europe too, other species are found, and I have been informed

*Verbascum of Linnaeus.

that our species is very rare in some parts of Germany, existing only by means of cultivation, in gardens.

Our plant is the *Digitalis purpurea*† of Linnaeus. It belongs to the 2d order of the 14th class, or the *Didynamia Angiospermia.* The *essential characters* of the genus are, *Cup with 5 divisions. Blossom bell-shaped, bulging. Capsule egg-shaped, 2-celled.—Linn.*

DIGITALIS purpurea. Little leaves of the empalement egg-shaped, sharp. Blossoms blunt; the upper lip entire. *Linn.*

. . . .

I have not observed that any of our cattle eat it. The root, the stem, the leaves, and the flowers have a bitter herbaceous taste, but I don't perceive that nauseous bitter which has been attributed to it.

This plant ranks amongst the LURIDAE, one of the Linnaean orders in a natural system. It has for congenera, *Nicotiana, Atropa, Hyoscyamus, Datura, Solanum,* etc. so that from the knowledge we possess of the virtues of those plants, and reasoning from botanical analogy, we might be led to guess at something of its properties.

I intended in this place to have traced the history of its effects in diseases from the time of Fuchsius, who first describes it, but I have been anticipated in this intention by my very valuable friend, Dr. Stokes of Stourbridge, who has lately sent me the following.

HISTORICAL VIEW OF THE PROPERTIES OF DIGITALIS

Fuchsius in his *hist. stirp.* 1542, is the first author who notices it. From him it receives its name of *Digitalis,* in allusion to the German name of *Fingerhut,* which signifies a finger-stall, from the blossoms resembling the finger of a glove.

Sensible Qualities. Leaves bitterish, very nauseous. *Lewis Mat. med.* I. 342.

Sensible Effects. Some persons, soon after eating of a kind of omolade, into which the leaves of this, with those of several other plants, had entered as an ingredient, found themselves much indisposed, and were presently after attacked with vomitings. *Dodonaeus pempt.* 170.

It is a medicine which is proper only for strong constitutions, as it purges very violently, and excites excessive vomitings. *Ray. hist.* 767.

Boerhaave judges it to be of a poisonous nature, *hist. plant.* but Dr. Alston ranks it among those indigenous vegetables, "which, though now disregarded, are medicines of great virtue, and scarcely inferior to any that the Indies afford." *Lewis Mat. med.* I. p. 343.

Six or seven spoonfuls of the decoction produce nausea and vomiting, and purge; not without some marks of a deleterious quality.—*Haller hist. n.* 330 from *Aerial Infl.* p. 49, 50.

---

†The trivial name *purpurea* is not a very happy one, for the blossoms though generally purple, are sometimes of a pure white.

The following is an abridged *Account of its Effects upon Turkeys.*

M. Salerne, a physician at Orleans, having heard that several turkey pouts had been killed by being fed with Foxglove leaves, instead of mullein, he gave some of the same leaves to a large vigorous turkey. The bird was so much affected that he could not stand upon his legs, he appeared drunk, and his excrements became reddish. Good nourishment restored him to health in eight days.

Being then determined to push the experiment further, he chopped some more leaves, mixed them with bran, and gave them to a vigorous turkey cock which weighed seven pounds. This bird soon appeared drooping and melancholy; his feathers stared, his neck became pale and retracted. The leaves were given him for four days, during which time he took about half a handful. These leaves had been gathered about eight days, and the winter was far advanced. The excrements, which are naturally green and well formed, became, from the first, liquid and reddish, like those of a dysenteric patient.

The animal refusing to eat any more of this mixture which had done him so much mischief, I was obliged to feed him with bran and water only; but notwithstanding this, he continued drooping, and without appetite. At times he was seized with convulsions, so strong as to throw him down; in the intervals he walked as if drunk; he did not attempt to perch, he uttered plaintive cries. At length he refused all nourishment. On the fifth or sixth day the excrements became as white as chalk; afterwards yellow, greenish, and black. On the eighteenth day he died, greatly reduced in flesh, for he now weighed only three pounds.

On opening him we found the heart, the lungs, the liver, and gall-bladder shrunk and dried up; the stomach was quite empty, but not deprived of its villous coat.—*Hist. de l'Academ.* 1748, p. 84.

Epilepsy.—"It hath beene of later experience found also to be effectual against the falling sicknesse, that divers have been cured thereby; for after the taking of *Decoct. manipulor. ii. c. polypod. quercin. contus. Ziv. in cerevisia,* they that have been troubled with it twenty-six years, and have fallen once in a weeke, or two or three times in a moneth, have not fallen once in fourteen or fifteen moneths, that is until the writing hereof."—*Parkinson,* p. 654.

Scrophula.—"The herb bruised, or the juice made up into an ointment, and applied to the place, hath been found by late experience to be availeable for the King's Evill."—*Park.* p. 654.

Several hereditary instances of this disease said to have been cured by it. *Aerial Influences,* p. 49, 50, quoted by *Haller, hist. n.* 330.

A man with *scrophulous ulcers* in various parts of the body, and which in the right leg were so virulent that its amputation was proposed, cured by *succ. express. cochl. i. bis intra xiv. dies, in ½ pinta cerevisiae calidae.*

The leaves remaining after the pressing out of the juice, were applied every day to the ulcers.—*Pract. ess.* p. 40, quoted by *Murray apparat. medicam. i.* p. 491.

A young woman with a *scrophulous tumour of the eye,* a remarkable *swelling of the upper lip, and painful tumours of the joints of the fingers,* much relieved; but the medicine was left off, on account of its violent effects on the constitution.—*Ib.* p. 42 quoted as above.

A man with a *scrophulous tumour of the right elbow,* attended for three years *with excruciating pains,* was nearly cured by four doses of the juice taken once a month.—*Ib.* p. 43. as above.

The physicans and surgeons of the Worcester Infirmary have employed it in ointments and poultices with remarkable efficacy.—*Ib.* p. 44. It was recommended to them by Dr. Baylies of Evesham, now of Berlin, as a remedy for this disease. Dr. Wall gave it a tryal, as well externally as internally, but their experiments did not lead them to observe any other properties in it, than those of a highly nauseating medicine and drastic purgative.

Wounds. In considerable estimation for the healing of all kinds of wounds.—*Lobel. adv.* 245.

Principally of use in ulcers, which discharge considerably, being of little advantage in such as are dry.—*Hulse,* in R. hist. 768.

Doctor Baylies, physician to his Prussian Majesty, informed me, when at Berlin, that he employed it with great success in caries, and obstinate sore legs.

Dyspnoea Pituitosa Sauvages I. 657.—"Boiled in water, or wine, and drunken doth cut and consume the thicke toughnesse of grosse, and slimie flegme, and naughtie humours. The same, or boiled with honied water or sugar, dǒth scoure and clense the brest, ripeneth and bring foorth tough and clammie flegme. It openeth also the stoppage of the liver spleene and milt, and of the inwarde parts."—*Gerarde hist.* ed. 1, p. 647.

"Whensoever there is need of a rarefying or extenuating of tough flegme or viscous humours troubling the chest,—the decoction or juice hereof made up with sugar or honey is availeable, as also to clense and purge the body both upwards and downwards sometimes, of tough flegme, and clammy humours, notwithstanding that these qualities are found to bee in it, there are but few physitions in our times that put it to these uses, but it is in a manner wholly neglected."—*Parkinson,* p. 654.

Previous to the year 1777, you informed me of the great success you had met with in curing dropsies by means of the fol. Digitalis, which you then considered as a more certain diuretic than any you had ever tried. Sometime afterwards, Mr. Russel, surgeon, of Worcester, having heard of the success which had attended some cases in which you had given it, requested me to obtain for him any information you might be inclined to communicate respecting its use. In consequence of this application, you wrote to me in the following terms.

In a letter which I received from you in London, dated September 29, 1778, you write as follows:—"I wish it was as easy to write upon the Digitalis—I despair of pleasing myself or instructing others, in a subject so difficult. It is much easier to write upon a disease than upon a remedy. The former is in the hands of nature, and a faithful observer, with an eye of tolerable judgement, cannot fail to delineate a likeness. The latter will ever be subject to the whims, the inaccuracies, and the blunders of mankind."

In my notes I find the following memorandum—"February 20th, 1779, gave an account of Doctor Withering's practice, with the precautions necessary to its success, to the Medical Society at Edinburgh."—In the course of that year, the Digitalis was prescribed in the Edinburgh Infirmary, by Dr. Hope, and in the following year, whilst I was Clerk to Dr. Home, as Clinical Professor, I had a favourable opportunity of observing its sensible effects.

In one case in which it was given properly at first, the urine began to flow freely on the second day. On the third, the swellings began to subside. The dose was then increased more than *quadruple* in the twenty-four hours. On the fifth day sickness came on, and much purging, but the urine still increased though the pulse sunk to 50. On the 7th day, a *quadruple* dose of the infusion was ordered to be taken every third hour, so as to bring on nausea again. The pulse fell to forty-four, and at length to thirty-five in a minute. The patient gradually sunk and died on the sixteenth day; but previous to her death, for two or three days, her pulse rose to near one hundred.—It is needless to observe to you, how widely the treatment of this case differed from the method which you have found so successful.

. . . .

AN ACCOUNT OF THE INTRODUCTION OF FOXGLOVE INTO MODERN PRACTICE

As the more obvious and sensible properties of plants, such as colour, taste, and smell, have but little connexion with the diseases they are adapted to cure; so their peculiar qualities have no certain dependence upon their external configuration. Their chemical examination by fire, after an immense waste of time and labour, having been found useless, is now abandoned by general consent. Possibly other modes of analysis will be found out, which may turn to better account; but we have hitherto made only a very small progress in the chemistry of animal and vegetable substances. Their virtues must therefore be learnt, either from observing their effects upon insects and quadrupeds; from analogy, deduced from the already known powers of some of their congenera, or from the empirical usages and experience of the populace.

The first method has not yet been much attended to; and the second can only be perfected in proportion as we approach towards the discovery of a truly natural system; but the last, as far as it extends, lies within the reach of every one who is open to information, regardless of the source from whence it springs.

It was a circumstance of this kind which first fixed my attention on the Foxglove.

In the year 1775, my opinion was asked concerning a family receipt for the cure of the dropsy. I was told that it had long been kept a secret by an old woman in Shropshire, who had sometimes made cures after the more regular practitioners had failed. I was informed also, that the effects produced were violent vomiting and purging; for the diuretic effects seemed to have been overlooked. This medicine was composed of twenty or more different herbs; but it was not very difficult for one conversant in these subjects, to perceive, that the active herb could be no other than Foxglove.

My worthy predecessor in this place, the very humane and ingenious Dr. Small, had made it a practice to give his advice to the poor during one hour in a day. This practice, which I continued until we had an Hospital opened for the reception of the sick poor, gave me an opportunity of putting my ideas into execution in a variety of cases; for the number of poor who thus applied for advice, amounted to between two and three thousand annually. I soon found the Foxglove to be a very powerful diuretic; but then, and for a considerable time afterwards, I gave it in doses very much too large, and urged its continuance too long; for misled by reasoning from the effects of the squill, which generally acts best upon the kidneys when it excites nausea, I wished to produce the same effect by the Foxglove. In this mode of prescribing, when I had so many patients to attend to in the space of one, or at most of two hours, it will not be expected that I could be very particular, much less could I take notes of all the cases which occurred. Two or three of them only, in which the medicine succeeded, I find mentioned amongst my papers. It was from this kind of experience that I ventured to assert, in the Botanical Arrangement published in the course of the following spring, that the Digitalis purpurea "merited more attention than modern practice bestowed upon it."

I had not, however, yet introduced it into the more regular mode of prescription; but a circumstance happened which accelerated that event. My truly valuable and respectable friend, Dr. Ash, informed me that Dr. Cawley, then principal of Brazen Nose College, Oxford, had been cured of a Hydrops Pectoris, by an empirical exhibition of the root of the Foxglove, after some of the first physicians of the age had declared they could do no more for him. I was now determined to pursue my former ideas more vigorously than before, but was too well aware of the uncertainty which must attend on the exhibition of the *root* of a *biennial* plant, and therefore continued to use the *leaves*. These I had found to vary much as to dose, at different seasons of the year; but I expected, if gathered always in one condition of the plant, viz. when it was in its flowering state, and carefully dried, that the dose might be ascertained as exactly as that of any other medicine; nor have I been disappointed in this expectation. The more I saw of the great powers of this plant, the more it seemed necessary to bring the doses of it to the greatest possible accuracy. I suspected that this degree of accuracy was not reconcileable with the use of a *decoction,* as it depended not only upon the care of those who had the preparation of it, but it was easy to conceive from the analogy of another plant of the same natural order, the tobacco, that its active properties might be impaired by long boiling. The decoction was therefore discarded, and the *infusion* substituted in its place. After this I began to use the leaves in *powder,* but I still very often prescribe the infusion.

Further experience convinced me, that the *diuretic* effects of this medicine do not at all depend upon its exciting a nausea or vomiting; but, on the contrary, that though the increased secretion of urine will frequently succeed to, or exist along with these circumstances, yet they are so far from being friendly or necessary, that I have often known the discharge of urine checked, when the doses have been imprudently urged so as to occasion sickness.

If the medicine purges, it is almost certain to fail in its desired effect; but this having been the case, I have seen it afterwards succeed when joined with small doses of opium, so as to restrain its action on the bowels.

In the summer of the year 1776, I ordered a quantity of the leaves to be dried, and as it then became possible to ascertain its doses, it was gradually adopted by the medical practitioners in the circle of my acquaintance.

In the month of November 1777, in consequence of an application from that very celebrated surgeon, Mr. Russel, of Worcester, I sent him the following account, which I choose to introduce here, as showing the ideas I then entertained of the medicine, and how much I was mistaken as to its real dose.—"I generally order it in decoction. Three drams of the dried leaves, collected at the time of the blossoms expanding, boiled in twelve to eight ounces of water. Two spoonfuls of this medicine, given every two hours, will sooner or later excite a nausea. I have sometimes used the green leaves gathered in winter, but then I order three times the weight; and in one instance I used three ounces to a pint decoction, before the desired effect took place. I considered the Foxglove thus given, as the most certain diuretic I know, nor do its diuretic effects depend merely upon the nausea it produces, for in cases where squill and ipecac have been so given as to keep up a nausea several days together, and the flow of urine not taken place, I have found the Foxglove to succeed; and I have, in more than one instance, given the Foxglove in smaller and more distant doses, so that the flow of urine has taken place without any sensible affection of the stomach; but in general I give it in the manner first mentioned, and order one dose to be taken after the sickness commences. I then omit all medicines, except those of the cordial kind are wanted, during the space of three, four, or five days. By this time the nausea abates, and the appetite becomes better than it was before. Sometimes the brain is considerably affected by the medicine, and indistinct vision ensues; but I have never yet found any permanent bad effects from it.''

''I use it in the Ascites, Anasarca, and Hydrops Pectoris; and so far as the removal of the water will contribute to cure the patient, so far may be expected from this medicine: but I wish it not to be tried in ascites of female patients, believing that many of these cases are dropsies of the ovaria; and no sensible man will ever expect to see these encysted fluids removed by any medicine.''

''I have often been obliged to evacuate the water repeatedly in the same patient, by repeating the decoction; but then this has been at such distance of time as to allow of the interference of other medicines and a proper regimen, so that the patient obtains in the end a perfect cure. In these cases the decoction becomes at length so very disagreeable, that a much smaller quantity will produce the effect, and I often find it necessary to alter its taste by the addition of Aq. Cinnam. sp. or Aq. Juniper. composita.''

''I allow, and indeed enjoin my patients to drink very plentifully of small liquors through the whole course of the cure; and sometimes, where the evacuations have been very sudden, I have found a bandage as necessary as in the use of the trochar.''

Early in the year 1779, a number of dropsical cases offered themselves to my attention, the consequences of the scarlet fever and sore throat which had raged so very generally amongst us in the preceding year. Some of these had been cured by squills or other diuretics, and relapsed; in others, the dropsy did not appear for several weeks after the original disease had ceased: but I am not able to mention many particulars, having omitted to make notes. This, however, is the less to be regretted, as the symptoms in all were very much alike, and they were all without an exception cured by the Foxglove.

This last circumstance encouraged me to use the medicine more frequently than I had done heretofore, and the increase of practice had taught me to improve the management of it.

In February 1779, my friend, Dr. Stokes, communicated to the Medical Society at Edinburgh the result of my experience of the Foxglove; and, in a letter addressed to me in November following, he says, ''Dr. Hope, in consequence of my mentioning its use to my friend, Dr. Broughton, has tried the Foxglove in the Infirmary with success." Dr. Stokes also tells me that Dr. Hamilton cured dropsies with it in the year 1781.

I am informed by my very worthy friend Dr. Duncan, that Dr. Hamilton, who learnt its use from Dr. Hope, has employed it very frequently in the Hospital at Edinburgh. Dr. Duncan also tells me, that the late very ingenious and accomplished Mr. Charles Darwin, informed him of its being used by his father and myself, in cases of Hydrothorax, and that he has ever since mentioned it in his lectures, and sometimes employed it in his practice.

At length, in the year 1783, it appeared in the new edition of the Edinburgh Pharmacopoeia, into which, I am told, it was received in consequence of the recommendation of Dr. Hope. But from which, I am satisfied, it will be again very soon rejected, if it should continue to be exhibited in the unrestrained manner in which it has heretofore been used at Edinburgh, and in the enormous doses in which it is now directed in London.

In the following cases the reader will find other diseases besides dropsies; particularly several cases of consumption. I was induced to try it in these, from being told, that it was much used in the West of England, in the Phthisis Pulmonalis, by the common people. In this disease, however, in my hands, it has done but little service, and yet I am disposed to wish it a further trial, for in a copy of Parkinson's Herbal, which I saw about two years ago, I found the following manuscript note at the article Digitalis, written I believe, by a Mr. Saunders, who practiced for many years with great reputation as a surgeon and apothecary at Stourbridge, in Worcestershire.

"Consumptions are cured infallibly by weak decoction of Foxglove leaves in water, or wine and water, and drank for constant drink. Or take of the juice of the herb and flowers, clarify it, and make a fine syrup with honey, of which take three spoonfuls thrice in a day, at physical hours. The use of these two things of late has done, in consumptive cases, great wonders. But be cautious of its use, for it is of a vomiting nature. In these things begin sparingly, and increase the dose as the patient's strength will bear, least, instead of a sovereign medicine, you do real damage by this infusion or syrup."

The precautions annexed to his encomiums of this medicine, lead one to think that he has spoken from his own proper experience.

I have lately been told, that a person in the neighborhood of Warwick, possesses a famous family receipt for the dropsy, in which the Foxglove is the active medicine; and a lady from the western part of Yorkshire assures me, that the people in her country often cure themselves of dropsical complaints by drinking Foxglove tea. In confirmation of this, I recollect about two years ago being desired to visit a travelling Yorkshire tradesman. I found him incessantly vomiting, his vision indistinct, his pulse forty in a minute. Upon enquiry it came out, that his wife had stewed a large handful of green Foxglove leaves in a half a pint of water, and given him the liquor, which he drank at one draught, in order to cure him of an asthmatic affection. This good woman knew the medicine of her country, but not the dose of it, for her husband narrowly escaped with his life.

It is probable that this rude mode of exhibiting the Foxglove has been more general than I am at present aware of; but it is wonderful that no author seems to have been acquainted with its effects as a diuretic.

. . . .

OF THE PREPARATIONS AND DOSES OF THE FOXGLOVE

Every part of the plant has more or less the same bitter taste, varying, however, as to strength, and changing with the age of the plant and the season of the year.

Root.—This varies greatly with the age of the plant. When the stem has shot up for flowering, which it does the second year of its growth, the root becomes dry, nearly tasteless, and inert.

Some practitioners, who have used the root, and been so happy as to cure their patients without exciting sickness, have been pleased to communicate the circumstance to me as an improvement in the use of the plant. I have no doubt of the truth of their remarks, and I thank them. But the case of Dr. Cawley puts this matter beyond dispute. The fact is, they have fortunately happened to use the root in its approach to its inert state, and consequently have not over dosed their patients. I could, if necessary, bring other proof to shew that the root is just as capable as the leaves, of exciting nausea.

Stem.—The stem has more taste than the root has, in the season the stem shoots out, and less taste than the leaves. I do not know that it has been particularly selected for use.

Leaves.—These vary greatly in their efficacy at different seasons of the year, and, perhaps, at different stages of their growth; but I am not certain that this variation keeps pace with the greater or lesser intensity of their bitter taste.

Some who have been habituated to the use of the recent leaves, tell me, that they answer their purpose at every season of the year; and I believe them, notwithstanding I myself have found very great variations in this respect. The solution of this difficulty is obvious. They have used the leaves in such large proportion, that the doses have been sufficient, or more than sufficient, even in their most inefficacious state. *The leaf-stalks* seem, in their sensible properties, to partake of an intermediate state between the leaves and the stem.

FLOWERS.—The petals, the chives, and the pointal have nearly the taste of the leaves, and it has been suggested to me, by a very sensible and judicious friend, that it might be well to fix on the flower for internal use. I see no objection to the proposition; but I have not tried it.

SEEDS.—These I believe are equally untried.

From this view of the different parts of the plant, it is sufficiently obvious why I still continue to prefer the leaves.

These should be gathered after the flowering stem has shot up, and about the time that the blossoms are coming forth.

The leaf-stalk and mid-rib of the leaves should be rejected, and the remaining part should be dried, either in the sun-shine, or on a tin pan or pewter dish before a fire.

If well dried, they readily rub down to a beautiful green powder, which weighs something less than one-fifth of the original weight of the leaves. Care must be taken that the leaves be not scorched in drying, and they should not be dried more than what is requisite to allow of their being readily reduced to powder.

I give to adults, from one to three grains of this powder twice a day. In the reduced state in which physicians generally find dropsical patients, four grains a day are sufficient. I sometimes give the powder alone; sometimes unite it with aromatics, and sometimes form it into pills with a sufficient quantity of soap or gum ammoniac.

If a liquid medicine be preferred, I order a dram of these dried leaves to be infused for four hours in half a pint of boiling water, adding to the strained liquor an ounce of any spiritous water. One ounce of this infusion given twice a day, is a medium dose for an adult patient. If the patient be stronger than usual, or the symptoms very urgent, this dose may be given once in eight hours; and on the contrary in many instances half an ounce at a time will be quite sufficient. About thirty grains of the powder or eight ounces of the infusion, may generally be taken before the nausea commences.

The ingenuity of man has ever been fond of exerting itself to vary the forms and combinations of medicines. Hence we have spirituous, vinous, and acetous tinctures; extracts hard and soft, syrups with sugar or honey, etc. but the more we multiply the forms of any medicine, the longer we shall be in ascertaining its real dose. I have no lasting objection however to any of these formulae except the extract, which, from the nature of its preparation must ever be uncertain in its effects; and a medicine whose fullest dose in substance does not exceed three grains, cannot be supposed to stand in need of condensation.

It appears from several of the cases, that when the Digitalis is disposed to purge, opium may be joined with it advantageously; and when the bowels are too tardy, jalap may be given at the same time without interfering with its diuretic effects; but I have not found benefit from any other adjunct.

From this view of the doses in which the Digitalis really ought to be exhibited, and from the evidence of many of the cases, in which it appears to have been given in quantities six, eight, ten or even twelve times more than necessary, we must admit as an inference either that this medicine is perfectly safe when given as I advise, or that the medicines in daily use are highly dangerous.

EFFECTS, RULES AND CAUTIONS

The Foxglove when given in very large and quickly repeated doses, occasions sickness, vomiting, purging, giddiness, confused vision, objects appearing green or yellow; increased secretion of urine, with frequent motions to part with it, and sometimes inability to retain it; slow pulse, even as slow as 35 in a minute, cold sweats, convulsions, syncope, death.*

When given in a less violent manner, it produces most of these effects in a lower degree; and it is curious to observe, that the sickness, with a certain dose of the medicine, does not take place for many hours after its exhibition has been discontinued; that the flow of urine will often precede, sometimes accompany, frequently follow the sickness at the distance of some days, and not infrequently be checked by it. The sickness thus excited, is extremely different from that occasioned by any other medicine; it is peculiarly distressing to the patient; it ceases, it recurs again as violent as before; and thus it will continue to recur for three or four days, at distant and more distant intervals.

These sufferings of the patient are generally rewarded by a return of appetite, much greater than what existed before the taking of the medicine.

But these sufferings are not at all necessary; they are the effects of our inexperience, and would in similar circumstances, more or less attend the exhibition of almost every active and powerful medicine we use.

Perhaps the reader will better understand how it ought to be given, from the following detail of my own improvement, than from precepts peremptorily delivered, and their source veiled in obscurity.

At first I thought it necessary *to bring on and continue the sickness in order to ensure the diuretic effects.*

I soon learnt that the nausea being once excited, it was unnecessary to repeat the medicine, as it was certain to recur frequently, at intervals more or less distant.

Therefore my patients were ordered *to persist until the nausea came on, and then to stop.* But it soon appeared that the diuretic effects would often take place first, and sometimes be checked when the sickness or a purging supervened.

The direction was therefore enlarged thus—*Continue the medicine until the urine flows, or sickness or purging takes place.*

---

*I am doubtful whether it does not sometimes excite a copious flow of saliva.

I found myself safe under this regulation for two or three years; but at length cases occurred in which the pulse would be retarded to an alarming degree, without any other preceding effect.

The directions therefore required an additional attention to the state of the pulse, and it was moreover of consequence not to repeat the doses too quickly, but to allow sufficient time for the effects of each to take place, as it was found very possible to pour in an injurious quantity of the medicine, before any of the signals for forbearance appeared.

Let the medicine therefore be given in the doses, and at the intervals mentioned above:—let it be continued until it either acts on the kidneys, the stomach, the pulse, or the bowels; let it be stopped upon the first appearance of any one of these effects, and I will maintain that the patient will not suffer from its exhibition, nor the practitioner be disappointed in any reasonable expectation.

If it purges, it seldom succeeds well.

The patient should be enjoined to drink very freely during its operation. I mean, they should drink whatever they prefer, and in as great quantity as their appetite for drink demands. This direction is the more necessary, as they are very generally prepossessed with an idea of drying up a dropsy, by abstinence from liquids, and fear to add to the disease, by indulging their inclination to drink.

In cases of ascites and anasarca; when the patients are weak, and the evacuation of the water rapid, the use of proper bandage is indispensably necessary to their safety.

If the water should not be wholly evacuated, it is best to allow an interval of several days before the medicine be repeated, that food and tonics may be administered; but truth compels me to say, that the usual tonic medicines have in these cases very often deceived my expectations.

From some cases which have occurred in the course of the present year, I am disposed to believe that the Digitalis may be given in small doses, viz. two or three grains a day, so as gradually to remove a dropsy, without any other than mild diuretic effects, and without any interruption to its use until the cure be completed.

If inadvertently the doses of the Foxglove should be prescribed too largely, exhibited too rapidly, or urged to too great a length; the knowledge of a remedy to counteract its effects would be a desirable thing. Such a remedy may perhaps in time be discovered. The usual cordials and volatiles are generally rejected from the stomach; aromatics and strong bitters are longer retained; brandy will sometimes remove the sickness when only slight; I have sometimes thought small doses of opium useful, but I am more confident of the advantage from blisters. Mr. Jones in one case, found mint tea to be retained longer than other things.

CONSTITUTION OF PATIENTS

Independent of the degree of disease, or of the strength or age of the patient, I have had occasion to remark, that there are certain constitutions favourable, and others unfavourable to the success of the Digitalis.

From large experience, and attentive observation, I am pretty well enabled to decide *a priori* upon this matter, and I wish to enable others to do the same: but I feel myself hardly equal to the undertaking. The following hints, however, aiding a degree of experience in others, may lead them to accomplish what I yet can describe but imperfectly.

It seldom succeeds in men of great natural strength, of tense fibre, of warm skin, of florid complexion, or in those with a tight and cordy pulse.

If the belly in ascites be tense, hard, and circumscribed, or the limbs in anasarca solid and resisting, we have but little to hope.

On the contrary, if the pulse be feeble or intermitting, the countenance pale, the lips livid, the skin cold, the swollen belly soft and fluctuating, or the anasarcous limbs readily pitting under the pressure of the finger, we may expect the diuretic effects to follow in a kindly manner.

In cases which foil every attempt at relief, I have been aiming, for some time past, to make such a change in the constitution of the patient, as might give a chance of success to the Digitalis.

By blood-letting, by neutral salts, by crystals of tartar, squills and occasional purging, I have succeeded, though imperfectly. Next to the use of the lancet, I think nothing lowers the tone of the system more effectually than the squill, and consequently it will always be proper, in such cases, to use the squill; for if that fail in its desired effect, it is one of the best preparatives to the adoption of the Digitalis.

A tendency to paralytic affections, or a stroke of the palsy having actually taken place, is no objection to the use of the Digitalis; neither does a stone existing in the bladder forbid its use. Theoretical ideas of sedative effects in the former, and apprehensions of its excitement of the urinary organs in the latter case, might operate so as to make us withhold relief from the patient; but experience tells me, that such apprehensions are groundless.

INFERENCES

To prevent any improper influence, which the above recitals of the efficacy of the medicine, aided by the novelty of the subject, may have upon the minds of the younger part of my readers, in raising their expectations to too high a pitch, I beg leave to deduce a few inferences, which I apprehend the facts will fairly support.

I. That the Digitalis will not universally act as a diuretic.

II. That it does do so more generally than any other medicine.

III. That it will often produce this effect after every other probable method has been fruitlessly tried.

IV. That if this fails, there is but little chance of any other medicine succeeding.

V. That in proper doses, and under the management now pointed out, it is mild in its operation, and gives less disturbance to the system than squill, or almost any other active medicine.

VI. That when dropsy is attended by palsy, unsound viscera, great debility, or other complication or disease, neither the Digitalis, nor any other diuretic can do more than obtain a truce to the urgency of the symptoms; unless by gaining time, it may afford opportunity for other medicines to combat and subdue the original disease.

VII. That the Digitalis may be used with advantage in every species of dropsy, except the encysted.

VIII. That it may be made subservient to the cure of diseases, unconnected with dropsy.

IX. That it has a power over the motion of the heart, to a degree yet unobserved in any other medicine, and that this power may be converted to salutary ends.

PRACTICAL REMARKS ON DROPSY, AND SOME OTHER DISEASES

The following remarks consist partly of matter of fact, and partly of opinion. The former will be permanent; the latter must vary with the detection of error, or the improvement of knowledge. I hazard them with diffidence, and hope they will be examined with candour; not by a contrast with other opinions, but by an attentive comparison with the phenomena of disease.

Anasarca

1. The anasarca is generally curable when seated in the sub-cutaneous cellular membrane, or in the substance of the lungs.

2. When the abdominal viscera in general are greatly enlarged, which they sometimes are, without effused fluid in the cavity of the abdomen; the disease is incurable. After death, the more solid viscera are found very large and pale. If the cavity contains water, that water may be removed by diuretics.

3. In swollen legs and thighs, where the resistance to pressure is considerable, the tendency to transparency in the skin not obvious, and where the alteration of posture occasions but little alteration in the state of distention, the cure cannot be effected by diuretics.

Is this difficulty of cure occasioned by spissitude in the effused fluids, by want of proper communication from cell to cell, or is the disease rather caused by a morbid growth of the solids, than by an accumulation of fluid?

Is not this disease in the limbs similar to that of the viscera (2)?

4. Anasarcous swellings often take place in palsied limbs, in arms as well as legs; so that the swelling does not depend merely upon position.

5. Is there not cause to suspect that many dropsies originate from paralytic affections of the lymphatic absorbents? And if so, is it not probable that the Digitalis, which is so effectual in removing dropsy, may also be used advantageously in some kinds of palsy?

Ascites

6. If existing alone (*i.e.*) without accompanying anasarca, is in children curable; in adults generally incurable by medicines. Tapping may be used here with better chance for success than in more complicated dropsies. Sometimes cured by vomiting.

Ascites and Anasarca

7. Incurable if dependent upon irremediably diseased viscera, or on a gouty constitution, so debilitated, that the gouty paroxysms no longer continue to be formed.

In every other situation the disease yields to diuretics and tonics.

Ascites, Anasarca, and Hydrothorax

8. Under this complication, though the symptoms admit of relief, the restoration of the constitution can hardly be hoped for.

Asthma

9. The true spasmodic asthma, a rare disease—is not relieved by Digitalis.

10. In the greater part of what are called asthmatical cases, the real disease is anasarca of the lungs, and is generally to be cured by diuretics. (See 1.) This is almost always combined with some swelling of the legs.

11. There is another kind of asthma, in which change of posture does not much affect the patient. I believe it to be caused by an infarction of the lungs. It is incurable by diuretics; but it is often accompanied with a degree of anasarca, and so far it admits of relief.

Is not this disease similar to that in the limbs at (3) and also to that of the abdominal viscera at (2)?

Asthma and Anasarca

12. If the asthma be of the kind mentioned at (9 and 11) diuretics can only remove the accompanying anasarca. But if the affection of the breath depends also upon cellular effusion, as it mostly does, the patient may be taught to expect a recovery.

Asthma and Ascites

13. A rare combination, but not incurable if the abdominal viscera are sound. The asthma is here most probably of the anasarcous kind (10);

and this being seldom confined to the lungs only, the disease generally appears in the following form.

Asthma, Ascites, and Anasarca

14. The curability of this combination will depend upon the circumstances mentioned in the preceding section, taking also into the account the strength or weakness of the patient.

Epilepsy

15. In epilepsy dependent upon effusion, the Digitalis will effect a cure; and in the cases alluded to, the dropsical symptoms were unequivocal. It has not had a sufficient trial in my hands, to determine what it can do in other kinds of epilepsy.

Hydatid Dropsy

16. This may be distinguished from common ascites, by the want of evident fluctuation. It is common to both sexes. It does not admit of a cure either by tapping or by medicine.

Hydrocephalus

17. This disease, which has of late so much attracted the attention of the medical world, I believe, originates in inflammation; and that the water found in the ventricles of the brain after death, is the consequence, and not the cause of the illness.

It has seldom happened to me to be called upon in the earlier stages of this complaint, and the symptoms are at first so similar to those usually attendant upon dentition and worms, that it is very difficult to pronounce decidedly upon the real nature of the disease; and it is rather from the failure of the usual modes of relief, than from any other more decided observation, that we at length dare to give it a name.

. . . .

Hydrothorax

18. Under this name I also include the dropsy of the pericardium. The intermitting pulse, and pain in the arms, sufficiently distinguish this disease from asthma, and from anasarcous lungs.

It is very universally cured by the Digitalis.

19. I lately met with two cases which had been considered and treated as angina pectoris. They both appeared to me to be cases of hydrothorax. One subject was a clergyman, whose strength had been so compleatly exhausted by the continuance of the disease, and the attempts to relieve it, that he did not survive many days. The other was a lady, whose time of life made me suspect effusion. I directed her to take small doses of the pulv. Digitalis, which in eight days removed all her complaints. This happened six months ago, and she remains perfectly well.

Hydrothorax and Anasarca

20. This combination is very frequent, and, I believe, may always be cured by the Digitalis.

21. Dropsies in the chest either with or without anasarcous limbs, are much more curable than those of the belly. Probably because the abdominal viscera are more frequently diseased in the latter than in the former cases.

Insanity

22. I apprehend this disease to be more frequently connected with serous effusion than has been commonly imagined.

. . . .

Nephritis Calculosa

24. We have had sufficient evidence of the efficacy of the Foxglove in removing the Dysuria and other symptoms of this disease; but probably it is not in these cases preferable to the tobacco.*

Ovarium Dropsy

25. This species of encysted dropsy is not without difficulty distinguishable from an ascites; and yet it is necessary to distinguish them, because the two diseases require different treatment and because the probability of a cure is much greater in one than in the other.

26. The ovarium dropsy is generally slow in its progress; for a considerable time the patient though somewhat emaciated, does not lose the appearance of health, and the urine flows in the usual quantity. It is seldom that the practitioner is called in early enough to distinguish by the feel on which side the cyst originated, and the patients do not attend to that circumstance themselves. They generally menstruate regularly in the incipient state of the disease, and it is not until the pressure from the sac becomes very great, that the urinary secretion diminishes. In this species of dropsy, the patients, upon being questioned, acknowledge even from a pretty early date, pains in the upper and inner parts of the thighs, similar to those which women experience in a state of pregnancy. These pains are for a length of time greater in one thigh than in the other, and I believe it will be found that the disease originated on that side.

27. The ovarium dropsy defies the power of medicine. It admits of relief, and sometimes of a cure, by tapping. I submit to the consideration of practitioners, how far we may hope to cure this disease by a seton or a caustic.

. . . .

28. When tapping becomes necessary, I always advise the adoption of the waist coat bandage or belt, invented by the late very justly celebrated

*See an original and valuable treatise by Dr. Fowler, entitled, *Medical Reports of the Effects of Tobacco.*

Dr. Monro, and described in the first volume of the Medical Essays. I also enjoin my patients to wear this bandage afterwards, from a persuasion that it retards the return of the disease. The proper use of bandage, when the disorder first discovers itself, certainly contributes much to prevent its increase.

Ovarium Dropsy With Anasarca

29. The anasarca does not appear until the encysted dropsy is very far advanced. It is then probably caused by weakness and pressure. The Digitalis removes it for a time.

Phthisis Pulmonalis

30. This is a very increasing malady in the present day. It is no longer limited to the middle part of life: children at five years of age die of it, and old people at sixty or seventy. It is not confined to the flat-chested, the fair-skinned, the blue-eyed, the light-haired, or the scrophulous: it often attacks people with full chests, brown skins, dark hair and eyes, and those in whose family no scrophulous taint can be traced. It is certainly infectious. The very strict laws still existing in Italy to prevent the infection from consumptive patients, were probably not enacted originally without a sufficient cause. We seem to be approaching to that state which first made such restrictions necessary, and in the further course of time, the disease will probably fall off again, both in virulency and frequency.

31. The younger part of the female sex are liable to a disease very much resembling a true consumption, and from which it is difficult to distinguish it; but this disease is curable by steel and bitters. A criterion of true phthisis has been sought for in the state of the teeth; but the exceptions to that rule are numerous. An unusual dilatation of the pupil of the eye, is the most certain characteristic.*

32. Sydenham asserts, that the bark did not more certainly cure an intermittent, than riding did a consumption. We must not deny the truth of an assertion, from such authority, but we must conclude that the disease was more easily curable a century ago than it is at present.

33. If the Digitalis is no longer useful in consumptive cases, it must be that I know not how to manage it, or that the disease is more fatal than formerly, for it would be hard to deny the testimony cited at [page 241]. I wish others would undertake the enquiry.

34. When phthisis is accompanied with anasarca, or when there is reason to suspect hydrothorax, the Digitalis will often relieve the sufferings, and prolong the life of the patient.

*Many years ago I communicated to my friend, Dr. Percival, an account of some trials of breathing fixed air in consumptive cases. The results were published by him in the second Vol. of his very useful *Essays Medical and Experimental,* and have since been copied into other publications. I take this opportunity of acknowledging that I suspect myself to have been mistaken in the nature of the disease there mentioned to have been cured. I believe it was a case of *Vomica,* and not a true *Phthisis* that was cured. The Vomica is almost always curable. The fixed air corrects the smell of the matter, and very shortly removes the hectic fever. My patients not only inspire it, but I keep large jars of the effervescing mixture constantly at work in their chambers.

35. Many years ago, during an attendance upon Mr. B----, of a consumptive family, and himself in the last stage of a phthisis; after he was so ill as to be confined to his chamber, his breathing became so extremely difficult and distressing, that he wished rather to die than to live, and urged me warmly to devise some mode to relieve him. Suspecting serous effusion to be the cause of his symptoms, and he being a man of sense and resolution, I fully explained my ideas to him, and told him what kind of operation might afford him a chance of relief; for I was then but little acquainted with the Digitalis. He was earnest for the operation to be tried, and with the assistance of Mr. Parrott, a very respectable surgeon of this place, I got an opening made between the ribs upon the lower and hinder part of the thorax. About a pint of fluid was immediately discharged, and his breath became easy. This fluid coagulated by heat.

After some days a copious purulent discharge issued from the opening, his cough became less troublesome, his expectoration less copious, his appetite and strength returned, he got abroad, and the wound, which became very troublesome, was allowed to heal.

He then undertook a journey to London; whilst there he became worse: returned home, and died consumptive some weeks afterwards.

Puerperal Anasarca

36. This disease admits of an easy and certain cure by the Digitalis.

37. This species of dropsy may originate from other causes than child birth. In the beginning of last March, a gentleman at Wolverhampton desired my advice for very large and painful swelled legs and thighs. He was a temperate man, not of a dropsical habit, had great pain in his groins, and attributed his complaints to a fall from his horse. He had taken diuretics, and the strongest drastic purgatives with very little benefit. Considering the anasarca as caused by the diseased inguinal glands, I ordered a common poultice and mercurial ointment to the groins, three grains of pulv. fol. Digitalis night and morning, and a cooling diuretic decoction in the day-time. He soon lost his pain, and the swellings gradually subsided.

THE END

1788

MATTHEW BAILLIE

DESCRIPTION OF A CASE OF CONGENITAL DEXTROCARDIA WITH COMPLETE SITUS-TRANSVERSUS

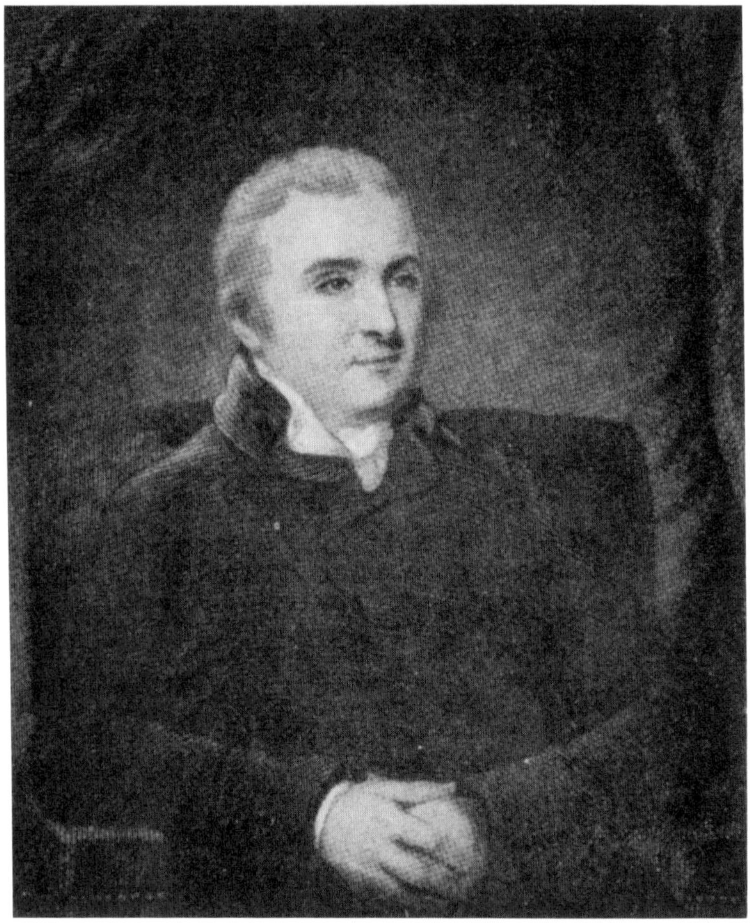

MATTHEW BAILLIE

From the portrait collection of Northwestern University Medical School

(Courtesy Petrolagar Laboratories.)

MATTHEW BAILLIE

(1761-1823)

IT IS of interest to note that Baillie wrote of the pertinent events concerning his own life, and the manuscript, in his own handwriting, is now in the Library of the Royal College of Surgeons of England. In 1896 it was printed in the "Practitioner." This illuminating account forms the basis for our brief discussion.

Matthew Baillie was born in the Manse of Shots and County of Lanark, Scotland, on October 27, 1761. His father, the Reverend Dr. James Baillie was, according to his son, "a man of the most respectable character." He ultimately became professor of divinity in the University of Glasgow.

Dorothea Baillie, the mother of Matthew, was a sister of William and John Hunter, the celebrated surgeons and anatomists; thus, early in life, Baillie received much genuine encouragement for his career in medicine.

Baillie's early education was obtained at Hamilton. There he studied first at the English School and later at the Latin School. At the age of thirteen, he became a student at the University of Glasgow. There he continued his study of Greek and Latin for a period of five years, receiving a thorough training in the classics and in philosophy.

In 1779, Baillie, acting on the advice of his uncle, Dr. William Hunter, decided to enter the profession of medicine. However, he had been appointed to an exhibition in Balliol College, Oxford, and for the next eighteen months he remained there, improving himself in the classics.

In 1780 he went to London to live with his uncle, Dr. William Hunter, and to attend his lectures in anatomy and dissections at the Great Windmill Street School. During the succeeding years he also studied chemistry, materia medica, and medicine under Dr. George Fordyce (1736-1802), who was, for several years, the most popular lecturer in London on these subjects. Baillie also attended the lectures on surgery given by his other uncle, John Hunter, and the lectures on midwifery which were given jointly by Dr. Thomas Denman (1733-1815) and Dr. William Osborne (1736-1808).

Dr. William Hunter died in March, 1783. He left Baillie a legacy of 5,000 pounds and a small estate in Scotland. Baillie, believing that his uncle, John Hunter, had a better claim to the estate, ceded it to him. Dr. Hunter had arranged through his will that Baillie should succeed him as lecturer in anatomy, in association with William Cumberland Cruikshank (1745-1800). At the Great Windmill Street School Baillie continued as lecturer in anatomy for fifteen years, in spite of the irascibility of his associate. Meanwhile, his private practice had increased and in 1799 he relinquished his anatomic lectures.

Shortly after his uncle's death, Baillie received the degree of Bachelor of Arts from Oxford University. He also received the degree of Bachelor of Medicine in 1786 and that of Doctor of Medicine in 1789, both from Oxford University.

In 1787 he was appointed physician at St. George's Hospital and in 1790 he received his fellowship in the Royal College of Physicians, London.

Baillie, in 1791, was married to Sophia, the youngest of twin daughters of Dr. Thomas Denman, under whom he had studied obstetrics. This marriage resulted in the birth of three children: James, Elizabeth Margaret, and William Hunter Baillie.

One of Baillie's patients was the celebrated Dr. David Pitcairn (1749-1809). When Pitcairn retired from the practice of medicine, because of ill health, he turned over much of his practice to Baillie.

Baillie's practice grew very rapidly and at length in order to attend all his patients he found it necessary to work from 6 o'clock in the morning until 11 o'clock each night. This state of practice lasted for a period of twelve years and was ruinous to Baillie's health. Soon he was obliged to confine his work to consultation.

In 1810, Baillie received the command of King George III to attend his daughter, the Princess Amelia, who died on November 2 of the same year. This was the beginning of his many attendances to the Royal family, for he was soon appointed physician extraordinary to the King.

In the summer of 1823, Baillie's health again failed, presumably because of continued overwork. A severe cough developed, apparently the result of an inflammation of the trachea. He died on September 23, 1823. A bust of him was made by Chantrey and placed in Westminster Abbey.

Baillie made important contributions to the medical literature. In 1788 and in 1789 he published two anatomic papers in the ''Philosophical Transactions'' of the Royal Society. The first of these was in the form of a letter to John Hunter entitled ''An Account of a Remarkable Transposition of the Viscera.'' This early observation of congenital dextrocardia with complete situs-transversus we are reprinting. According to Pettigrew, cases of a similar kind were recorded by Winslow, Sir Astley Cooper, Dr. Quain, Dr. Watson, and others. Baillie's second paper to the Royal Society was communicated by John Hunter. It was entitled ''An Account of a Particular Change of Structure in the Human Ovarium.'' In 1790, presumably because of these publications, Baillie was elected to the Royal Society.

In the year 1793 he published the first edition of his ''The Morbid Anatomy of Some of the Most Important Parts of the Human Body.'' During Baillie's lifetime this book went through several editions. In order to illustrate the subject of morbid anatomy on a systematic plan, Baillie began to publish ''fasciculi'' of engravings. Ten of these were published separately and in 1803 they appeared in book form. A second edition of this work appeared in 1812.

During his later years, Baillie contributed several articles to the ''Transactions'' of the Society for the Improvement of Medical and Chirurgical Knowledge and to the ''Transactions'' of the Royal College of Physicians.

In addition to membership in the Royal Society of London and the Royal Society of Edinburgh, Baillie was an honorary member of the Royal College of Physicians of Edinburgh, a Fellow of the Royal College of Physicians in London, a member of the Medico-Chirurgical Society in London, and an honorary member of the Medical Societies of Erlangen and Bonn.

OF A REMARKABLE TRANSPOSITION OF THE VISCERA*

By

MATTHEW BAILLIE

NOTHING tends more to illustrate the powers and the wisdom of nature than the investigation of the structure of animals. We there find a most wonderful delicacy of mechanism, and exquisitely adapted to a variety of purposes. This however is not to be better seen by following nature in her common track than by observing her wanderings. In these she often shows more particularly the extent of her powers, and throws light on her ordinary plans. Such circumstances give importance and value to the observation of singular phenomena. The variety in animal structure, an account of which is presented in this account, is a complete transposition in the human subject, of the thoracic and abdominal viscera, to the opposite side from what is natural. It is so extraordinary as scarcely to have been seen by any of the most celebrated anatomists, and indeed has been but very generally noticed at all. The circumstance has been mentioned, but it has not been particularly described so as to make it thoroughly known, or to establish its certainty. It was hanging in the minds of many as doubtful, whether such a variety did really exist. There is one circumstance that attends the account of the present case, which has not always happened in the record of singular phenomena, viz. that it has been examined by physicians and surgeons of the first reputation in this large town, and has been in some measure open to the gratification of public curiosity.

The person who is the subject of this paper was a male, nearly 40 years of age, somewhat above the middle stature, and of a clean active shape. He was brought for dissection in the common way to Windmill-street. On opening the cavity of the thorax and abdomen, the different situation of the viscera was so striking as immediately to excite the attention of the pupils who were engaged in dissecting it. I began immediately to examine every part of the change with considerable attention: for this purpose, after desiring a drawing to be made of the appearances as they were found on opening the body, I next day injected it.

The mediastinum, or anterior duplicature of the pleura, separating the 2 cavities of the chest from each other, was found to incline obliquely

*Phil. Tr. Roy. Soc., London **16**: 483-489, 1785-1790 (abridged 1809). (Original **78**: 350, 1788.)

downwards to the right side fully as much as it does commonly to the left side of the chest. The pericardium too inclined obliquely to the right side. On pressing it gently away from the lungs the phrenic nerves came distinctly into view, in their common situation; but the right phrenic nerve ran more obliquely, and was longer than the left. The lung on the right side was divided by a single oblique fissure into 2 lobes, having at the same time a deficiency opposite to the apex of the heart; and the lung on the left side was divided into 3 lobes, exactly contrary to what is found in ordinary cases.

On opening the pericardium the apex of the heart was found to point to the right side nearly opposite to the 6th rib, and its cavities as well as large vessels were completely transposed. What are commonly called the right auricle and ventricle were situated on the left side, and the left auricle and ventricle on the right. The pulmonary artery ascended towards the right side of the chest. The aorta was also directing its arch to the right; and the vena cava superior, as well as inferior, were seen opening into their auricle on the left side of the spine. There was nothing remarkable in the size or general figure of the heart. On the outside of the pericardium the transposition of the larger vessels was very striking. The longer subclavian vein was passing from the left side obliquely to the right before the branches which are sent off from the arch of the aorta. The left carotid and subclavian arteries were found to arise from the arch of the aorta by one common trunk; the right carotid and subclavian separately.

In the duplicature of the pleura behind, or what may be called the posterior mediastinum, there was a change corresponding to what we have already described. The descending aorta was found passing on the right side of the spine. The oesophagus was before it, inclining more and more to the right towards its lower extremity, and it at length perforated the diaphragm somewhat on the right side of the spine.* The thoracic duct was seen in the middle between the descending aorta and vena azygos, in some places forming a plexus of small branches, in another dividing itself into 2 branches, which afterwards re-united in a common trunk, and at length climbing up to terminate in the angle between the jugular and subclavian veins on the right side of the body. The recurrent nerve of the parvagum on the right side passed round the beginning of the descending aorta, and on the left passed round the common trunk of the carotid and subclavian arteries. The large intercostal nerves being exactly under the same circumstances on each side, it was impossible there could be any transposition in them. It appears then from the foregoing description, that every thing admitting of such a change was completely transposed in the thorax.

*The vena azygos was on the left side of the spine opening in the common way into the vena cava superior, which we formerly mentioned to be also transposed in its situation.—Orig.

The liver was situated in the left hypochondriac region, the small lobe being towards the right, and the great lobe in the left side. The ligaments uniting it to the diaphragm corresponded to this change, the right transverse ligament being longer, and the left being shorter, than usual. The suspensory ligament could undergo little change, except being pushed to the left side along with the liver. On pressing upwards the liver, so as to exhibit its posterior and under surface, the gall bladder was seen on the left side preserving its proper relative situation to the great lobe of the liver, and the vessels of the portae were found on dissection to be transposed corresponding to the change of circumstances. The hepatic artery was found climbing up obliquely from the right towards the left, before the lobulus spigelii, and entered at the portae into the substance of the liver by two or three branches on the right of the other vessels. The ductus communis cholidochus was on the left of the other vessels, being formed from the ductus hepaticus and ductus cysticus in the common way, and it passed obliquely downwards on the left, to terminate in the duodenum. What was most remarkable, it terminated in the fore part of the duodenum. The vena portarum passed behind the hepatic artery and ductus communis cholidochus, ascending obliquely towards the left side.

The spleen was situated in the right hypochondriac region, adhering to the diaphragm in the common way. There were 3 spleens, nearly of the size of a pullet's egg, found adhering to the larger spleen by short adhesions, besides 2 other still smaller spleens which were involved in the epiploon at the great end of the stomach. The pancreas was found on the right side behind the stomach, running obliquely from the spleen to the curvature of the duodenum, and had its duct entering in common with the ductus communis cholidochus into the cavity of that intestine. The splenic vessels were passing along the upper edge of the pancreas to the right side, corresponding to the change of situation in the pancreas and spleen.

The stomach was situated on the right side, partly hid by the small lobe of the liver passing to the left, and terminating in the pylorus, rather on the left side of the spine. The duodenum took a most singular course; it first passed to the right side, behind the small end of the stomach; it then turned on itself, towards the left side; it afterwards took its proper sweep to the right side, passing behind the superior mesenteric artery and mesaraica major vein. The mesentery began to be formed on the right side, instead of the left, as in ordinary cases. The ilium terminated in the great intestine on the left side, and there was in it a diverticulum of considerable size, a lusus not unfrequently occurring. The caecum was situated on the left psoas magnus and iliacus internus muscles. The transverse arch of the colon passed from the left to the right side of the body, and the sigmoid flexure crossed over the right psoas, to get into the cavity of the pelvis. The kidneys had their vessels transposed; the renal capsules had undergone no change, as no variety could be produced by a transposition.

The aorta passed between the crura of the diaphragm into the cavity of the abdomen, and adhered in its course to the spine on the right side of the vena cava inferior. Its branches were directed in their course corresponding to the peculiar situation of the viscera. The splenic and coronary arteries were passing to the right side, and the hepatic artery obliquely to the left. The superior and inferior mesenteric arteries were directed to the right side. There was no change in the spermatic arteries, any transposition in the testicles, if such a thing could take place, not being capable of affecting them. The lumbar arteries could also undergo little change, except that the left lumbar arteries must necessarily, from the peculiar situation of the aorta, be the longest. The vena cava inferior perforated the tendinous portion of the diaphragm, and adhered in its course to the spine on the left side of the aorta.

The right emulgent vein was much longer than usual, passing from the right kidney before the aorta to terminate in the vena cava superior; and the left emulgent much shorter, passing from the left kidney to the vena cava, which was situated on the left side of the spine. The right spermatic vein was found to open into the right emulgent, and the left into the vena cava inferior, about an inch under the left emulgent. The vena portarum was changed from its natural course, passing obliquely upwards to the left side, and its large branches, viz. the vena splenica, mesaraica major and minor, were all directed towards the right side of the spine. There was no change in the intercostal nerve within the cavity of the abdomen; nor does it seem to be capable of being affected by any transposition of parts. We see then, that there was a complete transposition of the abdominal viscera, each of them preserving its proper relative situation to the others. In the brain, organs of sense, of generation, the muscles, and blood vessels of the extremities, was found nothing remarkable.

The person seems to have used his right hand in preference to his left, as is usually the case, which was readily discovered by the greater bulk and hardness of that hand, as well as the greater fleshiness of the arm. It was not indeed to be expected he should be left handed. The person, while alive, was not conscious of any uncommon situation of his heart; and his brother has his heart pointing to the left side as in ordinary cases. Indeed, there was little reason to expect that we should meet with any thing particular in the account of his life. His health could not be affected by such a change of situation in his viscera; nor could there arise from it any peculiar symptoms of disease. Still less could there be any connection between such a change and his dispositions, or external actions. He might have known that his heart was directed towards the right side; but if we consider how little every person, especially those of the lower class, are attentive to circumstances not very palpable, it was scarcely to be expected he should know of it.

Notwithstanding the general similarity of parts in the same species of animals, there is no reason why nature should not sometimes deviate from her ordinary plans. Accordingly we find there is much variety in animal structure; but this does not commonly affect the animal functions. Under this restriction the variety is so great in the appearances of every part of an animal, that it is almost impossible to examine any 2 animals of the same species without remarking many differences. In the bony compages of an animal we find little variety in the extremities of bones where there is the apparatus of a joint, because a particular shape is best adapted to a particular kind or latitude of motion. In other parts of the bones, where a difference of features is not material, there is great variety, as in the foramina, depressions, ridges, and sutures of bones. The same general rule will apply to variety in muscles. The principal object is a certain insertion near a joint, so as to give a determined direction of motion. With respect to such insertions, there is, comparatively speaking, little variety; but there is a great difference in the bodies and connections of muscles, which have no share in the regulation of the motion.

There is no part of an animal where there is a greater latitude of variety than in the distribution of blood vessels. The reason of it is very obvious. The only object in the distribution of blood vessels is, to carry blood to every part of the body and bring it back to the heart. The parts of an animal, in order to be supported, must be visited by successive changes of fresh blood; but it surely cannot be an object of importance whether the blood passes by one route or another. Hence the variety of blood vessels is extremely great. Still, however, there is a method in the deviations of nature,—so that they may be marked or noted, the same varieties occurring in different animals.

It cannot be at all important to the function of a viscus, whether it be in one mass, or in separate portions. The structure being the same, the same action will take place. Hence we often find the two kidneys joined together, forming one mass; and not unfrequently two or three spleens, besides the common one. Neither can it be important whether a viscus should always be of the same shape, because its functions do not depend on shape, but on structure: we find accordingly, in this particular, much variety.

There are many of the viscera which are connected together in their functions, or by the junction of large blood vessels, in such a way as to require nearly the same relative situation among themselves. This becomes also necessary in order to preserve the general shape of the animal. Accordingly we find, that when any important viscus is changed in its situation, it affects the situation of other viscera, requiring in them a similar change. We saw in the person who is the subject of this paper, that a change in the situation of the heart and liver was accompanied with a change of situation in the stomach, spleen, pancreas and in short the whole abdominal viscera. This, however, is a great deviation in nature; for it is nothing less than changing almost the whole vital system in an animal, and therefore, it rarely happens. In such a change it does not appear that the functions can be affected, as they depend on structure and situation, which are both preserved. Hence the person who is the subject of this paper arrived at the age of maturity and might have continued to live to an extreme old age. The human machine might have been constructed in this way generally, and under such circumstances, what is now called the natural situation of parts would have been as singular as the present phaenomenon.

There appears to be less variety in the nervous system of animals of the same species, than in most parts of the body. There is scarcely any difference in the appearance of the brain, and much less in the distribution of the nerves than of the blood vessels. There is also little variety in the organs of sense: perhaps the mechanism in both these is nicer, so that a considerable deviation would interfere with their peculiar functions. The most common great deviations which nature produces in the structure of an animal, are various kinds of monstrosity, by which the animal becomes often unfit for continuing its existence. Why nature should in its greater deviations fall into a very imperfect formation, much below the standard of her common work, does not appear very obvious. It seems that there might have been many varieties where the functions could have been preserved. Perhaps it is with a view to check the propagation of great varieties, so as to preserve a uniformity in the same species of animals.

It has been much agitated, whether monstrosities depend on the original formation, or are produced afterwards in the gradual evolution of an animal. This does not appear to be a question of much importance; nor perhaps can it be absolutely determined. But on the whole it is more reasonable to think that the same plan of formation is continued from the beginning, than that at any subsequent period there is a change in that plan. It may be observed, that it is exactly the same creative action which produces the natural structure, or any deviation from it; for in cases of deviation the action is either carried too far, ceases too soon, or is diverted into uncommon channels. This will explain the various kinds of monstrosity from redundancy, deficiency, or transposition of parts.

1794

JOHN HUNTER

THE RECORD OF HIS CARDIAC HISTORY AS DETAILED BY HIMSELF AND LATER PUBLISHED BY HIS BROTHER-IN-LAW, EVERARD HOME

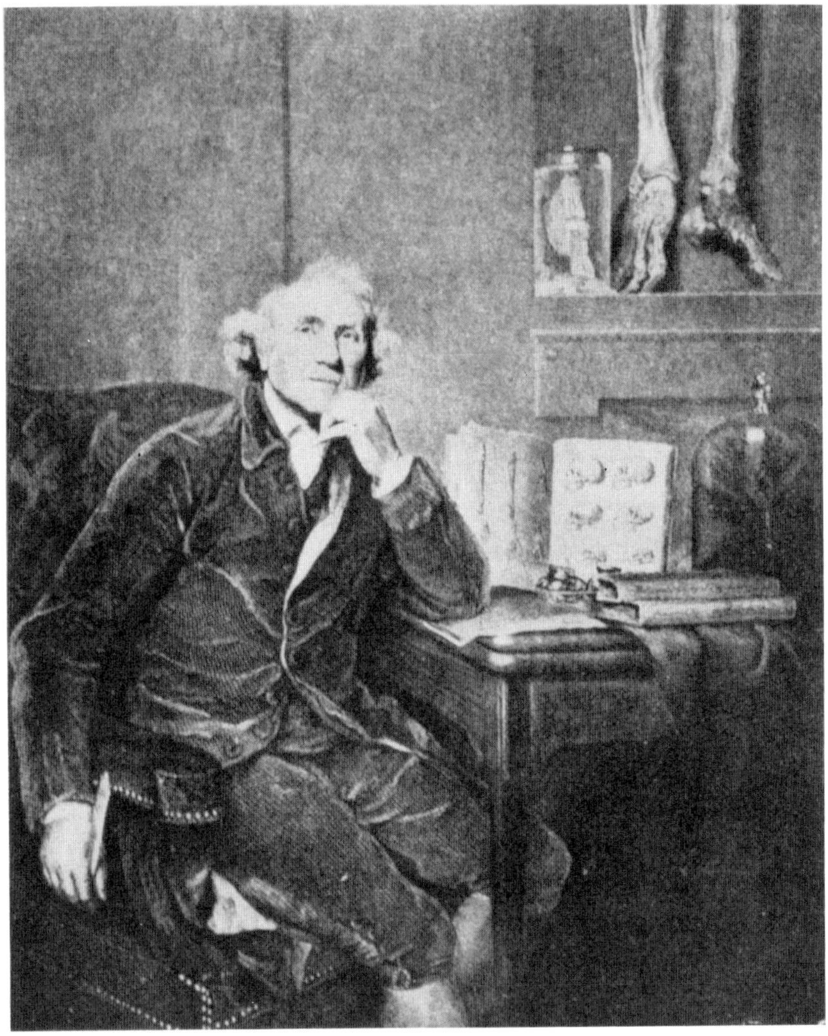

JOHN HUNTER

From a painting by Sir Joshua Reynolds

(Courtesy Medical Classics.)

JOHN HUNTER

(1728-1793)

"In the history of human progress there appears now and then a thunderbolt, and the thunderbolt of surgery is John Hunter."

—William Boyd.*

"Not Oxford with its intellectual store
Of Greek and Latin, but the open space
Of the wide firmament for him, to face
Nature herself and Universal Law.
He entered Truth's stout stronghold at the door
And, step by step, climbed up, with measured pace,
Until he reached a high embattled place
Where he remained and will, for evermore."

—T. W. Parry.

JOHN HUNTER was born at Long Calderwood, in the parish of East Kilbride, Lanarkshire, Scotland, on February 13 or 14, 1728, the youngest of ten children. Two of his brothers, James and William Hunter, also became physicians. His elder brother, James, died at the beginning of a most promising career, and to William fell the task of aiding John in an unparalleled career in medicine.

At the age of seventeen John Hunter was sent to live with his brother-in-law, a Mr. Buchanan, where he developed great mechanical skill as a carpenter in Buchanan's workshop. During this time his brother, William, had made a very successful start in the practice of medicine, and at the age of twenty John Hunter decided that he, too, would have a medical career.

He therefore wrote his brother William in London and offered his services as an assistant in William Hunter's dissecting laboratory. His offer was accepted and while in his brother's tutelage he was so successful that the next year he was to direct the dissections of the medical students.

Not long after he came to London, Hunter was introduced by his brother to the famous English surgeon, William Cheselden. He soon became a student of Cheselden, under whom he worked at Chelsea Hospital during the summer months of 1749 and 1750. On Cheselden's retirement in 1751, John Hunter became a surgical student at St. Bartholomew's Hospital. There he worked under the distinguished surgeon, Percival Pott.

In 1753 Hunter entered St. Mary's Hall, Oxford, as a student, at the suggestion, no doubt, of his brother, William. There he began to study the classics, but after a trial of two months dropped his course and determined to remain within the realm of surgery. In 1754 he became a surgical student at St. George's Hospital. Two years later he served there as house-surgeon.

In 1754, Hunter after making several dissections discovered the method of connection between the placenta and the uterus. This discovery twenty-five years later (1780) was to provoke a bitter public quarrel between the two brothers over the question of priority, and it is to be regretted that it was to dissolve their friendship. Both of the Hunters disputed with the Monros over priority in anatomic discoveries and later with Pott on the true nature of congenital hernia.

**Surgical Pathology,* ed. 4. 1938, p. 17.

In 1759 Hunter, having served a period of ten years in the study of human anatomy, in order to understand more clearly the human body and its functions, began the study of comparative anatomy. Because he worked very hard his health suffered and he was advised to seek the curative effects of a warmer climate. On this account he applied for an appointment with the army and was immediately made a staff surgeon.

During the Seven Years' War he accompanied the British expedition to Belle Isle in 1761. During that siege he found ample opportunity to treat gunshot wounds, a procedure for which he was later to become renowned. While he was thus engaged he found time to conduct investigations in experimental physiology. He studied the digestion in lizards and snakes during hibernation and among other things, the faculty of hearing in fishes.

By 1763 the war was terminated and Hunter returned to London. In order to increase his income he decided to teach anatomy in private classes. He conducted classes in anatomy for several years. During his spare time he continued his anatomic and physiologic investigations. To obtain specimens for this research he obtained the bodies of animals that had died in the zoos of London and elsewhere. He also purchased rare animals, when such a course was possible, spending money he could ill afford.

In 1767 Hunter was elected a fellow of the Royal Society. His election probably was the result of recognition of his devout interest in comparative physiology, an interest that had not been shown by the publication of original investigations, for he had not as yet begun his publications. Scientists in general in London already knew of his rapidly growing anatomic museum which, one day, was to become of national significance.

Hunter was appointed surgeon to St. George's Hospital in 1768, and soon afterwards he was chosen a member of the Corporation of Surgeons. Thereafter he obtained pupils on more advantageous terms. Among the most renowned of his students, according to Garrison, were Jenner, Astley Cooper, Abernathy, Cline, Clift, Parkinson, Blizard, Home, Alanson, Wright Post, and Physick.

In 1771, Hunter published the first part of his medical classic, ''The Natural History of the Human Teeth.'' This was followed in 1778 by the second part, ''A Practical Treatise on the Diseases of the Teeth.'' According to Garrison, Hunter was the first to study the teeth in a scientific manner and the first to recommend complete removal of the pulp before filling them.

Hunter's marriage to Miss Home, sister of Sir Everard Home, took place in July, 1771. They had four children, two of whom died when very young. In 1772, Hunter, being persuaded by Sir John Pringle, communicated his first paper to the ''Philosophical Transactions'' of the Royal Society. The work concerned the digestion of the stomach after death. In the fall of this year Sir Everard Home, his brother-in-law, became his student and afterward was to act as his assistant.

In 1776 Hunter was appointed surgeon-extraordinary to the King. That same year he was invited to deliver the Croonian Lectures before the Royal Society. For the subject of these lectures he chose ''Muscular Motion.'' In 1778 he was appointed surgeon to the new naval hospital at Plymouth. The Royal Society of Belles-Lettres of Gothenburg elected Hunter a fellow in 1781, and in 1783 he was elected to membership in the Royal Society of Medicine and the Royal Academy of Surgery of Paris.

Fordyce, Hunter, and others were instrumental in founding in 1783 the Society for the Improvement of Medical and Chirurgical Knowledge. Although this society had but a brief life, many valuable papers are included in its ''Transactions.''

In 1783, Hunter procured at a cost of 500 pounds the ''kidnapped'' body of the famous Irish giant, Byrne or Obrien. He disarticulated the skeleton and it occupied a prominent place in his Museum of Natural History. In the same year the Royal Society conferred upon him the Copley medal in recognition of his important discoveries in natural history.

In 1785, Hunter began to suffer from recurring attacks of angina pectoris. He, therefore, spent a holiday at Bath and during his convalescence entrusted his medical practice to his brother-in-law, for whose ability he had a high regard. In December of that year Hunter, feeling somewhat refreshed from his stay at Bath, established his famous operation for the cure of aneurysm. This consisted in tying the artery at a distance high in the healthy tissues by a single ligature.

Hunter was appointed deputy surgeon-general to the army in 1786. That same year he published his work on venereal disease.[1] Believing that syphilis and gonorrhea were identical he inoculated himself with spirochetes and subsequently thought he observed the symptoms of both diseases. This confirmed him in his belief that both diseases were identical. This erroneous conception was later demolished by Philippe Ricord (1800-1889) who proved the autonomy of these diseases (1831-1837). Hunter did, however, correctly differentiate between hard chancre and chancroid ulcer.

In 1786 Hunter also published his important work, ''Observations in Certain Parts of the Animal Oeconomy,'' which consisted of a revision and enlargement of many of his papers originally published in the ''Philosophical Transactions'' of the Royal Society.

In 1792, Hunter transferred his surgical lectures to his brother-in-law, Home, and devoted much of his time to the completion of his famous work, ''A Treatise on the Blood, Inflammation and Gunshot Wounds.'' This was not published until 1794, about a year after Hunter's death. From Home's account of the life of Hunter, which prefixes this work, we are reproducing Hunter's classic description of his own fatal illness, angina pectoris, as detailed to his brother-in-law.

Hunter had said that his ''life was in the hands of any rascal who chose to annoy and tease him.'' And there can be no doubt but that the violent disagreements he had with his colleagues at St. George's Hospital hastened his death, which occurred on October 16, 1793, following a meeting of the board of governors of St. George's Hospital, at which a colleague had directed some disparaging remarks to him.

The great monument to the fame of John Hunter is the Hunterian Museum of 13,000 specimens purchased by Parliament some time after his death for 15,000 pounds, a fraction of its cost, and presented to the Corporation of Surgeons, soon afterward to become the Royal College of Surgeons.

---

[1]Hunter, John: *A treatise on the venereal disease,* London, 1786, 398 pp.

A TREATISE ON THE BLOOD, INFLAMMATION, AND *GUN-SHOT WOUNDS*,

BY THE LATE

JOHN HUNTER.

TO WHICH IS PREFIXED

A SHORT ACCOUNT OF THE AUTHOR's LIFE,

BY HIS BROTHER-IN-LAW,

EVERARD HOME.

IN TWO VOLUMES, FROM THE LONDON QUARTO.

VOL. I.

PHILADELPHIA

PUBLISHED BY THOMAS BRADFORD, PRINTER

BOOK-SELLER & STATIONER,

No. 8,

South Front-Street,

1796.

A TREATISE ON THE BLOOD, INFLAMMATION, AND GUN-SHOT WOUNDS*

BY THE LATE JOHN HUNTER

A Short Account of the Author's Life†
By His Brother-in-Law
Everard Home

MR. HUNTER was a very healthy man for the first forty years of his life; and, if we except an inflammation of his lungs in the year 1759, occasioned most probably by his attention to anatomical pursuits, he had no complaint of any consequence during that period. In the spring of 1769, in his forty-first year, he had a regular fit of the gout, which returned the three following springs, but not the fourth; and in the spring of 1773, having met with something which very forcibly affected his mind, he was attacked at ten o'clock in the forenoon with a pain in the stomach, about the pylorus; it was the sensation peculiar to those parts, and became so violent that he tried change of position to procure ease, he sat down, then walked, laid himself down on the carpet, then upon chairs, but could find no relief; he took a spoonful of tincture of rhubarb, with thirty drops of laudanum, without the smallest benefit. While he was walking about the room he cast his eyes on the looking glass and observed his countenance to be pale, his lips white, giving the appearance of a dead man. This alarmed him, and led him to feel for his pulse, but he found none in either arm; he now thought his complaint serious; several physicians of his acquaintance were then sent for, Dr. William Hunter, Sir George Baker, Dr. Huck Saunders, and Sir William Fordyce, all came but could find no pulse; the pain still continued, and he found himself at times not breathing. Being afraid of death soon taking place if he did not breathe, he produced the voluntary act of breathing, by working his lungs by the power of the will; the sensitive principle, with all its effects on the machine not being in the least affected by the complaint. In this state he continued for three-quarters of an hour, in which time frequent attempts were made to feel the pulse, but in vain; however, at last, the pain lessened, and the pulse returned, although at first but faintly, and the involuntary breathing began to take place; while in this state, he took Madeira, brandy, ginger, etc. but did not be-

*The first English edition was published in 1794. We are reprinting from the first American edition, published in 1796.—F. A. W., 1940.

†Pp. xxiv-liii.

lieve them of any service, as the return of health was very gradual; in two hours he was perfectly recovered.

In this attack there was a suspension of the most material involuntary actions, even involuntary breathing was stopped, while sensation with its consequences, as thinking and acting with the will, were perfect, and all the voluntary actions were as strong as before.

Quere. What would have been the consequence of his not having breathed by means of the voluntary muscles? It struck him at the time that he would have died; but we cannot suppose that would have been the consequence, as breathing most probably is only necessary for the blood while circulating, and as the circulation was stopped, no good could have arisen from breathing.

. . . .

When he was at first attacked, the pulse was full and eight ounces of blood were taken away, but this did not appear to be of service; the day following he was cupped between the shoulders and had a large blister applied upon the part; he took an emetic, and several times purging medicines and bathed his feet in warm water, but nothing appeared to be of the least use. The purging and vomiting distressed him greatly, for both the stomach and intestines were so irritable that less than half the usual quantity had the desired effect. He took some James's powder,* and drank some white wine whey on account of the heat in the skin, especially in the feet and hands, which took it off and gave him for the first time a comfortable feel. At the end of ten days all his ideas of his present state became more natural, the strange deception concerning his own size was in part corrected, and the idea of suspension in the air became less; but for some time after, the fire appeared of a deep purple red. When he got so well as to be able to stand without being giddy, he was unable to walk without support, for his own feelings did not give him information respecting his centre of gravity, so that he was unable to ballance his body, and prevent himself from falling.

He gradually recovered from this state, and as soon as he was able went to Bath, where he staid some time and drank the waters, which were thought to be of service to him; but did not stay long enough to give them a fair trial; he returned to town much better, and in a few weeks got quite well. From this period to 1785, he had no particular indisposition, but certainly did not enjoy perfect health, for in 1785, he appeared much altered in his looks, and gave the idea of having grown much older than could be accounted for from the number of years which had elapsed.

About the beginning of April, 1785, he was attacked with a spasmodic complaint, which at first was slight, but became afterwards very violent,

*James's powder contained 1 part of antimonious oxide and 2 parts of calcium phosphate and was used as a diaphoretic.—F. A. W., 1940.

and terminated in a fit of the gout in the ball of the great toe; this, like his other attacks, was brought on by anxiety of mind; the first symptom was a sensation of the muscles of the nose being in action, but whether they really were or not, he was never able to determine; this sensation returned at intervals for about a fortnight, attended with an unpleasant sensation in the left side of the face, lower jaw, and throat which seemed to extend into the head on that side and down the left arm, as low as the ball of the thumb, where it terminated all at once; these sensations were not constant, but returned at irregular times; they became soon more violent, attacking the head, face, and both sides of the lower jaw, giving the idea that the face was swelled, particularly the cheeks, and sometimes slightly affected the right arm. After they had continued for a fortnight they extended to the sternum, producing the same disagreeable sensations there, and giving the feel of the sternum being drawn backwards toward the spine. . . .

. . . .

. . . I was with him during the whole of this attack, and never saw anything equal to the agonies he suffered; and when he fainted away, I thought him dead, as the pain did not seem to abate, but to carry him off, having first completely exhausted him.

He then fell asleep for half an hour, and awoke with a confusion in his head, and a faint recollection of something like a delirium; this went off in a few days.

The affections above-described were, in the beginning, readily brought on by exercise, and he even conceived that if he had continued at rest, they would not have come on; but they at last seized him when lying in bed, and in his sleep, so as to awaken him; affections of the mind also brought them on; but coolly thinking or reasoning did not appear to have that effect. While these complaints were upon him, his face was pale, and had a contracted appearance, making him look thinner than ordinary; and after they went off his colour returned, and his face recovered its natural appearance. On the commencement of the complaint, he suspected it to be rheumatism, and applied electricity to his arm, which took it off for the time only; he then, for two or three nights successively, took three grains of James's powder, without any abatement of the symptoms; he next had recourse to the camphorated julep, both at the commencement of the spasm, and while it was upon him, but obtained no relief; he tried Hoffman's anodyne liquor, in the dose of a tea-spoonful, and not finding it to answer alone, joined to it the camphorated julep, but the spasms seemed to be more violent; one night he took twenty drops of thebaic tincture, which made his head confused all the following day, but did not at all abate the spasms; the following day he took two tea-spoonfuls of the bark, which heated him, and gave him a head-ach, thirst, and dryness of his mouth, which prevented his continuing it. At the desire of Dr. David Pitcairn, he took the powder of valerian, an ounce a day, which seemed for the first two days to remove his spasms, but they returned on the third with more violence than usual, especially one evening at the Royal Society, which induced him to leave off the valerian, and he bathed his feet on going to bed in warm water, mixed with half a pound of flour of mustard, and took a tea-spoonful of tincture of rhubarb in ginger-tea; also wore worsted stockings all night.

On Friday morning, the twentieth of May, between six and seven o'clock, he had a violent spasm, attended with most violent eructations of wind from the stomach for nearly a quarter of an hour. Dr. Pitcairn, who was sent for upon this occasion, asked him, if there was any distress upon his mind that had brought on this attack; and he confessed his mind to have been much harrassed, in consequence of having opened the body of a person who died from the bite of a mad dog, about six weeks before, in doing which he had wounded his hand; and for the last fortnight his mind had been in continual suspense, conceiving it possible that he might be seized with symptoms of hydrophobia. This anxiety preying upon his mind for so long a time, there is every reason to believe was the cause of the present attack and probably had also brought on the former ones, which were all after the accident which had impressed his mind with this horrible idea.

At the desire of Dr. Pitcairn, he took at two doses in the forenoon, ten grains of asafoetida, and three grains of opium, and in the afternoon fifteen of asafoetida, and one of opium; in the evening he had a head-ach, which was supposed to be brought on by the opium, his bowels were loaded and oppressed with wind, and he endeavoured in vain to procure a motion by laxative clysters, although repeated, and ten grains of jalap were taken by the mouth; he passed a very restless night. On Saturday morning he was visited by Sir George Baker, Dr. Warren, and the late Dr. Pitcairn; he repeated the asafoetida twice in the course of the day, and two spoonfuls of the following mixture were taken every hour, without producing a motion till about half an hour after the whole was used.

Infusion of senna, six ounces;
Tincture of senna, one drachm and a half;
Soluble tartar, three drachms.

M.

In the afternoon he had another evacuation, soon after which, the most violent attack of spasm which he had experienced, came on; nothing was attempted internally during the attack, which lasted two hours; a bladder of hot water was applied to the heart, and afterwards to the feet, without any effect.

The asafoetida was now left off, and this evening he began the oleum succini in saline draughts fifteen drops every six hours. On Sunday morning he continued the oleum succini, but the saline draught was changed to cinnamon-water, and a large blister was put upon the back close to the neck; he continued pretty free from spasm. On Monday the blister was taken off, and the oleum succini continued; but about nine o'clock at night he had threatenings of spasm, with head-ach, and the feel of a load in his bowels; he had a pain in the left side and region of the stomach, with violent eructations of wind from the stomach, which lasted about two hours; he took thebaic tincture, twenty-five drops, in the warm tincture of rhubarb, and afterwards some baume de vie, but the eructations continuing, sinapisms were applied to the feet, after which they ceased, and the sinapisms were so troublesome that he had them taken off five hours after they were applied. On Tuesday morning he felt himself easier, the oleum succini was continued, five drops of laudanum being added to each dose; in the evening he bathed his feet in warm water, to clean them from the sinapisms, and both the great toes appeared a little inflamed, and very tender; they were more painful after being bathed, and were very troublesome all night. On Wednesday morning the inflammation and swelling in the great toes appeared evidently to be the gout, and the pain continued very acute till Thursday, when it began to abate: and on Friday was very much diminished: he continued the oleum succini on Wednesday, and took a bolus of aromatic species before each dose; but on Friday the oleum succini made him sick, and was left off. On Saturday he began the bark in tincture and decoction with the species aromaticae; Sunday continued the bark, and having eructations and flatulencies after his meals, he was ordered every day before dinner, rhubarb fifteen grains, ginger ten grains, in a bolus. He had no spasm after Monday the thirtieth of May; he however had threatenings, or slight sensations, similar to those which preceded the spasms, and occasional eructations. Although evidently relieved from the violent attacks of spasm by the gout in his feet, yet he was far from being free from the disease, for he was still subject to the spasms, upon exercise or agitation of mind; the exercise that generally brought it on, was walking, especially on an ascent, either of stairs or rising ground, but never on going down either the one or the other; the affections of the mind that brought it on were principally anxiety or anger: it was not the cause of the anxiety, but the quantity that most affected him; the anxiety about the hiving of a swarm of bees brought it on; the anxiety lest an animal should make its escape before he could get a gun to shoot it, brought it on; even the hearing of a story in which the mind became so much engaged as to be interested in the event, although the particulars were of no consequence to him, would bring it on; anger brought on the same complaint and he could conceive it possible for that passion to be carried so far as totally to deprive him of life; but what was very extraordinary, the more tender passions of the mind did not produce it; he could relate a story which called up all the finer feelings, as compassion, admiration for the actions of gratitude in others, so as to make him shed tears, yet the spasm was not excited; it is extraordinary that he eat and slept as well as ever, and his mind was in no degree depressed; the want of exercise made him grow unusually fat.

. . . .

In the autumn 1790, and in the spring and autumn 1791, he had more severe attacks than during the other periods of the year, but of not more than a few hours duration: in the beginning of October, 1792, one, at which I was present, was so violent that I thought he would have died. On October the 16th, 1793, when in his usual state of health, he went to St. George's Hospital, and meeting with some things which irritated his mind, and not being perfectly master of the circumstances, he withheld his sentiments, in which state of restraint he went into the next room, and turning round to Dr. Robertson, one of the physicians of the hospital, he gave a deep groan, and dropt down dead.

. . . .

At the time of his death he was in the 65th year of his age, the same age at which his brother, the late Dr. Hunter, died. Upon inspecting the body after death, the following were the appearances: the skin in several places was mottled, particularly on the sides and neck, which arose from the blood not having been completely coagulated, but remaining nearly fluid.

. . . .

The pericardium was very unusually thickened, which did not allow it to collapse upon being opened; the quantity of water contained in it was scarcely more than is frequently met with, although it might probably exceed that which occurs in the most healthy state of these parts.

The heart itself was very small, appearing too little for the cavity in which it lay, and did not give the idea of its being the effect of an unusual degree of contraction, but more of its having shrunk in its size. Upon the under surface of the left auricle and ventricle, there were two spaces nearly an inch and an half square, which were of a white colour, with an opaque appearance, and entirely distinct from the general surface of the heart: these two spaces were covered by an exudation of coagulating lymph, which at some former period had been the result of inflammation there. The muscular structure of the heart was paler and looser in its texture than the other muscles in the body. There were no coagula in any of its cavities. The coronary arteries had their branches which ramify through the substance of the heart in the state of bony tubes, which were with difficulty divided by the knife, and their transverse sections did not collapse, but remained open. The valvulae mitrales, where they come off from the lower edge of the auricle, were in many places ossified, forming an imperfectly bony margin of different thicknesses, and in one spot so thick as to form a knob; but these ossifications were not continued down upon the valve towards the chordae tendineae.

The semilunar valves of the aorta had lost their natural pliancy, the previous stage to becoming bone, and in several spots there were evident ossifications.

The aorta immediately beyond the semilunar valves had its cavity larger than usual, putting on the appearance of an incipient aneurism; this unusual dilatation extended for some way along the ascending aorta, but did not reach so far as the common trunk of the axillary and carotid artery. The increase of capacity of the artery might be about one-third of its natural area; and the internal membrane of this part had lost entirely the natural polish, and was studded over with opaque white spots raised higher than the general surface.

. . . .

From this account of the appearances observed after death, it is reasonable to attribute the principal symptoms of the disease to an organic affection of the heart. That organ was rendered unable to carry on its functions, whenever the actions were disturbed, either in consequence of bodily exertion, or affections of the mind.

The stoppage of the pulse arose from a spasm upon the heart, and in this state the nerves were probably pressed against the ossified arteries, which may account for the excrutiating pain he felt at those times.

The other symptoms may be explained from the defect in the valves and the dilatation of the aorta, which had lost its elasticity.

In the last attack the spasm upon the heart was either too violent in the degree of contraction, or too long continued to admit of relaxation, so that death immediately ensued.

His remains were interred in a vault under the parish church of St. Martin in the Fields, attended by a few of his oldest medical friends.

. . . .

1806

JEAN NICOLAS CORVISART

DESCRIPTION OF THE SIGNS OF CONTRACTION OF THE ORIFICES OF THE HEART, ETC.

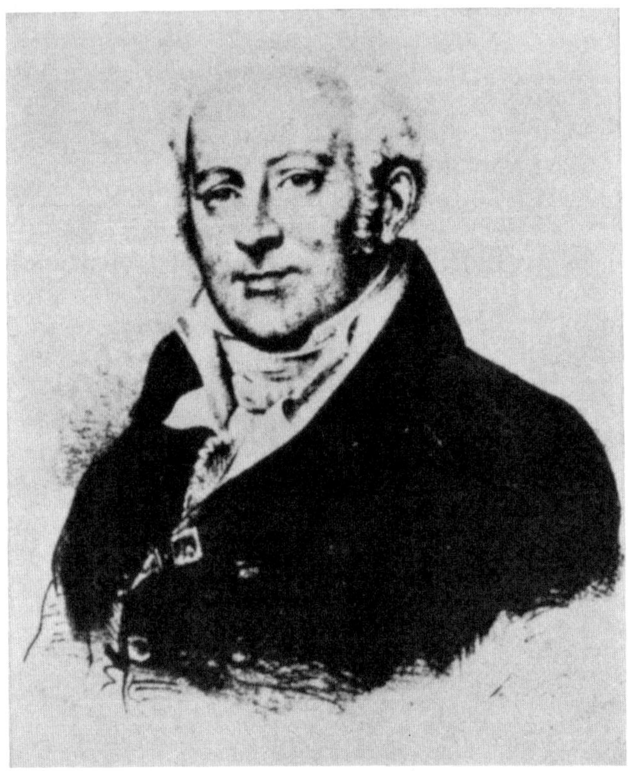

JEAN NICOLAS CORVISART

Portrait by Charles Bazin; etched by Delpech

(Courtesy Charles C Thomas.)

JEAN NICOLAS CORVISART

(1755-1821)

IN THE tiny French village of Dricourt, not far from Vouziers, Jean Nicolas Corvisart was born on February 15, 1755. As was to happen later to Laënnec, Corvisart early in life was sent to live with his uncle, who was the pastor of the parish at Vimille.

At the age of thirteen, Corvisart matriculated at the College of Saint Barbe. There he showed no signs of intellectual superiority, but, according to Beeson, was "lazy, mischievous, and quarrelsome." Originally it was intended that Corvisart was to become a lawyer, but while studying for the bar, he visited many hospital clinics in Paris. These visits made a profound impression on him, so he decided to forsake law for medicine.

This decision angered his father to such an extent that Corvisart was expelled from the paternal home. He immediately applied at the Hôtel-Dieu in Paris for a position which would insure his board and room. This he secured and with it came the splendid opportunity of studying medicine in one of the world's most famous institutions.

In 1785, the Paris Faculty of Medicine conferred upon him the degree of doctor-regent. Corvisart later became an associate to the chair of anatomy in the Hôtel-Dieu. He also assisted in the courses in operative surgery, obstetrics, and physiology.

On the death of Desbois de Rochefort in 1788, Corvisart succeeded him as physician to the Charité Hospital, and with the establishment of the medical school in 1795, Corvisart was chosen to occupy the chair of medicine. In 1797 he became professor of medicine at the Collège de France, and in 1799, Corvisart and Barthez became physicians to the government.

In 1804, Corvisart had the honor to become personal physician to Napoléon Bonaparte. He had known Napoléon at an earlier date, for in 1798 Bonaparte had presented him with a large carved mahogany chair which Corvisart had placed in his consulting rooms. This chair, now a highly valued antique, is still a cherished possession of the Corvisart family.

From all accounts, Napoléon and Corvisart greatly enjoyed each other's company, and many interesting anecdotes are told of their conversations. In one of these, it is said that the Emperor, who was in constant fear of being poisoned, literally rolled on the floor because of a slight attack of indigestion. Corvisart is supposed to have reproved him, saying, "Get up! What would be said if the master of the world were seen thus crushed by fear?"

Perhaps the most famous story is the reported conversation related by Beeson, between Corvisart and the Emperor following the birth of Napoléon's son, the King of Rome, in 1811.

"Sire," said the physician, "this child should fulfill your last wish. Consider from what a position you have arisen in less than ten years: lieutenant, captain, brigadier-general, general-in-chief, First Consul, Emperor, spouse of an Austrian Archduchess, and the father of a male child. You have reached the summit of the Wheel of Fortune and of great renown. Stop! Sire, or Destiny may desert you and then nothing remains but downfall and disaster."

''Well,'' replied the Emperor, ''that was such a speech as one would expect from a native of the Champagne.''

In reading the works of the famous Viennese physician, Max Stoll, Corvisart learned of Auenbrugger's treatise on percussion. He became very much interested in this new diagnostic procedure, and after practicing it for several years, translated Auenbrugger's treatise in 1808, adding several original observations. As we have mentioned in our biographic account of Auenbrugger, much credit is due to Corvisart for bringing into professional favor the discovery and use of percussion as an important aid in physical diagnosis.

Corvisart realized the importance of presenting to French medicine in translation the works of some of the important foreign physicians. In 1797 he translated Max Stoll's masterful work ''Aphorisms on the Knowledge and Cure of the Fevers.'' He also translated the aphorisms of the great Boerhaave in 1802. In this connection it is interesting to note that many years later a favorite pupil, Laënnec, published the aphorisms of his learned teacher, Corvisart.

The many contributions of Corvisart to cardiology are contained in his work entitled ''Essai sur les maladies du coeur et des gros vaisseaux,'' which was first published in 1806. Among the outstanding contributions to this field were his observations on the distinctions between cardiac and pulmonary disorders and the differences between functional and organic cardiac disease. Beeson wrote that Lassus was ''of the opinion that Corvisart's most important contributions to cardiology were: (1) the distinction between cardiac hypertrophy and dilatation, (2) the division of the clinical course of heart failure into three periods, and (3) the connection between cause and effect in valvular lesions and heart failure.'' We have chosen to reproduce from Gate's translation of the ''Essai,'' published in 1812, some of Corvisart's original observations.

During the peak of his career, Corvisart was physician to many distinguished women of the time, including the Empress Josephine, the Empress Marie Louise, Hortense de Beauharnais, who was Queen of Holland, the Queen of Spain, the beautiful Pauline Bonaparte, who like her mighty brother died of cancer, and Madame Walewska, whom he is said to have dearly loved.

In the short interlude of Napoléon's return to power before his defeat at Waterloo, Corvisart again served as physician to his old friend. Soon after the Emperor's final defeat, Corvisart retired, it is said, to Courbevoie near Paris. In 1815 he suffered a mild cerebrovascular seizure, following which he retired from the practice of medicine. On September 15, 1821, he suffered a final attack, which resulted in his death a few days later, approximately four months after the demise of the former Emperor at St. Helena on May 5.

AN

ESSAY

ON THE

ORGANIC DISEASES AND LESIONS

OF THE

HEART AND GREAT VESSELS.

FROM THE CLINICAL LECTURES OF

J. N. CORVISART,

First Physician of their Imperial and Royal Majesties; Officer of the Legion of Honor, Honorary Professor of the School of Medicine of Paris, and of the Imperial College of France; Physician in Chief of the Hospital of La Charite, &c. &c.

PUBLISHED, UNDER HIS INSPECTION, BY

C. E. HOREAU,

Doctor in Medicine, Surgeon of the Infirmary and House of the Emperor and King.

Hæret lateri lethalis arundo.
VIRG. ÆNEID.

TRANSLATED FROM THE FRENCH,

WITH NOTES,

BY JACOB GATES, M. M. S. S.

BOSTON

PUBLISHED BY BRADFORD & READ, AND BY

ANTHONY FINLEY, PHILADELPHIA.

1812.

ESSAY ON THE DISEASES AND ORGANIC LESIONS OF THE HEART*

THIRD CLASS, CHAPTER III, ARTICLE III

OF THE SIGNS PECULIAR TO THE CONSTRICTIONS OF THE ORIFICE†

THE cartilaginous or osseous induration of the orifices of the auricles and ventricles, of the mitral and tricuspid valves, of the aortic and pulmonary semi-lunar valves, and the vegetations, growing upon either the ventricular or arterial valves, tend principally to produce a more or less complete constriction of the orifices affected.

When these constrictions exist, the circulation is embarrassed, and its phenomena singularly perverted. By observing the disorder of the circulation, the practitioner may find, in the living man, I should presume, certain signs of this species of affection.

To point out with accuracy these signs, it is necessary to make a distinction between the different affections of which I have been speaking: 1st, those which produce a permanent obliteration of the orifices; 2d, those which form this constriction but momentarily.

In the first rank, must be placed the indurations, and ossifications of the circles and ventricular valves, as the effects of this permanent morbid state are the same in every instance, and are ever perceptible to the practitioner. In the second, must be placed the vegetations, or excrescences which are noticed upon the ventricular and sigmoïd valves, whose presence is known only at intervals, when these bodies, generally floating in the cavity of the ventricle, or vessel, appear at the orifice, and edge where their base is fixed.

The signs of constriction are commonly the more obscure, as the constriction is the more remote from the beginning of the general arterial system, because it is by considering attentively the derangements which obtain in the action of this system, that the knowledge of the signs is acquired. I will explain myself: the constrictions which are formed by the ossifications surrounding the orifices or valves of the right heart, as well as of the pulmonary artery, appear very difficult to comprehend on the living sub-

---

*Corvisart, Jean Nicolas: *Essai sur les maladies et les lésions organiques du coeur,* Paris, 1806. English translation by Jacob Gates, M.M.S.S., 1812, pp. 182-189 and 299-303.

†M. Corvisart planned his book on the basis of the medico-anatomic aspects of the heart. He used the word "class" instead of the usual "part" or "section," to indicate various portions of his work, beginning with "First Class" and ending with "Fifth Class" and "Corollaries." The portions reprinted herein are from the "Third Class" and the "Corollaries," respectively.—F. A. W., 1940.

ject. Where can we, in short, discover the signs proper to make them understood? The regular or perverted action of the right cavities of the heart are barely made sensible in the organs subordinate to the influence of the less circulation; likewise the disorder of the action of the left heart can be comprehended only in the nature of the arterial pulsation, or what amounts to the same, in the phenomena of the greater circulation.

Could we examine the pulsations of the pulmonary artery or its branches, as we do the pulsations of the aorta or its branches, we should recognize with equal ease, both the constrictions of the orifices of the right heart, and the same lesions when they obtain in the orifices of the left cavities; but such an investigation is impossible, and we are obliged, in this case, to examine the state of the lungs. Now, is it known, or shall we be ever able to know what disorder, or rather what modification respiration will undergo, when the lungs, from a constriction either of the ventricular orifice of the right side, or of the mouth of the pulmonary artery, will receive a less quantity of blood than what ought naturally to be conveyed to them, and upon which respiration exercises its vivifying influence? It is supposed that a particular modification of respiration must furnish the signs which I am endeavoring to discover; but such a modification is not sufficiently prominent, and striking, or rather we are not endowed with sufficient understanding, to recognize such a peculiar modification of respiration among the multitude of signs which this function evinces in the different affections of the lungs.

If we cannot comprehend the signs of the constrictions of the right orifices of the heart, can we expect to be more successful in a particular change of the phenomena of the greater circulation? The influence of one of the two circulations over the other is such, that, the one being disordered, it is impossible for the other not to partake of the disorder. But what can be the peculiar nature of the disorder which must exist? I doubt whether observation gives the practitioner a diagnosis subtile enough to discriminate the alteration of these orifices in the particular disorder of respiration, unless he be assisted by all the concomitant signs.

By reasoning physiologically, it may be advanced that the small quantity of blood conveyed from the right cavities of the heart, into the lungs, thence into the cavities of the left heart, and filling these cavities partially, will stimulate them imperfectly; that from this insufficient stimulus will arise feeble and slow contractions, which will induce debility, softness, and slowness of the pulse, etc. But in this case, as in various others, to how many gross mistakes, would not he be incessantly exposed who should so restrict the morbid phenomena to the opinions of physiology, and who should always find in these too often hypothetical opinions, the knowledge of the phenomena which are to characterize any such affection! How often does not clinical observation overturn such theoretical speculations, as it will subvert sooner or later many others, whose foundations appear as unstable as those too frequently established by the spirit of innovation!

Therefore the collection of a great number of symptoms would be necessary to elucidate the diagnosis of the constrictions of the right orifices; the countenance must appear of a livid hue, a more marked engorgement of the general venous system, and particularly of the liver, the size of this organ increased, the dyspnoea greater and longer continued, all the signs, in fact, which can point out the affection of the right cavities, which are usually dilated in consequence of constrictions of the right orifices, are joined to the character of the pulse, which, in this case, is less irregular than in the constrictions of the left orifices, but less regular however than natural.

The obscurity, involving the signs of the constrictions of the right orifices, is not entirely dissipated, when it is requisite to recognize the imperfect obliteration of the left auricle and ventricle. Beside the general signs of the diseases of the heart, which are ever found in this case as in the first, because an aneurismal complication generally obtains, some particular signs manifest the affections in question.

Of the preceding number of symptoms is a peculiar rushing like water, difficult to be described, sensible to the hand applied over the precordial region, a rushing which proceeds, apparently, from the embarrassment which the blood undergoes in passing through an opening which is no longer proportioned to the quantity of fluid which it ought to discharge. The same rushing is also recognized, though it is much less marked, by the hand that investigates the phenomena of the pulse. This character is not likewise the only one by which the pulse announces the existence of the contraction of the left orifice; it is effectually less regular than in the case of constriction of the right orifices, but less irregular than when the aortic orifice is deranged. Besides it presents neither impetus, hardness, nor fulness, because the quantity of blood which the left ventricle propels, is proportioned to what it receives from the auricle which is imperfectly emptied; moreover, the action of this ventricle cannot be vigorous, since it is feebly stimulated.

Notwithstanding the deficient excitement of the left ventricle, it must not be believed that in this case, the strokes and palpitations of the heart are continually weak and obscure. The right cavities, and the left auricle in particular, acquire very often a thickness and force which render the contractions extremely distinct; they may even become more violent in this case than in any other, as the strokes of the heart depend on the motion of the auricles which propels this organ, and the force of this motion of the auricles augments in proportion to the difficulty they encounter in driving the blood through their constricted orifice.

When the indurated and ossified semi-lunar valves of the aorta stop a portion of this vessel, the obstacle which they form breaks the wave of blood propelled by the heart into the artery; strong and frequent palpitations supervene, because the heart is easily filled, but is difficultly emptied; thence results a more protracted residence of the blood in the left cavities, a longer application of the stimulus of the blood on the parietes of the heart, in fact, a greater irritation of the organ. The pulse, in this case, may preserve a certain degree of hardness, and rigidity, but never much fulness or regularity. This continual irregularity, often increased by the frequency and force of the palpitations will always be sufficient to establish the precise diagnosis of the constriction of the aortic mouth, or the lesion of its valves. Here is no obscurity; the physician with practice and attention ought ever to pronounce with confidence, and his diagnosis can no longer be uncertain though he should have for a guide only this species of undulation, this rushing noise, dull trembling, the characters so manifest by the pulse in every case of this nature.

Case XL. A coachman, forty-eight years of age, robust, and of a sanguine temperament, had, three days before his admission into the hospital, suffered a very severe peripneumony, treated mostly by venesection. He was hardly convalescent, when he came to the hospital, May 28, 1800. I requested him to go into the Clinical Hall for the purpose of examining his pulse, which indicated an organic lesion of the heart.

The pulse was very full, and even rigid, on the right side; small, soft, obscure and scarcely sensible on the left; but irregular, *undulating* and *tremulous* on each side.

He was attacked with haemoptysis and very considerable suffocation; the suffocation appeared instant; the eyes were wild, the face injected; the thorax here and there painful did not sound toward the region of the heart and the lower part of the right side. The pulse preserved the same character.

From the effects of percussion, difficulty of breathing, haemoptysis, and characters of the pulse, I recognized the existence of hydrothorax which I judged to be subsequent to an organic lesion of the heart with constriction of the aortic orifice.

The patient, while he remained here, was bled several times, and obviously relieved, but greatly debilitated; an obstinate costiveness required the use of mild purgatives.

Sometime after the infiltration, which already existed, increased; diuretics, aperients, and anti-spasmodics, procured but very little relief. The patient had no rest, and was obliged to sit up night and day; when the hand was applied over the region of the heart, he was endangered with suffocation. He became a victim to this series of symptoms, 5th

June, eight days after his admission into the hospital, and four after the peripneumony with which he was affected.

On opening the body, there was much water in the right cavity of the thorax, but little in the left. The lungs were hard and adhering to the pleura. The pericardium contained no serum; the size of the heart was much enlarged; the right auricle and ventricle presented nothing remarkable. The left auricle was sound, with a large orifice, upon the valves of which was observed an incipient ossification. The left ventricle was hard, thick, and very fleshy; the tendons of the valves were nearly ossified. The aortic valves were ossified and united so closely that the end of the little finger could scarcely be introduced into the orifice of the aorta; this artery was dilated, rugous and thickened to the end of its curvature. The left subclavian artery was about an inch from its origin so constricted as scarcely to admit the head of a large pin. The constriction was owing to the osseous thickening of the arterial parietes.

The nearly complete obli eration of the left subclavian artery explains perfectly why the pulse was scarcely sensible on this side; but this singular character could not obscure the diagnosis sufficiently demonstrated by the other symptoms, and particularly by the continual irregularity of the pulse.

To conclude what I have to say on the signs of the constrictions, it remains for me to speak of the cases where the obliteration of the orifice is momentarily produced by the presence of an excrescence, vegetation, or polypous concretion on this part.

When these vegetations are found appended to the mitral valves, they are announced by all the signs peculiar to the constriction of the left auricular orifice, with this exception, that most of these signs are reproduced, in this last case, only at intervals more or less remote. Though, during the contractions of the left ventricle, these appendages, constantly floating at the aortic mouth, continue applied against the walls of the vessel, their effects are then very nearly the same as those produced by the simple ossification of the semi-lunar valves of the aorta, and the constriction which this ossification occasions in the aperature of the vessel; but do these excrescences, by their weight, or any other cause, compress the valves, and appear at the aortic orifice, during the contraction even of the ventricle, it is obvious that a momentary and nearly total obliteration of the aperture of the aorta will follow. This closure intercepts inperfectly, for some instants, the passage of the blood; thence the successive regularities and irregularities of the pulse, the frequent and partial syncopes; this momentary interruption of the circulation compels the heart to redouble its efforts to surmount the obstacle that opposes it; thence the repeated strokes and violent palpitations of this organ which cease as soon as the obstacle is removed, and which are renewed when it is reproduced; thence the impossibility, sometimes very protracted, of feeling the pulse, while within an instant, these pulsations return with momentary force, vivacity, frequency and regularity.

I have nothing to say of the signs of the pulmonary sigmoïd and tricuspid valves, as I have but seldom had the opportunity of observing them; besides, I think, as it has been already remarked, that, though this morbid state should be more frequent, it would be as difficult to indicate the particular signs of the kind of affection, as it is to distinguish the constrictions of these same orifices from those of the left cavities.

. . . .

COROLLARIES

ARTICLE IV

OF THE PROGNOSIS OF THE DISEASES OF THE HEART

When the diseases of the heart assume an acute or chronic character, the prognostic is always very perplexing. Nevertheless there are important modifications to make to the general proposition which I have just announced.

In order to establish, with exactness, the prognosis of the diseases of the heart, it is necessary to distinguish these diseases into several kinds: they may be divided, (1) into acute, (2) into chronic organic, and (3) into organic properly called.

1. The acute diseases of the heart cannot with propriety be inserted among organic diseases; those which come under this denomination, are acute *pericarditis,* and *carditis,* or inflammation of the substance of the heart.

In respect to the prognosis, these diseases follow the same order as do all acute inflammations in general; the greater danger that they bring with them, in many cases, is the only point in which the prognosis differs. It generally varies as do the same degrees of these inflammations.

When acute *pericarditis* is not announced in the beginning by strong symptoms, or severe accidents; and a marked disturbance in the action of the heart does not signify that the organ itself is sensibly affected; and the contiguous viscera, as the lungs, etc. seem not to participate of the inflammation; when the subject is besides, sound and well organized, then a pretty favorable prognosis may be formed; hence it is not extraordinary to see *pericarditis,* which is otherwise one of the severest affections, attain, by the combined efforts of nature and art, to a happy termination.

But the cases in which the solution of the disease is satisfactory, are not the most common; it seldom happens, therefore, that this inflammation is found distinct from those of the pleurae costales, diaphragmaticae, mediastinae, pulmonales, and from the same affection of a greater or less portion of the substance even of the lungs, and of the surface of the heart itself, which in every instance, is more or less inflamed; then, the disease either terminates in death, or is transformed into one of those alterations which I have designated under the name of *chronic organic,* according to the purulence of the pericardium, the adhesion of this membrane to the heart, its chronic inflammations, etc., etc.

The prognosis of the inflammation of the texture of the heart, or of *carditis* united with the same affection of the other viscera of the thorax, or destitute of complications, is always most perplexing, not to say mortal, in all cases. Seldom, therefore, does the inflammation of the parts, whose muscular substance constitutes the basis, obtain without its terminating in suppuration, and the suppuration of the organs contained in the great cavities of the body is generally mortal.

It is my belief that acute *carditis* has never been seen to reach a perfect solution; and when cases are quoted, all doubts are not removed; some very justly remain as to the actual seat of the inflammation, which cannot invariably be well ascertained.

Hence this inflammation almost always terminates fatally; but the death which it usually occasions may happen instantly or somewhat slowly. Thus *carditis* has been known to become fatal in a very few days; while in other instances, when the disease has attained to its highest degree, the most alarming symptoms partially disappear, and a sort of convalescence is established; sometimes even the patient is restored to apparent health; he then flatters himself with a near and perfect cure; but the more intelligent physician perceives only a transformation, or degeneration of the disease into another affection slower, but not less severe, as *a chronic organic* disease is then established, mortal in all cases.

Among the acute lesions of the heart, considered relatively to the prognosis, ought to be inserted the partial ruptures mentioned in this work, and the rupture of a fleshy pillar of the heart, and of the valvular tendons.

The rupture of the fleshy pillars of the heart (Case XLIV), seems to assume all the most sensible characters of an acute disease; this is at least the inference that must be drawn from the consideration of the assemblage of accidents to which the courier became the victim.

The prognosis in the cases where this lesion is manifest, will therefore be desperate, and the physician must announce the fatal event of the disease, which occasions death sooner, as the lesion happens suddenly in a sound organ.

The rupture of the valvular tendons appears, according to my observations, to be not so severe and so immediately fatal as that of a portion of the muscular substance. Hence in almost all cases in which this rupture has been observed, an organic disease of the whole of the heart has invariably followed, without any acute affection of this organ.

The prognosis of the entire rupture or laceration of one of the cavities of the heart is here omitted; such accidents are hardly ever known but from their effect, which is sudden death, or at least exceedingly quick.

2. The diseases of the heart to which I give the name of *chronic organic,* are almost all from the effects, consequences or degenerations of acute inflammations whose prognosis has just been mentioned; of this number are the serous or purulent effusions into the pericardium, the adhesions of this membrane to the heart, the ulcerations of the surface of this organ, its chronic inflammation, the softening of its texture, etc.

These various affections are almost all, let it be repeated, the results of acute inflammations of the heart. Thus, when *pericarditis* has reached so far that the symptoms usually become more moderate, the disease seems sometimes to lose its intensity; but it is evidently protracted farther than there was reason to expect; then the affection acquires different characters which, on account of their being less severe, are not less embarrassing to the eye of the experienced physician. The prognosis, at first uncertain, though always dangerous even in the beginning of the disease, less detrimental when the inflammation carried to its highest degree, is suddenly moderated; it becomes more and more unfavorable when the concurrence of particular signs announces that the disease is mistaken, that it degenerates, that a serous or purulent effusion is formed in the pericardium, or the disease assumes some other troublesome termination.

If the physician has not been able to decide as to the danger of the affection which has preceded that whose prognosis he wishes to establish, the inquiries which he will be obliged to make for the purpose of gaining a knowledge of the disease, will teach him also what prognosis he ought to form.

3. If, in order to treat of the prognosis of the diseases of the heart, I had divided them into curable and incurable; among the first, might have been inserted with the acute inflammations, most of the diseases *properly called beginning organic,* which would undoubtedly yield to care, and medical aid, were the first symptoms of these diseases, to the patients themselves, sufficiently evident and strong to induce them to apply for assistance on the first appearance of the disease; for as it has already been said, there are physical and moral signs, by the benefit of which the experienced and attentive physician may well suspect their formation.

But, if these organic lesions are old, if they have made evident progress, if all the functions which are connected with the circulation, suffer already from its alteration, then the prognosis is altogether desperate; the physician has no longer to estimate the danger of the disease; whenever he ascertains its existence, he recognizes a mortal affection; and his experience can enlighten him only in estimating the time that the patient will be able to lead a lingering life, and in the choice of the means capable of rendering it the most supportable.

It is from the character, intensity of the organic lesion, the constitution of the individual, his manner of living, etc., etc., that the physician can pronounce concerning the fatal, near, or more or less remote, period of the subject exposed to his observation.

If the attack of the organic disease has been sudden, if, from the beginning, it has assumed some dangerous symptoms, if a very great disturbance of the circulation announces a deep lesion of the principal organ of this function, the prognosis will be far more troublesome than had the disease been more moderate in its attack, and presented different or opposite symptoms.

Relatively to the constitution of the individual, if it is vigorous, if the subject is in the flower of his age, if he is free from the various degenerations of the humors, without violent passions, obedient to good advice, etc. it will be found that the termination is not so soon fatal as in the contrary conditions. Finally, as to the manner of living, if the patient is devoted to vice, debauchery, and every kind of excess; if, from his condition, he is exposed to hard labor, to the inclemency of the atmosphere, to laborious exercise, and to lively moral affections, etc., it will hasten so much the end of his life; while by the means of sobriety, temperance, and care, he will not only prolong his days, but will be able even to prevent, for years, the organic disease, to which sooner or later he will fall a victim.

1812

WILLIAM CHARLES WELLS

ONE OF THE EARLIEST CLINICAL REPORTS ON THE CARDIAC PARTICIPATION IN RHEUMATIC FEVER

WILLIAM CHARLES WELLS

(1757-1817)

WILLIAM CHARLES WELLS was born in Charleston, South Carolina, on May 24, 1757. His parents had emigrated from Scotland in 1753. His father was a bookseller who was also skilled in the art of bookbinding. As was the custom among Colonial booksellers, he owned a printing press and later undertook to publish a newspaper. The Wells family was firm in its loyalty to Great Britain. In keeping with the ideals of the Southern gentry, young William was sent across the sea to gain his preliminary education. He attended grammar school in Dumfries, Scotland, for two and a half years. At the end of that time he spent one year as an undergraduate in the University of Edinburgh.

In 1771, Wells returned to his native city and became apprenticed to Dr. Alexander Garden. Dr. Garden was not only Charleston's most prominent physician but also had a deep interest in zoology and botany. He was a member of the Royal Societies of Upsala and London, and corresponded in Latin with Linnaeus, who perpetuated Garden's name by the gardenia, which he called ''one of the most beautiful flowering shrubs in the world.''

With the outbreak of the War of Independence, Wells, whose sympathies were with the King, left for England to be with his father, who had returned to England a few months previously. In 1776 young Wells began the study of medicine at the University of Edinburgh. In 1778 he passed his preliminary medical examinations. He then went to London and there attended the lectures on anatomy and midwifery given under the able direction of Dr. William Hunter. Later he spent some time at St. Bartholomew's Hospital and then studied in Leyden for three months. Wells returned to Edinburgh and in June, 1780, received his medical degree.

To settle his father's business, which apparently had been mismanaged by an elder brother, Wells embarked on a trip to the Carolinas. When the Tories lost control of Charleston, Wells moved the printing press and stock to St. Augustine, Florida. There he had no time for the practice of medicine, but became printer, bookseller, merchant, and trustee. He also spent some time acting in a local theater company. On his return to Charleston, Wells was obliged to spend three months in prison because of some debts his brother had accumulated. After more difficulties which arose because of his loyalistic tendencies, he sailed for England in May, 1784.

On his return to London, Wells became acquainted with Matthew Baillie,[1] with whom he later became intimate. He also numbered among his close friends David Hume, Lord Glenlee, Robertson Barclay and William Lister. In 1785 he began the practice of medicine in London.

In 1788, Wells became a licentiate of the Royal College of Physicians, and in 1789 became physician to the Finsbury Dispensary, an appointment which he held for ten years. In 1795 he was elected assistant physician to St. Thomas' Hospital, and in 1800 he was promoted to the rank of physician.

---

[1]See pp. 255-256, biographic sketch of Matthew Baillie.

In 1792 he published the important work that has endeared him to ophthalmologists, his ''Essay on Vision.''[2] Therein he explained why objects are seen singly with the two eyes. Because of this contribution, presumably, he was elected to the Royal Society in 1793.

Another important work of Wells appeared in 1814. This was his ''Essay on Dew.''[3] Pleadwell suggested that it was the foundation stone of the modern science of ventilation. In 1814, also, Wells was elected a fellow of the Royal Society of Edinburgh.

That Wells anticipated Darwin in recognizing the principles of natural selection is suggested in his paper entitled: ''Account of a Female of the White Race of Mankind part of whose Skin resembles that of a Negro.'' This was published in 1818 in his collected works.

Wells' classic article on rheumatism of the heart, which it is our privilege to reproduce, was written, it must be remembered, before the time of the stethoscope. For this reason alone, his contribution to the study of this disease is remarkable.

It seems that David Pitcairn, the prominent English physician, who with Matthew Baillie had proposed Wells for fellowship in the Royal College of Physicians in 1797, with an unsuccessful result, was the first physician to express a knowledge of the relationship of rheumatism to heart disease. Matthew Baillie referred to Pitcairn's discovery of 1788, in the second edition of his work on ''Morbid Anatomy,'' published in 1797. Wells also referred to Pitcairn in his article. Unfortunately, Pitcairn did not publish his observations on rheumatism and heart disease.

On July 29, 1789, Edward Jenner is said to have read a paper before the Fleece Medical Society[4] on ''Remarks on a Disease of the Heart Following Acute Rheumatism.'' It is to be regretted that the manuscript of this paper was lost and that Jenner's observations were never published. Wells did not know of Jenner's work on this subject. Sir David Dundas[5] noted the disease in 1808 and in the same year, according to Keil, J. F. Davis made note of a colleague's observations on ''Acute Rheumatism Attacking the Heart.'' Wells' contribution, the first thorough treatise on this disease, was read in 1810 and published in 1812.

In 1800, at the age of forty-three, Wells began to suffer from apoplexy. The disease incapacitated him for several months. However, he placed himself on a limited diet and managed to remain in fairly good health until 1813. His health then became poor from general weakness, associated with shortness of breath and swelling of the ankles. Wells noticed in 1817 that he frequently made the sudden and deep inspirations which are suggestive of the disease John Cheyne was to describe a year later.

In August, 1817, his physicians, Lister and Baillie, who were also personal friends, abandoned hope for his recovery as did Wells, himself. He died in London on September 18 of that year.

---

[2]Wells, William Charles: *An essay upon single vision with two eyes; together with experiments and observations on several other subjects in optics,* London, T. Cadell, 1792, 144 pp.

[3]Wells, William Charles: *An essay on dew, and several appearances connected with it,* London, Taylor and Hessey, 1814, 146 pp.

[4]Keil, Harry: A note on Edward Jenner's lost manuscript on "Rheumatism of the Heart," Bull. Hist. Med. 7: 409-411, 1939.

[5]Dundas, David: An account of a peculiar disease of the heart, Med. & Chir. Soc. 1: 36-46, 1808.

ON RHEUMATISM OF THE HEART*

By

WILLIAM CHARLES WELLS

DR. DAVID PITCAIRN, about the year 1788, began to remark, that persons subject to rheumatism were attacked more frequently than others, with symptoms of an organic disease of the heart. Subsequent experience having confirmed the truth of this observation, he concluded, that these two diseases often depend upon a common cause, and in such instances, therefore, called the latter disease rheumatism of the heart. He communicated what he had observed to several of his friends, and to his pupils at St. Bartholomew's Hospital, to which he was then Physician; but no notice, I believe was taken of his remark in any book, before it appeared in the second edition of Dr. Baillie's *Morbid Anatomy*, which was published in 1797. No similar observation, as far as I know, is to be found in any book written before that time. Morgagni, indeed, and Dr. Ferriar of Manchester, had given cases of rheumatism existing with an organic disease of the heart, but it is evident that they considered the concurrence of the two diseases as merely accidental; and it is very probable, that similar cases occur in other authors who wrote before Dr. Baillie, though I have not met with them.

Since the appearance of Dr. Baillie's work, this disease has been treated of by Dr. Odier, of Geneva, in his *Manuel de Medicine Practique,* printed in 1803, and by Mr. David Dundas, Sergeant Surgeon to the King, in a Paper lately published in the *Transactions* of the Medical and Surgical Society of London. Dr. Odier's work is only a text-book for Lectures given by him on the Practice of Medicine, and as is common in such works, very few references are made in it to other authors. As he received, however, his professional education in this country, and has long conducted the medical department of the Bibliotheque Britannique, a literary journal printed in Geneva, he could not be unacquainted with Dr. Baillie's *Morbid Anatomy.* Mr. Dundas takes no notice in his paper of what had been said upon the subject of it, either by Dr. Baillie or Dr. Odier. He could scarcely, indeed, have seen the *Manuel* of Dr. Odier, and it is probable, that he had not read the account, which was given of it in the *Edinburgh Medical Journal,* for October, 1806; but there is a greater difficulty in sup-

*Read April 3, 1810. Published in Tr. Soc. Improv. Med. & Chir. Knowledge 3: 373-424, 1812.

posing, that he was ignorant of what had been mentioned, twelve years before, in Dr. Baillie's popular work, respecting Rheumatism of the Heart, on the authority of Dr. Pitcairn.

As I knew that Dr. Pitcairn did not mean to publish anything upon this disease, and as I had good reason to believe, that it was unknown to many practitioners of medicine in this country, I formed the design, about four years ago, of offering a Paper upon it to this Society. But very shortly after, I saw the article in the *Edinburgh Medical Journal,* which relates to Dr. Odier's book, and, in consequence, determined not to proceed, till I should see the work itself. In the meantime, Mr. Dundas's Paper appeared, and this I found to contain so much information upon the subject of which it treats, that I necessarily regarded the value of what I had collected myself as much diminished, and therefore abandoned the design of communicating it. But considering afterwards, that even a repetition of what had been already said might be useful, in exciting the attention of physicians to a disease hitherto little spoken of, I lately resumed my intention, and now offer, in the form of Cases, what I have acquired from other sources than Mr. Dundas's Paper, as our knowledge of the disease is still too imperfect, to admit the formation of a just history of it. I once expected that my Paper would be enriched by the contributions of my late most excellent friend Dr. Pitcairn; for although I knew that he had preserved no account in writing of what he had seen in this disease, yet I was confident, that the extent of his observation, for he had treated more than a dozen cases of it, and the accuracy of his memory, would enable him to afford me much valuable information. But I neglected to obtain this while the opportunity existed, and I now lament my indiscretion.

CASE I

Mr. T. M. came from Scotland in April, 1798, to reside in Berkshire, being then in his eighteenth year. He was of a fair complexion, short stature, and a habit rather full than muscular. From the age of nine years he had been every year attacked with acute rheumatism. Four of the attacks had been very severe, each of them confining him to bed for several weeks; the others seldom kept him at home longer than a week, though the redness, swelling, and pain of the joints did not leave him for two or three weeks more. While he was labouring under this disease, the pains often shifted in the most sudden manner; and, in the greater fits of it, he was often distressed with a sense of oppression in his chest, frightful dreams, and despondency of mind. In November, 1797, he had likewise had a slight spitting of blood.

Four weeks after he came to Berkshire, he fell into a small pond of water, while attempting to leap over it, and wetted his lower limbs as far up as the middle of his thighs. He pursued, however, his exercise, and suffered his clothes to dry upon him. The following day, while walking in the streets of Oxford, he was suddenly seized with trembling and coldness, principally affecting his lower limbs, with faintness, giddiness, sickness at the stomach, and a sense of oppression in his chest. He afterwards became warm, and then began to feel a palpitation of his heart, and a beating in his head. In the progress of his illness, he was frequently attacked with breathlessness, a sense of choking, and a feeling as if he were about to expire. In the night time he used to be warm, and to sweat. After he had been affected in this way about three weeks, he came to London and consulted me. At his first visit, I did not become acquainted with all the circumstances which I have mentioned; and as I found his pulse frequent, and tongue white, and was told by him, that he was worse every other day at ten o'clock in the forenoon, I thought it probable, that his disease was a tertian fever, which had not yet fully intermitted. As I learned, however, when I saw him next, that the beating in his chest was never absent, though at some times much greater than at others, and that he had been much subject to rheumatism, I began to suspect, that his disease might be rheumatism of the heart, of which I knew nothing, except what I had learned from Dr. Baillie's publication. I carried him therefore to Dr. Pitcairn, who confirmed my conjecture, and was fearful that he would not recover.

Mr. M. went again into the country; but I had frequent letters respecting him and once visited him there. I think it, however, unnecessary to say more upon his case, than, that, after he had laboured under the palpitation four months, he was attacked with pains, swellings, and redness of his joints, which continued about six weeks, but were not so severe as to confine him to bed; that during this time the palpitation began to lessen, but that it did not entirely leave him before the end of the second year from its commencement. Mr. M. during his illness was several times seen by Dr. Bourne of Oxford. He was seen also by Mr. James Russell, of Edinburgh, who had often attended him in sickness in Scotland, and having been called by business to Birmingham, had afterwards extended his journey to Berkshire to visit him.

Since his recovery I have met with him frequently, and have several times applied my hand to the region of his heart, without feeling there any unusual beating. But he says, that exercise is now more apt to excite palpitation than formerly, and that he sometimes experiences it without any apparent cause. He thinks too, that it occurs oftener while he is affected with rheumatism of the joints, which continues to attack him every year, than at any other time. Before the palpitation comes on, he is seized with a gnawing pain in the region of the heart, and a sense of suffocation. In two or three minutes these symptoms either disappear, or become less; the palpitation then begins, and lasts about the same time. Such attacks, however, do not happen oftener than twice or thrice in the year.

I may add, that in the course of my correspondence with the relations of Mr. M. I learned, that one of his uncles, whom he resembles in external appearance, after being severely afflicted with rheumatism, became, when about sixteen or seventeen years old, subject to violent palpitation of the heart, and some time after died suddenly; and that, his body being opened, the heart was found enlarged.

CASE II

Martha Clifton, aged nearly fifteen years, was admitted into St. Thomas's Hospital, on the 18th of February, 1802, after labouring under acute rheumatism about sixteen days. Her pulse was small, but the heart struck the ribs with such force, that its beats could be reckoned by applying the hand to the right side of the chest. About two or three years before, she had likewise been affected with acute rheumatism, during the presence of which she had been troubled also with a violent beating of her heart. In the interval between the two attacks of rheumatism, she had experienced no palpitation in her chest. The account of what I did not observe myself I received from the patient, and her mother; but those, who are conversant with the business of an Hospital, know that little dependence is to be placed upon the accuracy of patients or their friends, when they speak of symptoms which have formerly occurred. She remained in the Hospital eleven weeks, and was then taken away by her relations, for the purpose of being sent into the country. The pains in her limbs were nearly gone, and the palpitation of her heart was much diminished.

Many of the tendons of the superficial muscles in this patient were studded with numerous small hard tumours, an appearance I have observed only in one other person, a thin and feeble man forty-one years old, who also laboured under rheumatism.*

CASE III

Charles Williams, aged twenty years, was received into St. Thomas's Hospital the 21st of June, 1804, on account of painful swellings of his joints, under which he had laboured seven months. His pulse was quick, and his heart beat forcibly against the ribs. He had often, he said, in the course of the last eight years, been affected with a similar disease of the joints, during which he had always been troubled with a palpitation of his heart. After remaining a month in the Hospital, without receiving much benefit, he was discharged from it for disorderly conduct.

*Dr. Lister has informed me, that the superficial tendons of Salmon, the subject of the seventh case in this Paper, were similarly affected. As Salmon did not mention this to me, and as I did not discover it myself, the same symptom may have existed in several of my patients, labouring under rheumatism, besides those of whom I have spoken.

CASE IV

Mary Bond came into St. Thomas's Hospital on the 9th of January, 1806, labouring under acute rheumatism, which had seized her eight days before. She was then in her sixteenth year, had never menstruated, and since her ninth year had been frequently attacked with rheumatism. When she had been three months in the Hospital, I discovered, that her heart beat much too strongly, and I was afterwards informed by her mother, that this symptom had always been present, while she was afflicted with rheumatism, but at no other time. She staid in the Hospital nearly four months, in the whole, and during that time frequently complained of pains in her chest. These, in the month of April, were attended for ten days with cough, difficulty of breathing, and an increase of fever. When she left the Hospital, the pains in her limbs were not entirely gone, and her heart was still beating strongly. Possibly, however, as the pains of her limbs had lessened considerably in the time between her coming into the Hospital, and the discovery of the palpitation, this symptom had also diminished in the same interval. I learned its existence from inquiring, if she was affected with it.

CASE V

I visited Miss A. L. for the first time, on the 17th of September, 1806, at her father's house in Surrey, distant about eight miles from London. She was sixteen years old, tall, and thin, and had never menstruated. Several of her relations had died of pulmonary consumption, and she herself had laboured under an acute disease of the chest about four years before. From that time, however, to the commencement of the train of ailments which I am about to describe, she had enjoyed very good health, and had possessed a much greater degree of bodily strength, than was indicated by her appearance.

In the beginning of August, shortly after remaining some time in a cold cellar, she was seized with pains, swelling, and redness of her joints, and fever. These symptoms lasted only ten days. About a week after they had ceased, she walked about a mile from her father's house, assisted by an attendant, and, while returning, accidentally wetted her feet. In the evening of the same day, she was attacked with pains in her feet, which were not accompanied with swelling or redness. These pains remained only a day or two; immediately upon their ceasing, her heart began to beat with considerable violence. Her right hypochondrium soon after became painful, and about the same time she began to complain of a pain in the tops of her shoulders. Various other symptoms had also occurred; but as no regular history of them had been kept, and as the most important existed when I visited her, I shall proceed at once to give an account of the situation in which I found her, at the distance of nearly four weeks from the second attack of external pains.

The palpitation of the heart, which had never ceased from its first appearance, was distinctly felt in every part of the thorax, to which my hand was applied. In the arteries, only a shaking was perceivable, which could not be divided into distinct pulsations. The strokes of the heart were one hundred and ninety in a minute; they were equal in force, and the intervals, which were also equal, were so distinct, that I fancied I could have numbered the strokes, if two hundred and fifty, or even three hundred, had been given in the same time. Her breathing was not laborious, and she had no cough; but she frequently complained of a great and indescribable anxiety in her chest. This was always much lessened by her taking a few drops of laudanum and a drachm of vitriolic aether, although no change was ever induced by these medicines on the palpitation. The external jugular veins were swollen, and alternately rose and fell. She had a little headache, was often sick at the stomach, and sometimes puked; what was thrown up was for the most part green, and had a sour smell. Her appetite for food was, notwithstanding, far from being lost. The tongue was somewhat foul, and a small part of its middle was dry, but her thirst was inconsiderable. She had two or three stools daily; their colour had formerly been green, but was now natural. There was now no pain in her shoulders, nor any in her right hypochondrium, except it was pressed. On the day I visited her, the skin and eyes had begun to be a little yellow, and her urine, which was said to be sufficiently copious, now gave a slightly yellow tinge to white linen. On examining her feet, I found them oedematous. Her muscular strength was greater than might have been expected, considering the length and magnitude of her ailments.

I staid all night at her father's, and saw her early on the following morning, when I was astonished at learning, that soon after taking fifteen drops of laudanum, late in the evening, she had become quiet, had remained so the whole night, and had enjoyed much refreshing sleep. The urine, which was passed in the night, had a pink-coloured sediment. In the other symptoms there was no change.

On the evening of the 19th, I visited her again, and was accompanied by Dr. John Meyer, of New Broad-street. The day before, she had been thought better; but many things seemed now to indicate her speedy death. The sickness had increased; her face and hands were cold, the skin pale, the motion of the artery at the wrist scarcely perceptible, and the strokes of the heart against the ribs of much less force than formerly. Their number was a hundred and seventy in the minute. She shewed, however, no sign of weakness of mind or of delirium, and her tongue was moist and clean.

My last visit was on the 21st. Shortly after Dr. Meyer and I had left her on the night of the 19th, she had vomited a considerable quantity of a thin fluid, mixed with a less quantity of a thick and very black fluid, after which she became better. I could again distinctly perceive motions in the arteries, though they were not to be reckoned. The beats of the heart were one hundred and sixty in the minute, and were felt only in the left side of the chest. The skin of the whole body was warm and moist; that of the neck and chest was partially covered with a miliary eruption. Her bowels had been several days bound, except when loosened by glysters. The abdomen was somewhat swelled, and pressure upon it gave more pain than at my first visit. She was drowsy, but this was attributed to some laudanum which she had taken. She had lately spitten a little blood, but she was still without a cough. Respiration, likewise, was performed with little difficulty, and took place only twenty-five times in a minute.

On the following night, as I was afterwards informed, she was restless, which was attributed chiefly to the inflamed state of the skin of the chest, from a blister which had been applied several days before. She complained frequently in the night of pains in her legs and feet. She took, however, a considerable quantity of food; and her breathings, being reckoned, were found to be only twenty-two in a minute, although there was no diminution in the number of the beats of the heart. In the morning, she began to be inattentive to what was passing in her room, and to speak sometimes a little incoherently. At two o'clock in the afternoon she died suddenly.

I had previously requested a friend of the family to apply, when death should occur, for permission to me to inspect the body. Application was accordingly made, and permission obtained. But some mistake was committed with respect to informing me of what had happened; and the weather being warm, and the family anxious to have the examination over, this was performed by the apothecary who had attended the deceased, assisted by his partner, and another medical gentleman. Had I been present, the younger Mr. Cline would have conducted the examination, as he had been kind enough to promise to accompany me for that purpose. The following are the principal morbid appearances, which, as I was afterwards informed, were observed.

The pleura of the ribs, and that of the lungs, were inflamed, and in many places adhered to each other. The lungs felt firm and fleshy, from containing a quantity of coagulated blood. The whole of the internal surface of the pericardium was attached to the heart, by means of two distinct layers of solid matter, each having the thickness of a shilling; the outer resembled coagulated blood, while the inner was whitish, and sufficiently tenacious to permit its being torn. The surface of the heart was also inflamed, and, from the right auricle to the apex, black; its substance was flaccid, and appeared to be enlarged. About a pint of bloody serum was found in each cavity of the chest. A considerable quantity of fluid, slightly red, was likewise found in the abdomen. The right lobe of the liver was enlarged, and much inflamed, and, on its concave surface, black. The stomach, where in contact with the liver, was also black, and many parts of it had marks of inflammation. Many portions of the small intestines were inflamed, and the lower half of the rectum seemed to be gangrenous. I must remark, however, that what has been said of the stomach and intestines relates only to their external appearance, for no part of them was opened.

CASE VI

John Miller, a sailor aged thirty-six years, pale and thin from bad health, was admitted into St. Thomas's Hospital, on the 1st of June, 1809, on account of pains in his limbs, with which he had been afflicted five months. His pulse was frequent and rather feeble, and during the two last months he had felt a constant beating in his left side, which upon examination I found to depend upon the action of the heart. He remained in the Hospital two months, in which time he became free from pain in his limbs, and in a great measure recovered his flesh; but the pulsation in his side, which had never been very great, continued unchanged. He now thought himself sufficiently well to go to sea, and was discharged from the Hospital at his own desire.

CASE VII

George Salmon, at present in St. Thomas's Hospital, a domestic servant, nineteen years old, of a fair complexion, short stature, and while in health fresh-coloured, and inclined to be fat, but now pale and thin, became the patient of my colleague, Dr. Lister, on the 11th of January last. From the notes which Dr. Lister has been kind enough to communicate to me, and from my own examination of the patient, I have collected the following circumstances of his case.

In June, 1808, three days after being heated in a playhouse, and drinking while in this state a considerable quantity of porter, he was attacked with stiffness, pains, and weakness in his limbs, and with pains and swellings in the joints of his fingers. During this illness he also laboured, for a fortnight, under a pain of the right side of his chest, and a cough. In the course of three months the ailments in his joints became much less; but he did not entirely recover his health for nine months more, during which time he used to feel a beating in his forehead after running, and often had the joints of his fingers swelled for three or four days. He remained perfectly well to the middle of December, 1809, when he was seized with stiffness, and slight pain in his lower limbs, attended with a rash, and feverishness. The rash occupied various parts of his skin in succession, but was never very extensive, and receded in a week. It has since been several times present for a day, but has not appeared for the last six weeks. Shortly after the beginning of his illness, the joints of the fingers began to swell again, and to be painful when pressed, in which state they still continue. Sometimes they are slightly red, and the back of his right hand was lately swelled, and a little red, for a few days. The stiffness and pain of his lower limbs began to decrease soon after he came into the Hospital; the former is now nearly gone, and the latter has not been felt by him for a fortnight. In the first part of his stay in the Hospital, he was attacked with a pain in his left side, which was increased when he drew his breath; this remained about fourteen days, and he has lately been frequently troubled with a slight cough. Since his admission into the Hospital, it has been discovered, that his heart palpitates. He does not know that he laboured before under this symptom; but this seems no proof of its not having existed, for he is still scarcely ever conscious of it, from any internal feeling. While he is sitting or lying, the palpitation is often not to be perceived from applying the hand to his left side; but as soon as he rises it becomes very evident. The pulse varies in point of number very considerably, but is generally between ninety and a hundred. The strokes are full, but are easily made to vanish by pressure. Each stroke is given rapidly, as if with a jirk, forming, I think, what Morgagni calls the vibrating pulse, and which so frequently occurs in diseases of the heart, particularly at their commencement, and in acute rheumatism. His skin is cool, but at night, he says, his feet often burn. His tongue is a little white, his appetite much diminished, his bowels open; his urine is of a deep straw colour, but does not become turbid by cooling. He has no difficulty of breathing, except what he attributes to weakness, and his head is free from pain and uneasy feelings. He sleeps little, but is unable to assign any reason for it.*

Having finished the description of the cases seen by myself, which I think may be properly arranged under the title of rheumatism of the heart, I shall next relate several more, the knowledge of which I have derived from other sources.

CASE VIII

This has been furnished by Dr. Baillie, and will be given in his own words.

"March 25, 1807.

"A boy about ten years old, of a fair complexion, and irritable constitution, who had a scrophulous scar under the left side of the lower jaw, after labouring many months under rheumatism, was attacked with palpitation of the heart, and some time after died. He was attended by Dr. Vaughan, Dr. Reynolds, and myself. His body was examined, but I was not present. The heart, as I have been informed, was somewhat enlarged, and there was a strong adhesion of the pericardium to it. He had a few tubercles of the lungs, and I believe some of the glands of the mesentery were enlarged. The liver was also of a greater size than usual."

*This patient left the Hospital a day or two after his case was taken by me.

In another communication, dated in April, 1809, Dr. Baillie says—"I have known a good many instances of palpitation of the heart in children, and young people of both sexes. I cannot, however, now remember distinctly more than three or four, where this affection was preceded by rheumatism. But I can hardly doubt that several cases of this kind have been forgotten by me."

CASE IX

I received this from my colleague, Dr. Lister.

"Miss P--, thirteen years of age, became my patient on the 17th of May, 1807, at which time she laboured under a very considerable difficulty of breathing, and a palpitation of the heart so violent, that not only the motion it gave to her clothes might be seen at a distance, but her body itself was shaken by it. Both these symptoms were increased by the least exercise. She had a slight cough; her countenance discovered great uneasiness; her pulse beat a hundred and thirty-six times in a minute; the tongue was white; the appetite was less than natural; the bowels were confined; the urine was in the usual quantity. She was emaciated, and her emaciation was said to have taken place during her present illness. I was informed, that she had been attacked in the beginning of the preceding February with acute rheumatism, which lasted about a fortnight, and that, when this left her, the shortness of breath, palpitation and cough came on. At first the cough was very considerable. Her feelings became less uneasy, and her pulse slower, under the use of a spare diet, and of a blister applied to the region of the heart. The alleviation of symptoms occurred too quickly to have been the effect of digitalis, which she was taking at the same time. On the 25th, the feet began to be oedematous; on the 29th the abdomen was swelled, and a fluctuation was to be felt in it. On the 5th of June, the anasarca was general; the swelling of the abdomen was increased; the pulse intermitted, and was slower. On the 6th, in the morning, the swelling of the abdomen was lessened, and the patient thought herself much better. In the evening, she was suddenly seized with extreme difficulty of breathing, and an occasional suspension of breathing; while the breathing was suspended, the pulse either did not beat at all, or beat very slowly. On the 7th, at two o'clock in the morning, she died.

"Leave having been obtained for examining the body, the examination was made by my friend Mr. Smith, of Southampton-street, on the 8th of June, and the following is the account he was so good as to give me of the appearances he observed.

"The lungs adhered to the pleura costalis almost at every part. The left side of the chest contained about five ounces of water; in the right side there was about one ounce. The pericardium adhered to the whole surface of the heart; the adhesion was easily separable by means of the fingers. The heart was twice as large as natural; its muscular structure was increased in thickness, and all its cavities were very much loaded with blood. The cellular membrane of the lungs contained some water. In the cavity of the abdomen there was about a pint of water, in which were floating several portions of coagulable lymph. The viscera of the abdomen were free from disease.''

CASES X and XI

Both of these have been communicated to me by Mr. Benjamin Brodie, Assistant-Surgeon to St. George's Hospital.

''A girl, fourteen years of age, was admitted into St. George's Hospital, in the middle of April, 1807, with symptoms of acute rheumatism affecting the extremities. These symptoms in a short time subsided, but were immediately succeeded by pain in the chest, attended with a sense of oppression in breathing, palpitation of the heart, a quick feeble pulse, and general debility. On the 23d of May she died.

''On inspecting the body, the lung on each side was found adhering to the pleura lining the ribs, but the adhesions were not of a recent date.

''About twelve ounces of serous fluid were effused into the cavities of the chest.

''The pericardium was much inflamed, and the two folds of that membrane were united by a layer of coagulable lymph.''

''A woman, twenty-five years of age, was admitted into St. George's Hospital, under the care of Dr. Nevison, in July, 1807, labouring under dropsy of the abdomen, anasarca of the lower extremities, and a constant palpitation of the heart. She said, that some months previous to her admission she had been attacked with a rheumatic fever; that, on the fever subsiding, she was seized with the palpitation of the heart, which had continued ever since; and that the dropsical symptoms had appeared more lately. She died a few weeks after her admission.

''On inspecting the body, the lungs were found partially adhering to the mediastinum. There were adhesions every where between the two folds of the pericardium. On the internal surface of the left auricle of the heart, there was a space, of about an inch square, studded with very minute excrescences resembling small warts. Three excrescences of a larger size were found on the internal surface of the left ventricle, about an inch below the semilunar valves. One of these was so large, as to project about half an inch into the cavity of the ventricle. Two or three similar excrescences were attached to the mitral valve, and semilunar valves of the aorta.''

CASE XII

This case was originally published in the *London Medical Journal,* for April, 1803, by Mr. Wagstaffe of Southwark, in whose practice it had occurred. As it appears to me valuable, for this, among other reasons, that the body was examined after death by a teacher of anatomy, Mr. John Taunton, I shall here give an abridgment of the original account of it.

Miss M. aged about fourteen years, of a spare habit, sallow complexion, and active disposition, became the patient of Mr. Wagstaffe, in the middle of January, 1802, on account of her labouring under acute rheumatism. After continuing ill in town for nearly two months, she went into the country, whence she returned in a short time, apparently in good health. She remained well till the beginning of October, when she was again attacked with acute rheumatism. This disease disappeared in about a week, leaving a most distressing cough, an excruciating pain in the left side, palpitation of the heart, and difficult respiration, attended with great dread of suffocation. The pulse varied from a hundred to a hundred and forty in the minute; it was sometimes throbbing, at other times weak. Blood taken from the arm, at this period of the disease, exhibited but slight marks of inflammation. In a few days the respiration grew more difficult, and the patient now began to be sometimes affected with vomiting. Her situation afterwards became much less distressing, apparently in consequence of medical treatment; but the amendment did not continue long, and she died in great agony on the 23d of November.

On opening the body, strong and extensive adhesions were found between the lungs, and the adjoining parts; but the lungs themselves were sound. The pericardium was attached so closely to the heart, that it was very difficult in most places, and in some quite impossible, to separate them. The heart was enlarged, but its structure was natural. The abdominal viscera were in a healthy state.

. . . .

The preceding cases appear to me just instances of rheumatism of the heart. The two which follow are less so, but seem, notwithstanding, sufficiently connected with my subject, to excuse my relating them.

Philip Smith, aged fifteen years, feeble from his birth, became a patient in St. Thomas's Hospital, on the 9th of July, 1807. In 1804, he had laboured under acute rheumatism four months. Two years after this, he was seized with a fever, which lasted also four months. During the fever, his heart began to beat more strongly than formerly, and it continued to do so ever after. From the time of his recovery from the fever, he had often felt pains, chiefly at night, in his lower limbs. The front of his head almost constantly ached; and blood had twice lately flowed from his nostrils. His face was frequently flushed, and sometimes appeared to him a little swollen. After he had been a fortnight in the Hospital, he was attacked with a pain in his right side, and a cough. He was an only child, and his father was so unhappy while they were separated, that he took him home on the 30th of July.

Mr. E. of Canterbury, about twenty-four years of age, of a fair complexion, and stout make, after being long constantly afflicted with rheumatism, either in its acute or chronic form, became subject to attacks of extreme difficulty of breathing, and a sense of tightness across his chest, attended with a pulse always frequent and small, and sometimes irregular. These attacks had of late occurred about once a month. They were frequently preceded by a slight inflammation of the fauces, and were sometimes accompanied with inflammatory swellings of the joints, but never with cough, or pain in the chest. When the difficulty of breathing was most urgent, no motion was perceptible in the abdomen from respiration. Such was the account of Mr. E's disease, which I received in September, 1806, from his medical friends in Kent. By my own examination of him I learned, that in his best state he had a constant uneasiness under his sternum, which was increased by a deep inspiration; that he had often a beating of his heart while he was at rest, and always after he had walked a little quickly, when it was attended with breathlessness; that his pulse was frequent, and that his urine was highly coloured when first made, and became turbid on cooling. A month after he consulted me, I was informed by one of his medical friends that he was better; and the following year I was told, by a person whom he sent to me, that he was altogether well.

I think it proper also to mention here, that I have seen four persons die of peripneumony, which had supervened to acute rheumatism. The heart of one of them, a sailor boy, fourteen years old, beat with more than ordinary force, while he laboured under the disease of his chest. In another, a female servant, nineteen years of age, a patient of Dr. Lister's in St. Thomas's Hospital, the heart palpitated strongly in the beginning of the peripneumony. Her body being opened, along with other marks of disease in the contents of the chest, the pericardium was found to adhere in various places to the heart. The heart was not enlarged; but its muscular substance was in several places inflamed. Permission could not be obtained to examine the bodies of any of the other three patients. In all the four, the disease of the limbs either had become less, shortly before the accession of peripneumony, or was considerably diminished very soon after. Several other examples have been seen by me of an attack of peripneumony, in persons affected with acute rheumatism, but in these the patients recovered.

To render the historical part of my subject more complete, I shall add, that, in Mr. Burns' *Observations on the Diseases of the Heart,* there is an account of a girl affected with palpitation, who, among other symptoms, had frequently shifting pains in several of the large joints, and had formerly laboured under rheumatism; that, in the Nineteenth Number of the *Edinburgh Medical Journal,* an instance is related by Mr. Crowfoot of acute rheumatism, in a tall feeble man, about twenty-two years of age, being attended with symptoms of a diseased heart; and that of the three cases of carditis, which have been published by Dr. Davis, in his treatise on that disease, the first occurred in a girl twelve years old, who had laboured eight days under pains in her left shoulder, and insteps, before any symptom of a diseased heart appeared, and became free from those pains the second day after the accession of such symptoms; the second, in a boy seven years old, who suffered acute pains in the lower extremities, during different parts of his illness; and the third in a girl sixteen years of age, the disease of whose heart succeeded the sudden disappearance of inflammation in her feet and ancles.

. . . .

In regard to the treatment of rheumatism of the heart, the propriety of enjoining rest and low diet in the beginning of it, and, in every stage, of producing a discharge of serous or purulent matter from the integuments of the thorax in the neighbourhood of the heart, by the use of cantharides or other means, will, I believe, be admitted by every person. But, when the tender age of those most liable to it, and their frequent weakness, whether original, or consequential to the disease of the joints which had previously existed, are considered, it may often appear improper to bleed, even at its commencement. Besides, as it has been found, that in London bleeding is never necessary for the cure of acute rheumatism of the external parts, and sometimes proves highly injurious; and, as the translation of the disease to the heart seems analagous to the recession of gout from the extremities; additional arguments may hence be derived against the general practice of bleeding, even in the very onset of the disorder. My own opinion, however, is in favour of copious bleeding, in the beginning of the disease, notwithstanding the force of the arguments which I have related. When the disease of the heart has quickly followed the entire disappearance, or considerable diminution, of that in the joints, we may attempt to bring back the latter, or to imitate it, by inducing inflammation in their integuments. I followed this practice in the case of Miss A. L.; but she suffered so much distress from the stimulating substances, which were applied to her joints, that her mother soon removed them; and, as her situation had from the first appeared to me hopeless, I thought it cruel to urge their renewal. If the disease assumes a chronic form, and there be evident signs of an enlarged heart, it should, in my opinion, be treated, as if the enlargement had never been connected with external rheumatism; in which case, Dr. Ferriar of Manchester has experienced beneficial effects from the use of tonic remedies.

What has hitherto been said of the method of cure relates, chiefly, to the most considerable cases of the disease. In others of less magnitude, a different mode of treatment may sometimes, perhaps, be with propriety adopted, especially if they have been of long standing. In the second case, for instance, related by me, that of Martha Clifton, as I was informed that she had laboured under palpitation of the heart, in a former fit of rheumatism of the limbs, and that both diseases had left her at the same time, I applied myself solely to the removal of that in the limbs, expecting that the other would recede with it; and the event partly justified my practice, for they diminished together, though they both existed in some degree when she left the Hospital. I received similar information regarding the cessation of the internal and external disease in the former attacks, which had been suffered by the subjects of the third and fourth cases, and followed therefore a similar mode of practice. On the same grounds, I employed mercury in the treatment of John Miller, the subject of the sixth case, but unsuccessfully with respect to the removal of the palpitation.

To conclude, I take the liberty of calling to the recollection of the Society, that the bodies of six of the persons, whose cases I have related, were examined after death, and that in two of them the liver was found diseased. I had supposed this to arise from the impeded passage of the blood from the vena cava through the heart, and its consequent congestion in the vessels of the liver; but I have lately learned, that Dr. Odier has seen rheumatism translated from the joints to that viscus. The two instances, therefore, of disease in the liver, to which I have referred, may possibly have arisen from a common cause with the disease of the heart and not have been the effect of it.*

POSTSCRIPT

Read November 5, 1811

After the preceding Paper had been read to the Society, two further cases of rheumatism of the heart occurred to me, which seem worthy of being made known to it.

CASE XIII

Charles Mills, aged sixteen years, was admitted into St. Thomas's Hospital, on the 17th of August, 1810, after labouring three days under pains of his limbs. He was of a feeble appearance; and, four years before, his right leg had been amputated, in the same Hospital, on account of a long disease of the ancle. I saw him first at one o'clock in the afternoon of the 18th. His ancle was swelled, painful, and a little red. His pulse was frequent, and his face flushed; and both the latter symptoms were in a greater degree, as I then thought, than could be occasioned by the disease of the ancle, though he complained of nothing else. Three hours

*The following case, which I met with after the preceding Paper had been read to the Society, strengthens my former opinion.

A sailor boy, seventeen years old, was received into St. Thomas's Hospital, June 6, 1811, after he had laboured four months under a pain in the region of his heart, difficulty of breathing, and a slight cough. His pulse was frequent; his heart beat somewhat too strongly, especially when he stood or walked; and his lower limbs were a little dropsical. He remained nearly in the same state till about the middle of August. All the symptoms of the disease in his chest then increased, and he died on the 2d of September. I had never observed the beats of his heart and arteries to have, during any short space of time, unequal force, or to follow one another at unequal intervals. No disease of the limbs had preceded or accompanied that in his chest. His body was examined the day after his death. The pleura of the lungs adhered in many places to the pleura of the ribs, and, between other parts of those membranes were found about twelve ounces of a watery fluid. The heart was enlarged, but not considerably. The pericardium and the covering of the heart adhered every where so closely together, that they could not be separated, and scarcely any line of distinction could be perceived between them. The aortic valves were thickened. In other respects the heart was sound. Both the liver and spleen were enlarged, but their substance appeared to be without disease. The stomach and gallbladder were likewise large. A few ounces of a watery fluid were found also in the abdomen.

afterwards, he was attacked with a pain in his left side, difficulty of breathing, and a slight cough. In two hours more, the pain in his side was increased, but that of the ancle was nearly gone. At nine o'clock in the evening, the pain of the side, and the difficulty of breathing, having become greater, and his heart having begun to palpitate strongly, six ounces of blood were taken from his arm. After the bleeding, the symptoms were less for half an hour, at the end of which time they became as considerable, as they had been before. At four o'clock the next morning, the pain in the side was very great, and the palpitation violent. The patient frequently nearly fainted, and his pulse was one hundred and thirty in a minute. Eight ounces of blood being now taken away, the palpitation and pain became less. A blister was soon after applied to his left side. The occurrences after one o'clock on the 18th took place, while I was absent from the Hospital. I saw him again at one o'clock in the afternoon of the 19th. His breathing was then a little difficult, and his pulse one hundred and twenty in the minute, small, and hard; but the palpitation had ceased entirely, and the pain of his side had nearly ceased. On the 20th, his pulse was one hundred and twelve, and was softer and fuller than on the preceding day; he had no pain either in his side or ancle, and no cough. On the following day the palpitation was present several hours, and he complained of a feeling of tightness across his chest. Eight ounces of blood were in consequence taken from him, and it was directed, that the blistered part of his side should be dressed with the ointment of cantharides. From this time I scarcely ever observed the palpitation to be entirely absent. On the 28th his pulse was ninety-two, to which it had gradually fallen. He complained this day of a pain in the right side of his chest, and on the 4th of September of pain in his ancle and left shoulder; but, in both cases, the pain lasted only a day or two. The palpitation having increased considerably, and the pulse having become more frequent, eight ounces of blood were taken away on the 11th of September, though he had no pain in his chest. During the whole of his stay in the Hospital, he had been restricted to a low diet, and had taken as much tartarised antimony every six hours, as his stomach could bear without sickness being produced by it. When his bowels were costive, a little Epsom salts had been given to him. A discharge of serum or pus, from the skin of the left side of the thorax, had always been preserved. On the 15th of September, the antimonial medicine was omitted, and he was ordered to take ten drops of the tincture of digitalis three times a day. He used the digitalis for more than three weeks, and during this time the pulse was mostly as slow as it is in a healthy person, and sometimes intermitted; but the palpitation of the heart was scarcely lessened in force. On the 11th of October he left the Hospital. I saw him three months afterwards, at which time the strokes of his heart against the ribs were more frequent, and much stronger, than they ought to have been, if he had been entirely well. His external appearance, however, was nearly that of a healthy person. He said, that he had now no ailment, and that, for the most part, he did not feel any beating at his heart; but that shortly after he went from the hospital he had been seized with a pain in his chest, which, however, left him soon, without his using any medicine. I saw him again a few days ago, about a twelvemonth after he went from the Hospital. He has become taller, and more robust, and has the look of being in perfect health, and this he said he enjoys. But I found his pulse to be one hundred and ten in a minute, and his heart to beat strongly against the ribs. The beating he imputed to his surprise at seeing me; and he assured me, that now he almost never experiences the slightest degree of it. As I staid with him, however, half an hour, and during the whole of that time perceived alteration in the action of the heart, I must conclude, at least, that a small degree of surprise produces a greater effect upon it, than would happen, if there did not exist in it some remnant of an organic disease.

CASE XIV

Anne Warwick, a nursery maid, in the twenty-first year of her age, was received into St. Thomas's Hospital, on the 14th of March, 1811, being then affected with acute rheumatism, which had attacked her a month before. She had also pains in her chest, which I supposed to be seated in the external muscles, and a headach. In the course of the two preceding years, she had twice laboured under acute rheumatism, in a more considerable degree than at present, but at both those times she was free from ailment in her chest. The day after she came into the Hospital, she was seized with a pain in the region of the heart, on account of which a blister was applied to her left side. The following day I found her heart to beat strongly, which she said it had done nearly two days. Her breathing was also difficult, but she had no cough. Ten ounces of blood being taken from her arm, the symptoms of the disease in her chest were lessened; they encreased, however, on the morrow, and again became less, after a blister had been applied over the sternum. Her pulse was one hundred and forty in a minute, and she had now no pain in any limb except the right leg. On the evening of the 18th, she was breathless, and had a great tendency to faint; but she did not complain of pain in her side or palpitation. The disposition to faint was, indeed, always present, when the disease of the chest was urgent, and at such times she frequently did faint. Twelve ounces of blood were drawn from her arm, and she soon became better. On the 21st, the difficulty of breathing and palpitation returned, but ceased almost immediately after she lost ten ounces of blood. I here mean by palpitation such a degree of beating of the heart against the ribs, as excited the patient's attention, and was uneasy to her. For I believe, that the heart, from the time of the first attack of the pain in her side, had always beat much more strongly in her, than it ordinarily does in a person in health. She remained free from uneasy feelings in her chest till the 28th, when she was attacked again with pain in the left side, and palpitation of the heart, both of which ceased on the following day, within two hours after twelve ounces of blood were taken from her. The pain of her side never returned; but she was often afterwards breathless and disposed to faint, particularly when in an erect posture; but, as her strength had been much reduced by bleeding and other circumstances, these symptoms were probably occasioned only in part by the disease of her heart. On the 31st, about an ounce of blood flowed from her nose, soon after which her headach ceased, which had been almost constantly present from the day of her admission, into the Hospital. She continued long feeble, and suffered much from various ailments, during the rest of her stay in the Hospital, which lasted till the 1st of the following June. When she went away, she complained of nothing; but she was still weak, and her heart still beat strongly. One of the nurses of the Hospital saw her about a month afterwards, at which time she appeared to be altogether well. I have no doubt, however, but that the action of her heart was then too great.

I shall now mention several things respecting this patient, which I have hitherto omitted speaking of, in order that the narration of the chief circumstances of her case might not be interrupted.

1. For the first four weeks, the only medicines she took internally were lemon juice, neutralised by salt of tartar, and infusion of senna with Epsom salts. During the same time, a constant discharge, either of serous or of purulent matter, from the skin of the left side of her chest, was procured by means of cantharides; but when she became feeble, the discharge was allowed to cease, as the cantharides irritated her then considerably. At the commencement of the fifth week, she began to take the tincture of digitalis thrice a day, in doses of twenty drops, and she continued its use eight days. It seemed to produce no effect, either upon her pulse or her stomach.

2. Her pulse, during the whole of her stay in the Hospital, except upon one day, was very frequent; once, while she was in bed, it was a hundred and forty-four in the minute; but its strokes and intervals were always equal, except on the day to which I have just alluded. It was then only seventy-six in the minute, and both the strokes and intervals were very unequal. It was felt while she was in a sitting posture; and she had not taken digitalis for five weeks.

3. I have said that, in the first attack of the disease of her heart, she had no cough, no cough ever occurred in the progress of that disorder; from which it seems probable, that the inflammation did not affect any portion of the lungs.

4. After she had been a month in the Hospital, I discovered an eruption on the skin of her chest, arms, and hands, which I pronounced positively to be the itch. It went away, however, in three weeks, without any means being employed to remove it.

5. Five weeks after she came into the Hospital, she complained of her throat being painful. A few days afterwards, I perceived her breath to smell, as if she were in a salivation from the use of mercury; her tongue at the same time felt sore, and had white spots upon it. Saliva also ran from her mouth, though in no great quantity. She had used no mercury, in any form, while in the Hospital. This state of her mouth lasted nearly three weeks, and caused her to become feeble, chiefly by preventing her from taking food. Small doses of Peruvian bark were now prescribed for her; and she was allowed a little porter. Hitherto she had been kept on a low diet, and had been debarred the use of all fermented liquors.

6. Immediately after her mouth had become well, and as her strength was returning, her feet and legs began to be dropsical; but her progress towards recovery did not seem to be retarded by this event, and the swellings disappeared in the space of ten days. While they were present, she took Griffith's mixture of iron, myrrh, and salt of tartar.

7. The pains in her limbs, which were said to have nearly ceased at the time she was first seized with the pain in her side, never returned with any violence. Indeed, while the disease of her chest was most considerable, they were sometimes entirely absent. They increased a little, when the disease of the chest became less, but left her altogether a few days before she went out of the Hospital.

In both of the preceding cases, the general health of the patients seems to have suffered from the means which were employed to overcome the internal inflammation; but, I shall not hence be deterred, from using the same means in an equal degree, in any similar case that may hereafter occur to me. The palpitation, which remained in both patients so long after the violence of the disease had been subdued, probably depended, in part, upon some relic of inflammation in the immediate covering of the heart, and, in part also, upon the heart being irritated by the adhesion of the pericardium to it. As the palpitation, however, entirely ceased, in the course of time, in Mr. T. M. the subject of the first Case in the foregoing Paper, it is to be hoped, and perhaps expected, that time will produce a similar effect in the subjects of the two last cases.

1818

JOHN CHEYNE

DESCRIPTION OF THAT PERIODIC TYPE OF RESPIRATION LATER TO BECOME KNOWN AS THE CHEYNE-STOKES TYPE

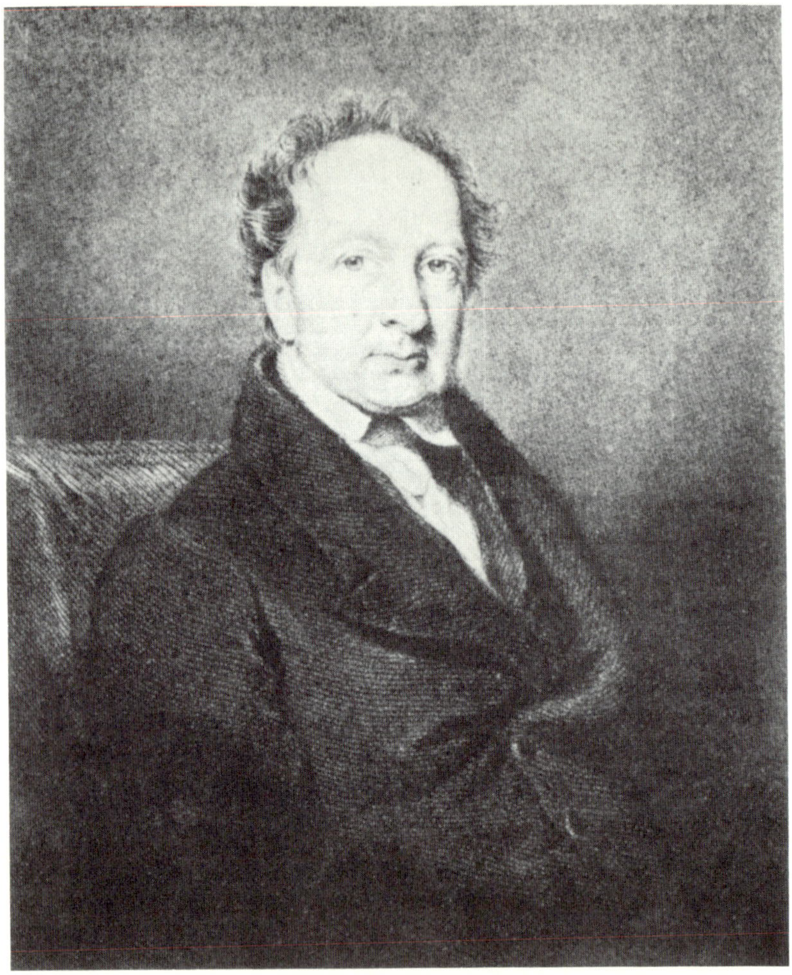

JOHN CHEYNE

(Courtesy Medical Classics.)

JOHN CHEYNE

(1777-1836)

JOHN CHEYNE was born on February 3, 1777, at Leith, the seaport of Edinburgh. His father was a physician and, according to Pettigrew, was a man of great cheerfulness, benevolence, good sense, and singleness of mind. Cheyne's mother was the daughter of William Edmonston, a fellow of the Royal College of Surgeons (Edinburgh).

Young Cheyne's education began with four years at the grammar school at Leith. When he was ten years of age he was sent to the high school at Edinburgh. There he was placed under the care of Dr. Adam, rector and headmaster. This seems to have been an ill-advised step, for Cheyne was not yet ready for high school and was consequently unable to keep up with the required pace. In general, he was very unhappy while he was at school.

Soon he left high school and was tutored by a clergyman of the Episcopal Church of Scotland. Under his new instructor he studied Greek and Latin for a period of two years, but again, as at high school, he apparently profited little from this contact.

When he was twelve years old he made his acquaintance with the practice of medicine by assisting his father in caring for the elder Cheyne's charity patients. It was his duty to supply these patients with medicine, to bleed them when necessary, to dress their wounds, and to report their conditions to his father.

In 1792, Cheyne began to attend the medical lectures at the University of Edinburgh. His contacts with his father's patients, effects of medical lectures he had heard, the boarding-house jargon of medical students, his frequenting a club of students who alternately examined each other in the required medical subjects, and the assistance of the celebrated ''grinder,'' Mr. Caudlish, all combined to aid Cheyne when he took his examination in 1795. This he passed without difficulty, and obtained his medical degree.

Following graduation, Cheyne left Edinburgh for Woolrich, where the Royal Regiment of Artillery was quartered. There he was appointed to the medical corps as assistant surgeon. He served with the army in various parts of England until 1797, in which year he was elevated to the rank of surgeon. He accompanied a brigade of home artillery to Ireland, and was in action in the campaign against the rebels at Ross and Vinegar Hill in 1798.

Cheyne left the army in 1799 and returned to Scotland. On his return he was placed in charge of the Ordnance Hospital at Leith Fort. He also assisted his father in medical practice. At this time he was fortunate in making the acquaintance of Charles Bell (1774-1842), the leading British physiologist of the day, who later was knighted for his researches in the field of neurology. Bell assisted Cheyne in making dissections and taught him the rudiments of pathologic anatomy.

Cheyne had in 1795 published his first work, ''De rachitide,'' which no doubt was his doctorate thesis. He continued his studies of pediatrics and between 1801 and 1819 published several essays on the diseases of children.

In 1809 Cheyne left Scotland and after visiting Dublin, decided to practice medicine there. His first two years in Dublin were rather unproductive so far as patients were concerned. But in 1811 he was appointed physician to the Meath Hospital, and the appointment seemed to be the turning point in his career. He soon was called on to lecture on military medicine at the Irish College of Surgeons, and his private practice began to increase. In 1815 he was appointed one of the physicians to the House of Industry.

The Dublin hospital reports for 1818 contain Cheyne's classic paper, ''A Case of Apoplexy, in which the fleshy part of the Heart was converted into fat.'' In his historic account, which we are reprinting, Cheyne mentioned the unusual type of breathing now known as the ''Cheyne-Stokes respiration.'' Stokes, as we shall show, put more emphasis on the diagnostic value of this symptom, but Cheyne was the first accurately to describe it.

In 1820 Cheyne was appointed physician-general to the Army in Ireland. This was the highest medical rank in Ireland. With this rank and with a highly successful medical practice, he felt he had fully attained the object of his ambition.

Cheyne's health had never been robust and his medical practice fatigued him to such an extent that he soon found it necessary to limit its scope. He gradually declined the responsibilities of private practice and limited his work to that of a consultant. In 1825, at the age of forty-nine, he was afflicted with a type of ''nervous fever.'' This deprived him of much of his remaining strength and he sought relief by spending a few months in England. He later returned to Dublin, where he continued some professional activity until 1831. Then he decided to retire. He moved to a country town, Sherrington, in England. He did not give up his interest in medicine, but gladly undertook to contribute articles for the ''Cyclopaedia of Practical Medicine.''[1]

In 1833 a cataract formed in his right eye, depriving him of the sight of that organ, and in 1835 gangrene developed in one of his limbs. He died on January 31, 1836.

[1]*The Cyclopaedia of Practical Medicine; comprising a treatise on the nature and treatment of diseases, materia medica and therapeutics, medical jurisprudence, et cetera,* edited by John Forbes, Alexander Tweedie, and John Conolly, London, Sherwood, Gilbert and Piper, 1833, 4th vol.

A CASE OF APOPLEXY, IN WHICH THE FLESHY PART OF THE HEART WAS CONVERTED INTO FAT*

By

J. CHEYNE

DOUBTS having been entertained of the conversion of the fleshy part of the heart into fat, and only one dissection,† in so far as I know, having been published illustrative of that very curious morbid alteration, the following case and dissection have been thought of sufficient importance to meet the public eye.

In this dissection, although no chemical experiment was made in proof of the matter into which the heart was converted being fatty, I have no doubt that it was so. Placed along side of the fat which lay over the ribs, I could perceive no difference, save that it was softer and more easily torn, and rather of a deeper yellow; the substance in question communicated a greasy stain to paper, and the animal oil in viscous drops adhered to the knife used in dissecting the heart. I was not, at the time of dissection, aware that the morbid change was so uncommon, or that the specimen which lay before me was perhaps the most complete exemplification ever witnessed of the conversion of the flesh of the heart into fat.

The patient certainly died of apoplexy; and apoplexy in this case must have depended upon increased action of the vessels of the head. The heart itself was apparently incapable of communicating much impetus to the circulating mass.

Certainly the dissection would have been more complete had the liver been examined: at the same time I may observe, that although the function of the liver had frequently been disordered during the last ten years of the patient's life, I should not have been surprised had that viscus been found apparently sound. I am persuaded that diseases of the liver, which do not end in structural changes, often produce the greatest disturbance of the constitution, laying the foundation of fatal diseases of distant organs.

A. B., sixty years of age, of a sanguine temperament, circular chest, and full habit of body, for years had lived a very sedentary life, while he indulged habitually in the luxuries of the table.

---

*Published in Dublin Hospital Reports 2: 216-223, 1818. We reprint from Medical Classics 3: 705-709, 1939.—F. A. W., 1940.

†See a dissection, illustrative of this morbid change, in an elaborate paper on inflammation of the heart, by Dr. Duncan, jun. See Edin. Med. and Surgical Journal, Jan. 1816.

This gentleman having had several attacks of the gout in his feet, began a course of magnesia in the year 1813, after which he had only one regular attack of the gout. For many years he had been subject to severe attacks of catarrh, which ended without much expectoration. He had long been subject to oedema of the ankles in the evening; for two or three years before his death (the time could not be ascertained) he had remarked an occasional intermission in the pulse of his heart.

In the latter end of January 1816, he consulted me for a pain in his right side under the false ribs, for which he took calomel at bedtime, and salts in the morning, repeating these once or twice; but he neglected my directions with regard to diet; nay, his appetite being remarkably keen, he ate more than usual, and took at least a pint of port wine or Madeira daily, as was his habit, and this notwithstanding a hard frequent cough, which came on after I was consulted by him.

On the third of February he had walked a good many miles and came home exhausted, with a fluttering or palpitation of his heart, for he could not well say which, in a degree he had not felt before. He ate as usual, and drank six or seven glasses of wine, which he thought relieved the fluttering. He was sitting at tea about nine o'clock when he was attacked with a severe fit of coughing, during which he fell from his chair insensible. I saw him in three or four minutes after his fall, and found him with a contusion on the upper and left side of the frontal bone; he was confused, and unable to recollect himself; he was conscious that some accident had befallen him, the exact nature of which he declared himself incapable of understanding. His pulse was extremely irregular and unequal. It bounded quickly for several pulsations, then it paused and went on more quickly, but with less force. He was pale, but none of the muscles were affected with palsy. I lost no time in having blood drawn from his arm to the amount of nearly a pound. He gradually became more collected, but his pulse continued irregular and unequal; his countenance became flushed, the cough occurred in suffocative fits, and he complained of pain on either side of the tuberosity of the occipital bone. Twelve ounces more of blood were drawn about an hour after the first blood-letting, after which the pulse, though it continued equally irregular, was much softer. He complained of the contusion, and of considerable pain behind his ears. He was removed to bed, the heat of the extremities was restored, and fifteen leeches were applied over the contusion, and he took two pills consisting of two grains of James's powder, three of calomel and four of compound extract of colocynth.

On the 4th of February he had several large bilious stools; his understanding was unimpaired, his recollection restored, and he seemed to comprehend the nature of his illness, and he had a sense of fulness in his head, which led me to order him to lose a few more ounces of blood. It would be tedious and unprofitable to particularize the medicines which were ordered from day to day for this patient; they consisted of a mild mercurial every second or third day, and squills with ammoniacum, etc. These were indicated by the loaded tongue, scanty high coloured urine and dry cough. The expectoration being restored, the squills were laid aside on the 15th of February, as they produced nausea and extreme depression of spirits, and bitter infusion with tincture of cardamoms and soda was prescribed. On the 19th a horse-radish bath was ordered, in consequence of some slight demonstration of gout. On the 21st he had some smart pain, with slight inflammation in the ball of the left great toe. About this period he submitted with so much dissatisfaction to a reduced diet, and declared himself so much better after food, that we were induced to allow him a couple of glasses of wine, and to encourage him to take carriage exercise. The irregularity in his pulse never ceased. On the 1st of March he had a return of the suffocative cough and flushing, with some wheezing, which again seemed to demand blood-letting, which was practised with immediate relief. At this period a blister was applied over the region of the heart, which had become the seat of considerable increase of pain, and a discharge was maintained from the blistered surface, by means of ointment of savine and cantharides; about the 4th of March, the sputa became free and concocted. His tongue at this period was for many days furred and of a dark brown colour, as if it had been sprinkled with ground coffee; it was expanded, and its edge was moist. On the 25th of March he began to complain of wheezing, more particularly after exertion, but it sometimes attacked him when he was at perfect rest; his legs and ankles became oedematous, the urine very scanty, much loaded, but without being coagulable by heat. At no period of his illness did his pulse beat more than twelve, or fifteen strokes in regular succession. Various diuretics were given; the digitalis was proposed, but he refused to take it. Crystals of tartar, the extractum lactucae virosae, nitrous aether, etc., were tried without any benefit.

The symptoms of dropsy rapidly increasing, on the 9th of April, he took a draught of infusion of senna, tincture of jalap and Rochelle salts, which operated largely. On the 10th of April he was found in bed flushed, speechless, and hemiplegiac. How long he had been in that state could not be ascertained, as he had peremptorily ordered his servant not to remain in the chamber with him, and not to come to him in the morning till called. All attempts to relieve him were unavailing; his right side continued powerless, and his attempts to articulate were vain. The only peculiarity in the last period of his illness, which lasted eight or nine days, was in the state of the respiration: For several days his breathing was irregular; it would entirely cease for a quarter of a minute, then it would become perceptible, though very low, then by degrees it became heaving and quick, and then it would gradually cease again: this revolution in the state of his breathing occupied about a minute, during which there were about thirty acts of respiration.*

The Dissection was made by Mr. Crampton, the Surgeon General, and witnessed by Mr. John Moor and myself.

There was nothing remarkable in the configuration of the body but the great depth of the chest; the anasarcous swelling of the inferior extremities was considerable.

The scalp was bloodless. The arachnoid membrane was slightly opaque; there was some fluid between it and the pia mater, and the vascularity of the latter was increased, more particularly over the middle and posterior lobes of the cerebrum on the left side, where, in a large patch, it was thickened and of a deep red colour. The brain was firm, its cortical substance of a pale drab colour. There were between three and four ounces of fluid in the ventricles.

There were not more than two ounces of fluid in the pericardium. The heart was about three times its natural size. The lower part of the right ventricle was converted into a soft fatty substance; the upper part was remarkably thin, and it gradually degenerated into this soft fatty substance. The cavity of the left ventricle was greatly enlarged. The whole substance of the left ventricle, with the exception of the internal reticulated structure and carneae columnae, was converted into fat. The valves were sound. The aorta was studded with steatomatous and earthy concretions.

*The same description of breathing was observed by me in a relative of the subject of this case, who also died of a disease of the heart, the exact nature of which however I am ignorant of, not having been permitted to examine the body after death.

1819

RENÉ THÉOPHILE HYACINTHE LAËNNEC

THE INTRODUCTION OF THE STETHOSCOPE AND AUSCULTATION

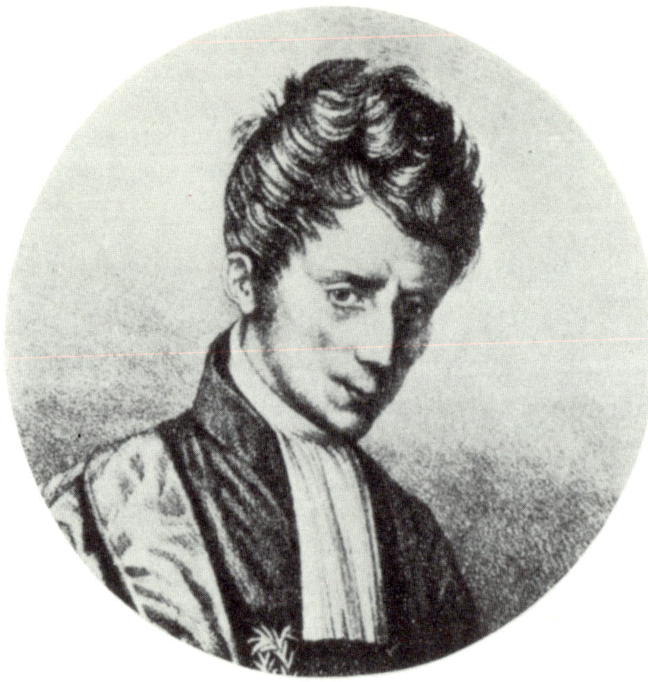

RENÉ THÉOPHILE HYACINTHE LAËNNEC

(Courtesy Annals of Medical History.)

RENÉ THÉOPHILE HYACINTHE LAËNNEC

(1781-1826)

"I profess free medicine, I am not with the ancient nor with the modern, but seek the truth in each, and test everything by repeated trial."

—Laënnec's credo from his doctoral thesis, after Webb.

WHILE Auenbrugger, long past his prime, was leading a retired life in Vienna, a child of sickly appearance was born of a probably tuberculous mother at Quimper in Lower Brittany, one of the most beautiful districts in France. His name was René Théophile Hyacinthe Laënnec.

The other immediate members of the family were a boy, Michel, who was born in 1782, and a girl, Marie, born in 1785. Another girl was born in 1786, but she lived only a few days and the death of the brave mother of this family occurred shortly afterward. The father was a lawyer and to judge by subsequent records, was not a very successful one. He also wrote poetry and that not too well.

After the death of the mother, the father, seemingly unable to accept the responsibilities of rearing his sons, sent the two boys to live with their paternal uncle, Michel, the rector of a parish in Elliant. This clergyman shortly afterward became one of the émigrés to England. And so in 1788, after spending about a year with Uncle Michel, the boys were sent to their other and more famous uncle, Guillaume-François Laënnec, a former pupil of John Hunter and professor of medicine at the University of Nantes. Dr. Guillaume Laënnec was interested in many things besides medicine. He enjoyed the humanities, was proficient in the Greek classics, derived pleasure from writing and was an effective speaker. René profited much from this association and indeed his physician uncle was more than a father to him.

For three years the two boys studied at L'Institution Tardivel, and in 1791, René was placed in the Collège d'Oratorie. There he studied religion, political science, orthography, grammar, geography, Latin prose and verse.

Contrasted to the peaceful life René was leading as an individual was the turmoil in which his country was embroiled. For by this time the French Revolution was in full sway. The new powers, Mirabeau, Danton, Robespierre, Marat and Carnot, were reshaping the destinies of millions. Even the son of sixty kings, now Citizen Louis Capet, was on his way to the guillotine. René, himself, must have felt the horror of this bloody revolution for he had seen several heads drop from the guillotine which was stationed in the square outside of his home in Nantes. His uncle was imprisoned for six weeks on suspicion of being out of sympathy with the contemporary government.

Despite the political confusion and chaos caused by the Revolution, the education of Laënnec was not neglected. In 1793 he entered the National Institute. In 1795, encouraged by his uncle, Laënnec began the study of medicine at the early age of fourteen and a half years. L'Hôtel Dieu at Nantes, where he began his study, was a large hospital, containing 400 beds. His uncle had charge of 100 beds; most of these were occupied by sailors suffering from tropical diseases. Besides medicine, Laënnec studied botany and he also found time for the study of Greek at L'École Centrale.

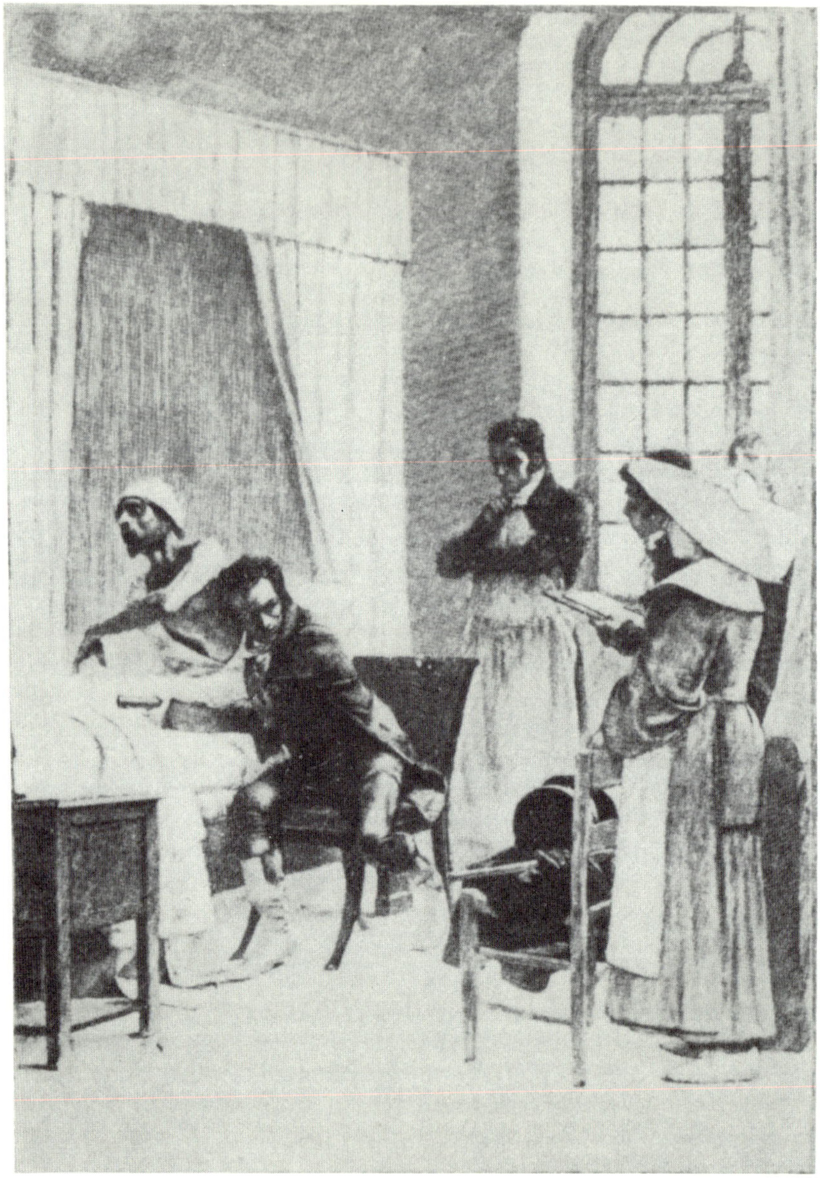

THÉOPHILE LAËNNEC ON HIS ROUNDS IN THE NECKER HOSPITAL IN PARIS

From a painting by Chartrau

(Courtesy Roche Review.)

After spending five years at Nantes, Laënnec, at the insistence of his uncle, was sent by his father to Paris. There he immediately enrolled at L'École de Médecine, which at that time was championed by the great Jean Nicolas de Corvisart. Corvisart was the founder of French clinical medicine, and when Napoleon by chance became Corvisart's patient, the Emperor singled him out to be his personal physician. It was Corvisart, also, as we have shown, who caused Auenbrugger's discovery of percussion to be broadcast throughout the medical world. From all accounts, Laënnec got along well with his famous teacher and received much genuine encouragement from the master on the theories that he advanced. It is interesting to note in this connection that at some time later, the aphorisms of Corvisart were published by Laënnec, who had collected and preserved them during his residency in Paris.

Other famous teachers of Laënnec were Marie François Xavier Bichat (1771-1802), whose work in physiology and medicine resulted in the founding of pathologic anatomy and scientific histology, and Baron Guillaume Dupuytren (1778-1835), whom Garrison described as "the ablest and best trained French surgeon of his time."[1] Dupuytren tolerated no rivals and consequently he and Laënnec did not get along.

In 1802 Laënnec observed, during necropsy on the body of a patient who had had cardiac disease, ossification of the mitral valves and dilatation of the ventricle. His report of the case constituted his first published work. Laënnec's lecture in March, 1804, on tuberculosis, delivered shortly before his graduation, established the fact that phthisis was simply tuberculosis of the lungs. From that time onward the disease was called "pulmonary tuberculosis."

Laënnec received his doctor's degree in June, 1804. His thesis was entitled "Propositions on the doctrines of Hippocrates in regard to the practice of medicine."

For five years after graduation Laënnec busied himself lecturing on pathologic anatomy, doing what private practice he could, and contributing several articles to medical journals, and to the medical dictionaries and encyclopedias which were then in fashion. Many of his articles were published in the "Journal de Medecine" of which he was an editor from 1805 to 1808. It is apparent from some of his notes and editorials published therein that he was violently opposed to the nebulous theories of John Brown (1735-1788) and François J. V. Broussais (1772-1838). Brown's therapeutic ideas, according to Baas,[2] destroyed more people than did the French Revolution and the Napoleonic wars combined. Broussais thought that life depended on irritation and that disease owed its existence to localized irritation of the affected part. Broussais felt that nature had no healing power and therefore his therapy consisted of starving the patient and applying leeches over various parts of the body. Broussaism was such a popular doctrine that seven years after Laënnec's death (1833) 41,500,000 leeches were imported into France to be used for the purposes of bleeding.

In 1812 Laënnec was appointed physician to the Beaujon Hospital. During this time he especially interested himself in diseases of the chest and, of course, he employed percussion in his diagnosis as he had learned it from his master, Corvisart.

Laënnec became associated with the Necker Hospital in 1816. It was at this time, also, that he developed the art of auscultation. The story of his discovery is admirably told in his own words in the introduction to the second part (diagnosis) of his famous book, "De l'auscultation médiate."

---

[1]Garrison, F. H.: *An Introduction to the History of Medicine.* Ed. 4. Philadelphia, W. B. Saunders Company, 1929, p. 488.

[2]Quoted by Garrison, p. 315.

''In 1816, I was consulted by a young woman labouring under general symptoms of diseased heart, and in whose case percussion and the application of the hand were of little avail on account of the great degree of fatness. The other method just mentioned being rendered inadmissible by the age and sex of the patient, I happened to recollect a simple and well-known fact in acoustics, and fancied at the same time, that it might be turned to some use on the present occasion. The fact I allude to is the augmented impression of sound when conveyed through certain solid bodies, as when we hear the scratch of a pin at one end of a piece of wood, on applying our ear to the other. Immediately, on this suggestion, I rolled a quire of paper into a sort of cylinder and applied one end of it to the region of the heart and the other to my ear, and was not a little surprised and pleased, to find that I could thereby perceive the action of the heart in a manner much more clear and distinct than I had ever been able to do by the immediate application of the ear. From this moment I imagined that the circumstance might furnish means for enabling us to ascertain the character, not only of the action of the heart, but of every species of sound produced by the motion of all the thoracic viscera.''

With the stethoscope René Laënnec first heard the language of pathology. Lesions within the thorax that for centuries had been inaudible now announced their presance. At first, Laënnec's discovery was treated with indifference by his immediate colleagues. But although even his book met with a cold reception from these men, the first edition of 3500 copies was soon exhausted, and his deserved fame as a clinician and his pathologic work placed him on a firm footing. His foreign colleagues greeted his discovery with much enthusiasm and soon physicians from all over Europe crowded into the Necker Hospital to hear his ideas on auscultation. At last his own colleagues were convinced of the validity of Laënnec's discovery. Laënnec was made professor of medicine in the Collège de France in 1822 and simultaneously became a member of the Academy of Medicine of France. A year later he succeeded his teacher, Corvisart, in the College. He also at that time was appointed physician to the Duchess of Berry. In 1824 Laënnec was made a knight of the Legion of Honor.

That same year Laënnec married a widow, Madame Argou. It was a marriage of convenience, not of love. The widow, who had been his housekeeper, was about forty-five years of age and ill health made her look older. Laënnec, himself, presented an emaciated appearance, suffering as he was from asthma.

In 1826 Laënnec published the second edition of his work on mediate auscultation. This entailed considerable hard work and his health, which had never been robust, broke down. In April of 1826, he contracted a severe cold. This was accompanied by infection of the throat, high fever, and thoracic pains. From that time onward his health became progressively worse. He died on August 13, 1826.

Except for his treatise on auscultation (1819), Laënnec's most important contributions to medicine were produced during the beginning of his career. They included his description of the pathologic appearance of peritonitis (1803) and a description of the capsule of connective tissue investing the liver (1803). In 1806 Laënnec published the first accurate account of melanosis, and in 1812 he described an extraperitoneal type of hernia. He was also the first to describe chronic diffuse interstitial hepatitis.

The ''Boston Medical and Surgical Journal'' recorded in 1867 that 20,000 francs had been raised during that year for a monument to Laënnec, the money having been raised chiefly in France, but in part by the Medico-Chirurgical Society of London and also by physicians in Scotland, Ireland, Prussia and Austria. Modelled by Lequesne and cast by Ducel, the monument was exhibited at the Paris Exposition and was dedicated in May of 1868.

A

TREATISE

ON THE

DISEASES OF THE CHEST,

IN WHICH THEY ARE DESCRIBED

ACCORDING TO THEIR

ANATOMICAL CHARACTERS.

AND THEIR

DIAGNOSIS

ESTABLISHED ON A NEW PRINCIPLE

BY MEANS OF

ACOUSTICK INSTRUMENTS.

With Plates.

TRANSLATED FROM THE FRENCH OF

R. T. H. LAENNEC, M. D.

WITH

A PREFACE AND NOTES,

BY JOHN FORBES, M. D.

PHYSICIAN TO THE PENZANCE DISPENSARY, SECRETARY OF THE ROYAL GEOLOGICAL SOCIETY OF CORNWALL, &C. &C.

FIRST AMERICAN EDITION.

PHILADELPHIA:

JAMES WEBSTER, 24 S. EIGHTH STREET.

William Brown, Printer.

1823.

TREATISE ON MEDIATE AUSCULTATION*

PREFACE

I BEGAN, three years since, the researches of which I now publish the results. Although these have not reached the degree of perfection which longer experience would have conferred on them, I have thought it advisable for many reasons, to communicate them to the public. Among those reasons I may mention—the incorrect accounts of my discoveries that have found their way into the journals of the day; the favourable report of the Academy of Sciences;† and the hope and conviction that the mode of exploration detailed in this work will be confirmed and extended by other observers.

It will be found that of the facts narrated in my treatise, I have given some as certain, others as doubtful, and a few merely as problematical. Of the first class, if future experience should invalidate any, I may venture to believe that the number will be few; and I am even convinced that the greater part of those which I have stated as doubtful, will be found by further observation to be constant and certain.

In respect of the pathological details, which constitute so large a portion of the work, I think it necessary to make a few observations. The great attention that has been paid to morbid anatomy, since the commencement of the present century, throughout Europe, and more especially in Paris, has been productive of many improvements and discoveries which are but imperfectly known; and, indeed, many of which have not at all been communicated to the public, at least by their discoverers. On this account, the present state of our written knowledge is obviously behind our actual knowledge; and if, in the present work, I had contented myself with merely describing the signs of the organic lesions, without describing the lesions themselves, I should have often

*Laënnec, R. T. H.: *Traité de l'auscultation médiate.* The first French edition was published in 1819. We are reprinting from the first American edition, published in 1823.—F. A. W., 1940.

†Extract from the Report of the Academy of Sciences (drawn up by M. Percy, and signed by him, and MM. Portal and Pelletan, 29th June, 1818), on a Memoir of M. Laënnec respecting the use of Auscultation, more particularly in Phthisis Pulmonalis.

"The Cylinder, applied to the chest of a healthy person who sings or speaks, produces a sort of vibration, which is more distinct in some places than others. But when there exists an ulcer in the lungs, the patient's voice then, instead of being heard in the usual manner by the exposed ear, reaches the other entirely through the tube of the instrument. We have ourselves verified this fact on several consumptive patients; it appeared to us striking, and well fitted for furnishing a certain and easy sign of certain morbid conditions of the lung, which, in the present state of medicine, can only be suspected to exist. . . .

"We have also examined, by means of the cylinders, the respiration in different parts of the chest of a healthy person, and found it very distinctly audible in every point of this cavity which corresponded with the lungs. We have also found that the motions of the heart were equally perceptible; and it has, consequently, appeared to us, that the assertions of the author, of the possibility of obtaining, through these two kinds of auscultation, certain signs of the several diseases of the heart and lungs, were, at least, extremely probable."

run the risk of being not understood at all, or (what is worse) of being misunderstood. I have, therefore, felt that the only means left of escaping this danger, was to give an anatomical description of all the diseases of which I have noticed the symptoms. In fulfilling this task I have endeavoured to render my descriptions concise, yet, at the same time, sufficiently exact and complete to characterise the objects.

Another motive has contributed to strengthen this resolution:—viz. the conviction of the practical utility of my mode of diagnosis, and the belief that the surest way of procuring its more general adoption was to associate the exposition of its principles with a description of the diseases which it indicates, more exact than any that yet exists.

Many reasons have induced me to prefer the anatomical to the more symptomatical description of diseases. The former method has the advantage of brevity, perspicuity and certainty. It is, for example, much easier to describe tubercles and detail the signs of these, than to define the disease by the external symptoms only, and to arrange its varieties according to their *causes*. Emphysema of the lungs consists in an alteration of parts which can be described in a few words, and of which the signs can be easily recognised; while in studying asthma, according to the method of Sauvages, we shall require to write a volume on generalities before we can arrive at anything positive.

It will, perhaps, be objected that the anatomical method has the disadvantage of founding its species on distinctions, the chief characters of which can only be obtained after death: but this objection scarcely merits refutation. We might as well say that it is useless for surgeons to make any distinction between dislocation of the femur, and fracture of its neck; or that it is useless to separate bronchitis from peripneumony.

The morbid alteration in the affected organ is, unquestionably, the least variable and most positive of the phenomena of local disease; it is on the nature and extent of this alteration that the danger and curability of diseases always depend; and it is this, consequently, that ought to be considered as characterising them. On the contrary, the derangement of functions which accompanies these alterations is extremely variable: it is often the same under circumstances entirely different; consequently, it can rarely serve to discriminate different diseases.

Besides, it is a mistake to consider the recognition of nosological species, founded on the data of morbid anatomy, as impracticable before death: on the contrary, they are often more readily recognised during life, and certainly present to the mind something much clearer and more positive, than any nosological distinction founded on the symptoms merely. Peritonitis, for example, is assuredly a disease easily distinguished during life; and out of twenty medical men acquainted with morbid anatomy called to see a case of it, not one will make a mistake

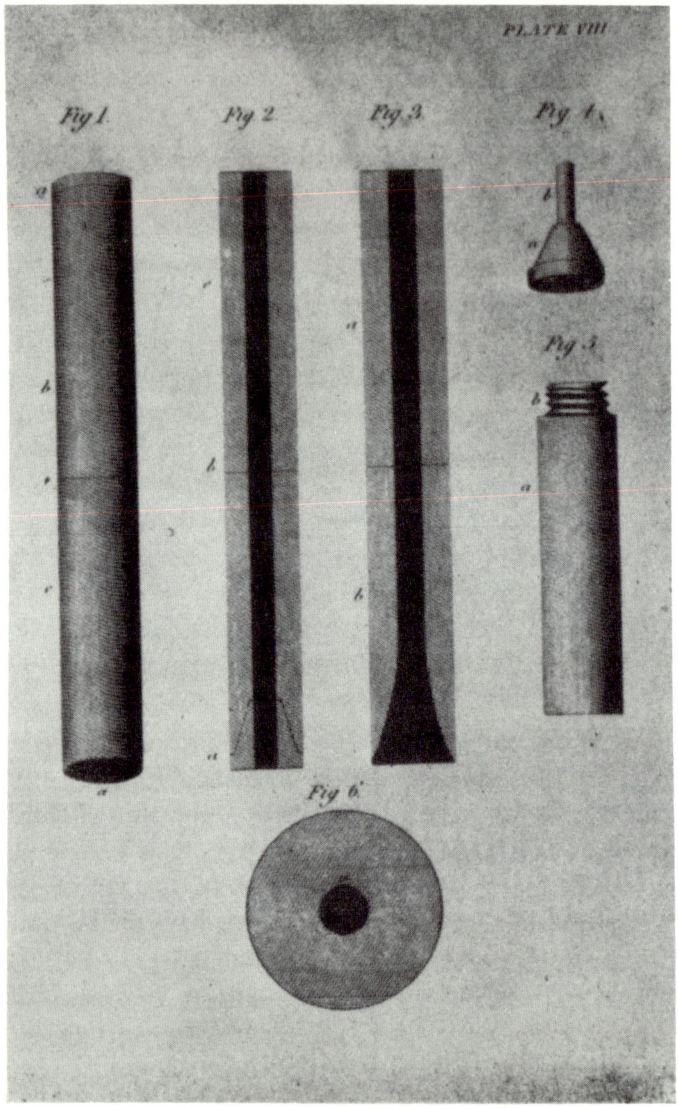

PLATE VIII

Fig. 1. The Stethoscope or Cylinder, reduced to one-third its actual dimensions. *a.* Stopper. *b.* The lower end. *c.* The upper half. *d.* The auricular or upper extremity.

Fig. 2. Longitudinal section of the same. *a.* The stopper. *b.* Point of union of the two parts. *c.* The upper half.

Fig. 3. The same section, with the stopper removed.

Fig. 4. The stopper. *a.* The body of it, formed of the same wood as the rest of the instrument. *b.* Small brass tube traversing the stopper, for fixing it in the tube of the stethoscope.

Fig. 5. Upper half of the stethoscope. *a.* Body of it. *b.* Screw (in the wood) for fixing the two portions together.

Fig. 6. Actual diameter of the stethoscope.

N.B. Any turner will be able to make the instrument, from the above description. —*Trans.*

concerning its nature or name. But will this be the case with those who are accustomed to see in diseases nothing but symptoms? Of the twenty shall we not find one considering the affection as *ileus,* another as *hepatic colic,* a third as *puerperal fever,* and so on? The same thing may be said of peripneumony, nephritis, hepatitis, etc.; and I hope that the work now submitted to the public will enable us to say the same thing of most of the diseases of the lungs, pleura and heart.

Morbid anatomy must, then, I think, be considered as the surest guide of the physician, as well to the diagnosis as to the cure of diseases. But it must not be forgotten that it has also its obscure points. It is, no doubt, an easy matter to distinguish striking changes of structure; but there are many slighter alterations, among which it is difficult to ascertain what is healthy and what diseased; what cause and what effect; and, lastly, whether the appearances are truly the effect of disease, or merely an accident of assimilation, or circulation, that has taken place in articulo mortis, or even after death. In these cases we must content ourselves with what is clear and distinct; never forgetting in practice the principle of Hoffman—*Nunquam aliquid magni facias ex mera conjectura aut hypothesi;* and sedulously guarding against the error of believing that the mere knowledge of the seat and nature of the disease can justify our neglecting its individual character, as influenced by external circumstances or personal idiosyncrasy.

From the foregoing observations it will be seen that this work is not, like that of Auenbrugger, a simple exposition of new means of diagnosis. Neither can it be considered as a monography of the diseases of the chest,—since I have taken little notice of the ordinary and more general symptoms of the diseases, and have not at all touched upon their treatment.

In the construction of my treatise I have quoted but two authors. The chief object of my researches was, in a great measure, new; and for the facts already known respecting the diseases of the lungs and heart, I have thought it unnecessary to go beyond the works of M. Corvisart and Bayle.* If I have occasionally differed from these distinguished authors, I trust no one will misinterpret my motives. No one can be more sensible of their merits, both as men and Physicians, than myself. At the very time I question their opinions, I most willingly confess my great obligations to them. It is much easier to improve a field already cultivated, than to reclaim a wild and barren soil. In respect of the works of M. Corvisart, more particularly, it is to be regretted that those of them published by others, are far from giving a just idea of the

***Essai sur les maladies et les lésions organiques du coeur, etc.* par J. N. Corvisart. Translated by Hebb. London, Underwood, 1813.

Nouvelle méthode pour reconnoitre les maladies internes de la poitrine par la percussion de cette cavité, par Auenbrugger, ouvrage traduit du latin et commenté, par J. N. Corvisart. Paris, 1808.

Recherches sur la Phthisie pulmonaire, par G. L. Bayle. Paris, 1810. Translated by Barrow. 1815.

author's merits. The uncertainty of the signs of diseases, and the vagueness of description in these, appears peculiarly striking to those who, like myself, were his pupils, and habitual witnesses of the boldness and precision of his diagnostics. This defect, no doubt, partly depends on the incommunicable tact of the physician, which forms so great a part of the art, and which M. Corvisart possessed in the highest degree.

I have hopes that the advantages of my method of diagnosis may be extended, in some degree, to veterinary medicine. Many reasons, however, exist, why this art must derive inferior benefit from it. Among these I may mention the absence of the voice;—the comparative inaccessibility of the region of the heart; and, lastly, the great indistinctness of respiration in the horse, and probably all herbivorous animals. In cases of disease, however, the respiration will be more audible in the sound portions of the lungs; as I found in a case of peripneumony in a cow, which I recognised during the animal's life, as easily as in the human subject. In the dog, and cat, and probably in all carnivorous animals, the sound of respiration is as distinct as in man. Notwithstanding these difficulties, I have no doubt that further experience will prove the utility of mediate auscultation in the disease of animals, especially, if combined with percussion of the chest.*

OF THE ACTION OF THE HEART IN GENERAL, IN HEALTH AND DISEASE†

Before entering upon the diagnostic signs furnished by the stethoscope in particular diseases of the heart, it will be necessary to examine the general results afforded by it, as well in the sound as diseased state of that organ. I shall do this under four principal heads, viz. 1st, the extent of the heart's action, as ascertained by the cylinder; 2nd, the shock or impulse communicated; 3rd, the nature and intensity of the sound; and 4th, the rythm of its actions.

I. Of the Extent of the Pulsation of the Heart

This must be considered in two points of view:—first, the sensation conveyed by the instrument when applied to the region of the heart; and, secondly, the parts of the chest (other than this region) in which its action can be perceived.

*The author further suggests the probable utility of the stethoscope in the instruction of the deaf and dumb, by applying one end of it to the trachea of the speaker and the other to the ear of the pupil:—but surely this must be fanciful—or at least of inferior value to other means.—*Trans.*

†Laënnec's work in the translation by John Forbes is composed of three books, Book First, Book Second and Book Third. We have reprinted portions of Book Third, which deals first, with diseases of the heart, and second with diagnosis of diseases of the heart. Excerpts from these two parts of Book Third are not reprinted in the sequence in which they appear in Forbes' translation. To aid the reader in distinguishing the two parts of Book Third, a star has been appended to the titles of all paragraphs taken from the first part of Book Third (on diseases of the heart). Paragraphs *not* marked with a star have been taken from the second part of Book Third (on diagnosis of diseases of the heart).—F. A. W., 1940.

1. In the natural condition of the organ, the heart, examined between the cartilages of the fifth and sixth ribs, and at the lower end of the sternum, communicates, by its motions, a sensation as if it corresponded evidently with a small point of the thoracic parietes, not larger than that occupied by the end of the stethoscope. Sometimes, it appears as if it were placed deep in the mediastinal cavity, leaving a vacant space between it and the sternum: in this case its movements, even when pretty energetic, appear to communicate no vibratory impulse to the neighbouring parts. In other cases, again, the heart seems entirely to fill the cavity of the mediastinum, and to extend much beyond the point on which the instrument rests; and, in this case, its contractions, even when slow and noiseless, seem to elevate, to a considerable extent, the thoracic parietes before them, and to displace the adjacent viscera within. This difference of sensation seems, in a word, to convey the impression of the action of a smaller or a larger heart; and, generally speaking, this indication is sufficiently correct, when the organ is examined in the state of quietude which results simply from repose of body.

2. The second point is of more practical importance. In a healthy person, of moderate fulness, and whose heart is well proportioned, the pulsation of this organ is only perceived in the cardiac region, that is, in the space comprised between the cartilages of the fifth and seventh ribs, and under the lower end of the sternum. The motions of the left cavities of the heart are chiefly perceptible in the former position, those of the right cavities in the latter. This is so much the case, that, in disease of one side of the heart only, the pulsation in these two situations gives quite different results. When the sternum is short, the pulsations extend to the epigastrium. In very fat subjects, the pulsation of whose hearts is quite imperceptible to the mere touch, the space in which it can be detected by the cylinder is sometimes not more than an inch square. In thin persons, in the narrow-chested, and, also, in children, the pulsation is more extended; being perceptible over the lower third, or even three-fourths, of the sternum, and sometimes even over the whole of this bone; also at the superior part of the left side, as high as the clavicle, and sometimes, though feebly, under the right clavicle.

When the pulsations are confined to the places above mentioned, in subjects of the kind noticed, and when they are much weaker below the clavicles than in the region of the heart, we may conclude that this viscus is well proportioned.

When the pulsations of the heart become more extended, they are heard successively in the following places:—1st, the whole left side of the chest, from the axilla to the stomach; 2nd, the whole of the right sides; 3rd, the posterior part of the left side of chest; and, 4th, the posterior part of the right side. This last is rare. In these cases the intensity of the sound is progressively less in the succession mentioned. This succession has appeared to be constant, and may be taken as an index of the extent of pulsation. For instance, if this be perceptible on the right side, we may be assured that it will be equally so over the whole sternum, under both clavicles, and over the left side; but we are not sure that it will be so on the back. But if it be perceptible on the back on the right side, we may calculate on its being still more audible in every other part of the chest.

Several circumstances unconnected with the state of the heart may derange the order above mentioned, and augment the extent of the pulsation. This latter effect is produced by a hepatized or compressed lung, and also by a part containing tuberculous excavations. In every case the heart gives two distinct pulsations for one beat of the arterial pulse. In my examinations of several hundred individuals, I have only met with one in whom the pulsation of the subclavian arteries could be heard by the stethoscope; and I may state it is an almost universal fact, that neither the pulsation of this artery, nor of the aorta, can be mistaken for that of the heart.

When the pulsation of the heart is heard over a greater extent than what is above stated to be the range of a well proportioned organ, the individual rarely enjoys good health. If he has not formal dyspnoea, he has, at least, shorter breath than usual, is put more easily out of breath, and is more subject to palpitation. This state, however, which is that of many asthmatics, may remain stationary many years, and does not always prevent the attainment of an advanced age.

With regard to the relation between the state of the heart and the extent of its pulsation, I think it may be taken as a general fact, that the extent of pulsation is in the direct ratio of the thinness and weakness of the heart, and consequently, inversely as its thickness and strength. The size of the organ must also be considered as affecting the extent of its pulsation.

In explanation of what has been just stated; we may presume, when the pulsation extends over all the places above mentioned, that the heart is increased beyond the natural size, and that this increase is owing to the dilatation of one or both ventricles. This presumption will be strengthened, if the pulsation is as great under the clavicles or in the axilla, as in the region of the heart. If the pulsation is perceived neither in the back nor right side, but only in the other points mentioned, and if its intensity is nearly equal in all these, we may conclude that the ventricles are moderately dilated, and that the parietes of the heart are naturally thin. On the contrary, when there is very strong pulsation in the region of the heart, and none or very little under the clavicle, we may be assured (if the patient has other general symptoms of diseased heart) that the disease is hypertrophia of the ventricles. If the patient has never experienced any marked disorder of the circulatory organs, we may be certain that the parietes of the left ventricle are much thickened, though still not sufficient to constitute disease.

Generally speaking, then, it may be taken for granted that a great extent of pulsation is a mark of thin parietes of the heart, more particularly of the ventricles; and that a confined range of pulsation coincides with an increased thickness of these. Some accidental causes may augment for a time the extent of the heart's pulsation, such as nervous agitation, fever, palpitation, haemoptysis, and, in general, whatever increases the frequency of the pulse.

II. Of the Impulse Communicated to the Ear by the Action of the Heart

In investigating this we must be careful not to confound with the action of the heart, the rise of the thoracic parietes during inspiration. This caution is more particularly necessary when the respiration is very short and frequent.

The degree of impulse communicated by the cylinder to the ear, is, in general, inversely as the extent of the pulsation of the heart, and directly as the thickness of the walls of the ventricles. In a person whose organs of circulation are well proportioned, this impulse is very little perceptible, often quite imperceptible, especially if the individual is rather fat. When the parietes of the heart are unnaturally thick, the impulse is usually so great as very sensibly to elevate the head of the observer, and sometimes to give a disagreeable shock to the ear. The more intense the hypertrophia, the longer time the impulse is perceptible. When the disease exists in a high degree, we feel as if the heart, in dilating, first comes in contact with the thoracic parietes in one point only, and then with its whole surface, and that it contracts and falls back all at once. The impulse of the heart is only felt during the systole of the ventricles; or if, in some rare cases, an analogous phenomenon accompanies the contraction of the auricles, this is easily distinguished from the former. In fact, when the systole of the auricles is attended by any sensible action, this is perceived to have its seat much deeper; and most commonly it consists merely of a sort of vibration. In any case, it is very little marked as compared with the sensation produced by the contraction of the ventricles, when these are of a good degree of thickness.

When the parietes of the heart are thinner than usual, no impulse is communicated, even when the pulsation is the greatest; and, in this case, the alternate contraction of its cavities is only distinguished by the sound these produce. A strong impulse, therefore, must be regarded as the chief sign of hypertrophia; and the absence of all impulse as the characteristic of dilatation of the heart. The correctness and constancy of this result have been confirmed to me by many examples.

The impulse of the heart's action is usually perceptible only over the region of the heart, or, at most, over the inferior half of the sternum. When very great, it extends to the epigastrium in cases where the sternum is short. In simple hypertrophia, it is usually perceived in no other part;

but when this is conjoined with a certain degree of dilatation, it is sometimes distinctly perceived under the clavicles, and in the right side of the chest. The impulse of the heart's action is, of course, diminished by whatever debilitates the general strength of the system.

III. Of the Sound Produced by the Action of the Heart

The alternate contraction of the different parts of the heart produces a peculiar sound, of which the individual is himself sensible during palpitation and in fever. In certain states of disease it can be heard at some distance from the patient; but this is a very rare case. The sound is the only phenomenon usually observable in any other part of the chest beside the precordial; the impulse of its action being confined, as already observed, to that part.

The sound produced by the action of the heart is great in proportion as the parietes of the ventricles are thin and their impulse feeble: consesequently, it cannot be attributed to the percussion of this organ against the side. In a moderate degree of hypertrophia, the contraction of the ventricles yields only a dull sound, like the murmur of inspiration, and the auricle, in like manner, a much less noise than in the natural state. In a high degree of hypertrophia, the contraction of the ventricles produces merely a shock without any sound, and the sound of the auricles is scarcely audible. On the other hand, when the ventricular parietes are thin, the noise produced by their contraction is clear and loud, approaching to that of the auricles; and if there be a marked dilatation of the ventricles, the sound becomes very similar, and almost as strong as that of the auricles.

In the state of health the sound of the contractions of the heart is nowhere heard so strongly as in the region of the heart. In certain states of disease it may be heard more distinctly in other places.

The softening of the substance of the heart deadens the sound of its contractions; as does also any impediment of the circulation, whether caused by too much blood, or by an obstacle in the auriculo-ventricular orifices. This latter state, further, gives rise to a dull rustling sound, very like the noise of bellows, or (when stronger) like that produced by the action of a file on wood. The particular orifice affected is, in this case, indicated by the place and time in which the sound is observed. When the orifice is on the left side, we can sometimes feel with the hand a sort of vibratory sensation like that produced by the purring of a cat. In this case, the noise produced by the contraction of the cavity having the obstructed orifice is not only duller, but much more prolonged than in the natural state.

IV. Of the Rythm of the Pulsations of the Heart

By rythm I understand the order of the contractions of different parts of the heart, and their relative duration and succession, as detected by the cylinder. Before entering on this subject I think it necessary to notice the relative proportions of the heart to the body of the individual, and of the different parts of the heart to each other, in a state of health, and in a well proportioned subject.

The heart, including the auricles, ought to be of a size equal to the closed hand of the subject, or only a little less or greater than it. The walls of the left ventricle ought to be of a thickness somewhat more than double that of the right. The texture of the left ventricle, firmer and more compact than that of the muscles, ought to keep it from collapsing when laid open. The right ventricle ought to be a little larger than the left, with columnae carneae of greater size, and ought to collapse on being cut into. In a heart so proportioned, the alternate contractions of the ventricles and auricles, as examined by the cylinder, and the pulse as examined by the finger, afford the following results:—

At the moment of the arterial pulse, the ear is slightly elevated by an isochronous motion of the heart, which is accompanied by a somewhat dull, though distinct sound. This is the contraction of the ventricles. Immediately after, and without any interval, a noise resembling that of a valve, or a whip, or the lapping of a dog, announces the contraction of the auricle. (I make use of these trivial expressions because they appear to me to express better than any description, the nature of the sound in question.) This noise is accompanied by no motion perceptible by the ear, and is separated by no interval of repose from the duller sound and motion indicative of the contraction of the ventricles, which it seems, as it were, to interrupt abruptly. The duration of this sound, and consequently the period of contraction of the auricles, is less than that of the ventricles,—an incontestible fact of which Haller entertained doubts. Immediately after the systole of the auricles there is a very short, yet well-marked interval of repose, subsequently to which we feel the ventricles swell anew, with the dull sound and gradual progression which characterise their action; then follows the quick and sonorous contraction of the auricles, and again the renewed but momentary immobility of the heart. This state of quietude after the contraction of the auricles does not appear to have been known to Haller as a natural condition. The relative duration of the contractions of the auricles and ventricles, appears to me to be as follows: Dividing the whole into four parts, a fourth (or third) belongs to the systole of the auricles, a fourth (or somewhat less) to the state of quiescence, and two-fourths to the systole of the ventricles.—These observations are most conveniently made when the pulse is slow.

From the foregoing observations it appears that the heart, far from being in a state of constant action, as is usually supposed, presents alternations of action and respose, the sum of which does not differ from those of many other muscles, more especially the diaphragm and intercostal muscles. From the proportions above stated it follows that in twenty four hours the ventricles have twelve, and the auricles eighteen hours of quiescence. In persons whose pulse is habitually below 50, the repose of the ventricles is more than sixteen hours in the four-and-twenty.

Hypertrophia of the ventricles, when in a moderate degree, presents, in some respects, an exaggeration of the natural rythm of the heart's action. The contraction of the ventricles becomes less noisy, and more readily distinguishable from that of the auricles. After the latter, the interval of quiescence is well-marked and contrasts very sensibly with the sound that precedes, and the motion which follows it. But in hypertrophia carried to a very high degree the rythm of the heart is singularly changed.

In this case, the contraction of the ventricles is greatly prolonged. This at first is perceived as a profound and obscure motion, which gradually augments, elevates the applied ear, and then terminates in producing the impulse or shock. This contraction is unaccompanied by any noise, or, if this exists, it is merely a sort of murmur like that of respiration.

The contraction of the auricles is extremely short, and almost, or altogether, without sound; and in some cases the systole of the ventricles seems scarcely over before they begin to swell afresh.

In extreme cases there is no sound distinguishable but the murmur above mentioned, and we merely recognise an elevation of the heart corresponding to each beat of the pulse. In these cases the increased brevity of the auricular contraction is not the consequence of their diminished contractibility merely, but, also, of their contraction commencing before that of the ventricles has entirely ceased.

When the walls of the left ventricle are naturally thin, or have become so from dilatation, the rythm of the heart's actions is quite different. In this case, the interval of repose after the contraction of the auricles is no longer perceptible. The contraction of the ventricles is more sonorous, more resembling that of the auricles, and more approaching the latter in duration. In this condition of the heart, there is as already observed, a less degree of impulse during the contraction of the ventricles, and a greater extent in the pulsation of the heart. This condition of the organ of circulation is congenital in many cases. It does not necessarily abridge life, but is usually conjoined with a delicate constitution.

Actual dilatation of the heart produces merely an increase of all the characters which indicate a heart with thin parietes. The contraction of the ventricles becomes as short and noisy as that of the auricles; the pulse, consequently, becomes very frequent; and the isochronism of the arterial pulse and the contraction of the ventricles becomes quite indistinguishable. In addition to these signs we must add—the absence of any sensible impulse; the extension of the heart's pulsation over the whole or greater part of the chest; and the existence of this in as great force under the clavicles and the axilla as in the region of the heart itself. This last character, particularly, may be regarded as pathognomonic, if the patient is not phthisical and pectoriloquous in the places mentioned.

V. Of Palpitation of the Heart

By palpitation of the heart is meant, in the common language of medicine, every beating of the heart which is sensible and unpleasant to the individual, and, at the same time, more frequent than natural. When this affection is studied by the aid of the cylinder, we find that there are many varieties of it, all of which appear to have merely this one character in common, viz. that the individual is sensible of the heart's action. Frequently, also, the patient *hears* the pulsation, especially when in the horizontal posture. In the upright position, the contraction of the ventricles only is heard; while, when lying on the side, the individual is sensible of a pulsation of his ear double that of the pulse, viz. the alternate contraction of both the ventricles and auricles. In many cases there is merely an increased frequency of pulsation, although the patient imagines, from his sensations, that there is also great increase of force. This species of palpitation is most common in dilatation of the ventricles, and lasts the longest of any. I have known it continued eight days; the pulse remaining, through the whole of this time, extremely small and weak, and between 160 and 180.

Another variety consists in an increase both of frequency and force of pulsation. This is what arises in healthy persons from great exertion or from moral causes; it also accompanies slight degrees of hypertrophia. In simple hypertrophia in a high degree, the ventricles are found to contract with great force, and to elevate the thoracic parietes in an extent and to a height much greater than natural. The noise, however, produced by their contraction is much duller and more indistinct than usual; the extent of thorax over which the pulsation is perceptible is not increased; and, notwithstanding the increase of the heart's power to double or triple its ordinary force, the pulse is, almost always, two or three times more feeble and smaller than in the natural condition of the circulation. In hypertrophia with dilatation, the impulse, noise, and extent of the heart's action, are usually equally increased.

VI. Of Irregularity of the Heart's Action

Irregularity in the pulsation of the heart may exist without palpitation. In old persons this is often met with without any perceptible alteration of the general health. The irregularity which occurs in palpitation consists usually in mere variations in the frequency of the heart's pulsation. Sometimes this variation is almost constantly recurring; at other times it is at longer intervals, and consists only of a few contractions longer or shorter than the rest. These irregularities occur most frequently in cases of dilatation.

In hypertrophia, and during the existence of palpitation, the contractions of the ventricles are so quick, and so much prolonged, that those of the auricles cannot be perceived. It sometimes, though very rarely, happens during palpitation, that each contraction of the ventricles is followed by several successive contractions of the auricles, so quick as only to equal in point of time one ordinary contraction. Sometimes these contractions are two or four, but most frequently three.

VII. Intermission of the Pulsation of the Heart

By intermission, we usually understand a sudden and momentary suspension of the pulse, during which the artery is no longer perceptible beneath the finger. The duration of the intermission is very variable, and may serve to divide this affection into well-marked varieties. Sometimes the intermission is shorter than one arterial pulsation; sometimes it is equal; and sometimes it is longer.

The first kind of intermission is the most common; it is frequent in old age, even during health. At other periods of life, it is only observed in certain diseased states of the heart, particularly hypertrophia. By means of the stethoscope we ascertain that this species of intermission always succeeds the contraction of the auricles. It, therefore, only differs from the natural quiescence after this contraction, in the irregularity of its recurrence. The duration and recurrence of this species of suspension of the heart's action are very variable. This, the real intermission, must be distinguished from the false intermission, already noticed, produced by the variation of the duration and strength of the heart's contractions. This can easily be done by the cylinder. The species of intermission which consists in the absence of one complete pulsation, returning sometimes with an exact periodicity at longer or shorter intervals, constitutes the sign deemed by Solano indicative of the approach of critical diarrhoea. The third variety is accompanied by a state of fulness of the artery during its continuance.

Many considerations, some of which have been stated, prove that the mere examination of the pulse is insufficient to inform us of the true state of the circulation; and must often lead us into error.—To notice only the indications afforded by it as to blood-letting, to prognosis in all diseases, and to diagnosis in several:—

We have seen, that, in peripneumony and pleurisy, the absence of fever and a perfectly natural state of the pulse, frequently accompany an incurable disease. In diseases of the heart, the pulse is often feeble, sometimes even almost imperceptible, although the heart's contraction, that especially of the left ventricle, is much more energetic than natural. In apoplexy, on the contrary, we often meet with a very strong pulse in persons in whom the impulse of the heart's action is scarcely observable. These two opposite facts may easily be verified by the use of the cylinder; I have myself done so, perhaps more than a thousand times, within the last three years. They appear quite inexplicable, unless we admit the arteries to possess a power of action independent of that of the heart.

It would seem to be proved, also, by many other facts, that the different systems subservient to the circulation, although necessarily and reciprocally dependent, have still, in other respects, a particular or individual existence, which, in certain states of the disease and in certain individuals, is more marked and isolated than in ordinary cases and circumstances. This view of the case is supported by the observations of practitioners, in all ages, of the different effects of bleeding, according as it is general or local, venous or arterial, depletive or derivative. The same is shown by the great benefit of a natural hemorrhage of a few ounces only, and the inefficacy of copious venesection in the same case; and by the trifling degree of exhaustion produced sometimes by very profuse hemorrhage, compared with the great collapse occasioned by the bleeding of a few leeches in the same person. These facts prove, I think, that the capillary circulation is in some sort independent of the general. The influence of the latter on the former seems very inconsiderable indeed in certain hemorrhages from the uterus, bowels, nose or lungs, which are found to be very little affected by the most copious venesection.

The mere state of the pulse, then, is far from indicating the state of the circulation in general; it does not even certainly indicate its condition in the whole heart, as it merely corresponds with the contraction of the left ventricle, which may be regular at the time when that of the auricles and right ventricle is irregular. In like manner, the state of the pulse fails to be a sure guide as to the expediency of blood-letting. Every one knows that in certain cases, for instance in apoplexy, peripneumony, pleurisy, and inflammatory affections of the abdomen, the weakness and smallness of the pulse do not always contra-indicate venesection; on the contrary, that the artery, in such cases, recovers its force and fulness after the loss of blood. The recognition of this kind of pulse (*fictitite debilis*) is one of the most important and difficult points in the treatment of the acute diseases, as an error in respect of it may be fatal. In cases of this sort, the stethoscope affords a rule much surer than the pulse. Whenever the contraction of the ventricles is energetic, we may bleed without fear,—the pulse will rise; but if the contractions of the heart are feeble, although the pulse still retains a certain degree of strength, we must be cautious respecting the employment of venesection. When the pulse is very strong, and the contractions of the heart moderately strong (as is frequently the case in apoplexy), we may still bleed with advantage as long as there is not a marked diminution in the noise and impulse of the heart's actions. But when both the pulse and the heart are feeble, we must not open a vein, whatever be the *name* of the seat of the disease, as such practice must infallibly destroy the few resources still left to nature. The most we can do, in such a case, if there be any local congestion, is, to try, by the application of a few leeches, if the patient can bear the subtraction of blood from the capillaries.

The certainty and facility with which the cylinder indicates the propriety of blood-letting in such cases as those above mentioned, (which have been hitherto considered among the most difficult in practical medicine,) appears to me to be the greatest advantage to be derived from the employment of this instrument.

After what has been said, and after its general uncertainty avowed by the most experienced practitioners, it may seem surprising that the practice of feeling the pulse has been so generally followed in all ages. The reason of this practice is, however, sufficiently obvious: it is of easy performance, and gives little inconvenience either to the physician or patient; the cleverest, it is true, can derive from it but a few indications and uncertain conjectures; but the most ignorant can, without exposing themselves, deduce from it all sorts of indications. Its very uncertainty gives it a preference with persons of inferior qualifications, over means quite certain in their nature, and which enable the non-professional observer to judge of the skill of the physician by the correctness of his diagnosis and prognosis.

The facts above stated relative to the discordance existing between the pulsation of the heart and of the arteries,—more especially as to strength, are contrary to the more general opinion of modern physiologists, who consider the action of the arteries as entirely dependent on that of the heart. Bichat himself has fallen into this error.*

. . . .

OF SYMPTOMS COMMON TO ALL THE DISEASES OF THE HEART

These are an habitually short and difficult respiration; palpitations and oppression constantly produced by the action of ascending, by quick walking, by emotions of mind,—or without any perceptible cause; frightful dreams, and sleep frequently disturbed by sudden starts; a cachectic paleness and a tendency to anasarca which, indeed, comes on after the disease has persisted some time. To these symptoms is frequently added the *angina pectoris*,—a nervous affection characterised by a sense of oppression, constriction and oppression in the region of the heart, and a pain or numbness of the arm, more commonly of the left, sometimes of both at once. When the disease has reached a high degree it is recognised at a single glance. The patient, unable to bear the horizontal posture, remains night and day seated in his bed, with the face more or less swollen, sometimes very pale, but more commonly of a deep violet tint, either over the whole or only on the cheeks. The lips are swollen and prominent, of a deeper violet than the rest of the face, or of this hue when it is quite'pale. The whole body is more or less anasarcous. The congestion and lentor of

*Anat. Gener. 1're part. tom. II, page 371.

the capillary circulation are further shown by affections of the internal organs; for instance—haemoptysis, pains of the stomach, vomiting, apoplexy (which frequently terminates such affections), and most of all, dyspnoea, which last symptom has been the cause of confounding such diseases (with many others) under the name of *Asthma*. Emphysema of the lungs likewise bears much resemblance to some varieties of disease of the heart, but the following marks will distinguish them from each other.

In disease of the heart, the patient, although with the respiration habitually short, does not usually experience the feeling of oppression and dyspnoea, except when walking rather quick, or using much exertion, or, more particularly, when ascending an elevation.

On the other hand, the individuals affected with emphysema, become oppressed on the breath when they are quite still: and these attacks recur without any known cause, or from a slight change of the weather. Moderate exercise seems often to relieve them, if the disease has not reached a great degree of intensity.

In diseases of the heart the general circulation is not always so much affected as the capillary. Sometimes the pulse is almost natural, but is often irregular.—At all events, it is evident that none of the general symptoms already mentioned suffice to characterise disease of the heart; and that for a certain diagnosis we must recur to mediate auscultation. It is necessary here to remark that the study of the physiological conditions of the heart, by means of the cylinder, requires much more time and application than that of the voice and respiration. In hospital practice, also, owing to our general ignorance of the anterior history of patients, we are liable to be led into error by its use, without proper care. For example, we may, in some cases, consider a patient as labouring under hypertrophia or dilatation of the heart, when he is merely affected with nervous palpitations. Another, and more insidious cause of mistake, arises in diseases which diminish the extent of respiration; for instance, peripneumony, emphysema, and more particularly chronic pleurisy. In cases of this kind I have sometimes found the heart enormously dilated and thickened after death, although, during life, its contractions had been perfectly natural in respect of sound, impulse and rythm. It would seem as if the diminished capacity of the lungs produced a diminished action of the heart.

. . . .

*OF HYPERTROPHIA, OR SIMPLE ENLARGEMENT OF THE HEART**

By Hypertrophia I mean simple increase of the muscular substance of the heart, without a proportionate dilatation of its cavities, or even with a diminution of these. This affection is by no means common, and appears to have escaped the notice of M. Corvisart, as, through his whole work, he

*Book Third, Chapter 1, Section First. See note on page 332.—F. A. W., 1940.

seems to consider enlargement of the parietes of the heart, as being uniformly accompanied by a proportionate dilatation of the cavities of that organ.

This enlargement of the heart is always attended by a considerable increase of its consistence, except when conjointed with another affection of this organ, to be noticed presently, viz: *softening of the heart.*

Hypertrophia may exist in one or both ventricles, with or without a similar affection of the auricles. Most commonly the auricles are not affected, but occasionally they are so, while the ventricles are sound.

When affecting the left ventricle, I have seen its parietes more than an inch thick at the base, that is, double that of its sound state. Commonly, this morbid thickening diminishes insensibly from the base to the apex of the ventricle, where it is scarcely perceptible; sometimes, however, the apex partakes in the enlargement; as I have seen it from two to four lines thick, which is double or quadruple the natural size. The columnae carneae of the ventricle and of the valves acquire a proportionate enlargement. The septum between the two ventricles becomes also notably thickened in the disease of the left ventricle, (which fact seems to mark it as belonging to this rather than the other ventricle,) but never so much so as the other parts.

The muscular substance in these cases is of a degree of consistence sometimes double the natural, and is of redder colour. The cavity of the ventricle appears to have lost in capacity what its parietes have gained to thickness. Sometimes I have found this so small, in hearts twice the size of the fist of the individual, as scarcely to be capable of containing an almond in its shell. The right ventricle, in such cases, is flattened along the septum, and does not extend to the apex of the heart. In extreme cases, it seems as if it were merely included within the parietes of the left ventricle.

In hypertrophia of the right ventricle the appearances are somewhat different. The thickening is here more uniform, and never so great as in the other: I have never found it greater than four or five lines. It is always a little greater in the vicinity of the tricuspid valves, and at the origin of the pulmonary artery. The columnae carneae are much enlarged, considerably more so, in proportion, than those in the left, in disease of that side. Simple enlargement of the right ventricle, without dilatation, is much rarer than that of the left. When this disease affects both ventricles at the same time, the only difference from the description just given is, that each side assists to form the apex of the heart.

. . . .

HYPERTROPHIA OF THE LEFT VENTRICLE

It is to this variety of the disease, especially, that the symptoms attributed by M. Corvisart to *active aneurism* of the heart, must be referred.

These are,—a strong full pulse, strong and obvious pulsation of the heart, absence or diminution of the sound afforded by percussion on the region of the heart, and a tint of complexion rather red than violet. None of these symptoms, however, are constant; and it is not uncommon to find the disease in persons who have none of them. The pulse, in particular, is very deceptive, being almost as frequently weak as strong, in such cases.

The cylinder furnishes signs which are much more constant and positive. The contraction of the left ventricle, examined between the cartilages of the fifth and sixth ribs, gives a very strong impulse, and is accompanied by a duller sound than natural; it is more prolonged in portion as the thickening is more considerable. The contraction of the auricle is very short, productive of little sound, and, consequently scarcely perceptible in extreme cases. The pulsation of the heart is confined to a small extent, being, in general, scarcely perceptible under the left clavicle, or at the top of the sternum; sometimes it is confined to the point between the cartilages of the fifth and seventh ribs. In this disease the patient experiences, more constantly than in any other, the sensation of the action of the heart; but he is less subject to violent attacks of palpitation, except from accidental causes, such as moral affections and violent bodily exertion. In this case, during the palpitations, irregularity and intermission of the pulse are uncommon: There is rather increase of the power of the ventricles than of the noise produced by their action.

. . . .

HYPERTROPHIA OF THE RIGHT VENTRICLE

According to M. Corvisart, the symptoms are the same as when the disease is on the other side, only that respiration is more oppressed, and the colour of the face is deeper. Lancisi has mentioned the swelling of the external jugular veins, with a pulsation analogous to that of an artery, as a sign of the aneurism of the right ventricle. M. Corvisart has rejected this symptom, because, he says, ''it has been found in cases where the left side of the heart was dilated, and because the pulsation may be confounded with that of the carotids.'' In this opinion I differ from M. Corvisart. I have uniformly found this symptom in every case of this kind, of any degree of severity; and I have never met with it in hypertrophia of the left ventricle unless there existed, at the same time, a similar affection of the right. I think a very little attention must distinguish this pulsation from that of the carotids. I would, therefore, be disposed to regard this symptom as one which ought to lead us to suspect the existence of the thickening of the right ventricle.

The contractions of the heart, as explored by the cylinder, give the same results nearly, whether the hypertrophia be on the right or left side; only, in the former case, the shock of the heart's action is greater at the bottom of the sternum than between the cartilages of the ribs, which is the reverse of what happens when the disease is in the left side of the organ. In most men, in health, the heart is heard equally in both these places; and I am disposed to believe, when heard better below the sternum, we may suspect an incipient hypertrophia or dilatation of the right ventricle. When both ventricles are affected, the symptoms of both co-exist, only those of the right side are almost always more marked.

. . . .

OF DILATATION OF THE VENTRICLES*

This disease of the heart, which has been named *passive aneurism* by M. Corvisart, consists in dilatation of the cavities of the ventricles, with decreased thickness of their parietes. With these conditions there are commonly conjoined a notable degree of softening of the muscular substance, and a colour, either more violet, or paler, than natural. Sometimes the softness is so considerable, especially in the left ventricle, that the muscular substance can be destroyed by mere pressure between the fingers; and the parietes of the same ventricle may be so much diminished in thickness, as to be only two lines in the thickest point, and scarcely half a line at the apex, while the right ventricle is sometimes so completely extenuated, as to appear merely composed of a little fat and its investing membrane. The columnae carneae, particularly of the left ventricle, are more remote than in the natural condition of the part. The septum between the ventricles loses less of its thickness and of its consistence than the rest of the parietes.

Dilatation may be confined to one ventricle, although it more commonly affects both at the same time. When one only is affected, the apex of it extends below the other, but not in so remarkable a degree as in the case of hypertrophia. The augmentation of the cavity seems to be more in its breadth than length. This is particularly observable when both the ventricles are dilated at the same time, as in this case, the heart assumes a rounded shape, being nearly as wide at the apex as at the base.

. . . .

DILATATION OF THE LEFT VENTRICLE

The symptoms of this affection, according to M. Corvisart, are—"a soft and weak pulse, and feeble palpitations:—the hand applied to the region of the heart feels as if a soft body elevated the ribs, and did not strike these with a sharp and distinct stroke."

The only certain sign of the existence of this disease is that given by the stethoscope, viz. the clear and sonorous contractions of the heart between the cartilages of the fifth and seventh ribs. The degree of dis-

*Book Third, Chapter 1, Section Second. See footnote on page 332.—F. A. W., 1940.

tinctness of the sound, and its extent over the chest, are the measure of the dilatation: thus,—when the sound of the contraction of the ventricle is as clear as that of the contraction of the auricle, and if it is, at the same time, perceptible on the right side of the back, the dilatation is extreme.

. . . .

DILATATION OF THE RIGHT VENTRICLE

According to M. Corvisart, the state of the pulse and the pulsation of the heart are very nearly the same as in dilatation of the left ventricle, only that the action of the heart is heard somewhat better towards the bottom of the sternum than in the region of the heart. More certain symptoms he considers to be—a greater degree of oppression, more marked serous diathesis, more frequent haemoptysis, and a more livid state of the countenance,—than in the affection of the left ventricle. With regard to the swollen state of the jugulars without pulsation, which M. Corvisart considers of little importance, I am disposed to look upon it as the most constant and characteristic of the *equivocal* signs of this affection. The only constant and truly pathognomonic symptom, however, is the loud sound of the heart perceived at the bottom of the sternum, and between the cartilages of the fifth and seventh ribs of the right side. The degree of dilatation is measured by the extent of the action of the heart over the chest. The palpitations which accompany this affection consist principally, in an increase of the frequency and sound of the contractions, while, at the same time, the impulse of the heart's action is frequently feebler than in the ordinary state of the patient.

. . . .

OF DILATATION COMBINED WITH HYPERTROPHIA OF THE VENTRICLES*

This reunion, which constitutes the *active aneurism* of M. Corvisart, is extremely common; much more common than simple dilatation, and still more so than simple thickening without dilatation. This complication may exist in one or both ventricles. In the latter case the heart acquires a prodigious size, sometimes more than triple that of the hand of the individual. As the augmentation of volume is here the effect of dilatation and thickening, the muscular substance acquires the great firmness already described. The apex of the heart becomes blunter, but this is rarely so great as to give to the organ the rounded form noticed in the case of simple dilatation.

Dilatation of one ventricle is sometimes conjoined with hypertrophia of the other, but this is not so common as the complication in individual ventricles. I have met with the following varieties of this complication: 1st, Hypertrophia with the dilatation of the left ventricle, and simple dilatation of the right; 2nd, Hypertrophia with dilatation of the left ventricle,

*Book Third, Chapter 1, Section Third. See footnote on page 332.—F. A. W., 1940.

and simple hypertrophia of the right; 3rd, Hypertrophia with dilatation of the right, and simple dilatation of the left; 4th, Hypertrophia of the right, with dilatation of the left: this last is the rarest. I do not remember to have met with hypertrophia of the left ventricle (with or without dilatation) complicated with dilatation of the right. I would even be disposed to consider such a union as impossible.

In this case there is a combination of the symptoms of two affections. The contractions of the ventricles yield at the same time a strong impulse and a very marked sound, and they are felt widely over the chest. When palpitation is present, the hand applied to the region of the heart is forcibly raised. Even in the absence of palpitation, if we observe the patient, we find his head, limbs, and even his bed-clothes shaken at each contraction of the heart. The beating of the arteries is often visible.

. . . .

DILATATION OF ONE OF THE VENTRICLES WITH HYPERTROPHIA OF THE OTHER

The signs of this complication are—a mixture of those common to each affection, with predominance of those belonging to the one of greater intensity. They are to be discovered by comparing the two sides of the heart together. In this case, however, the indications of the cylinder must be taken in conjunction with those of the general symptoms of disease, else we shall be led into error.

. . . .

*DILATATION OF THE AURICLES**

Dilatation of the auricles is an extremely rare disease, and it appears still more so compared with the frequency of the same affection of the ventricles. Sometimes we find in subjects affected with hypertrophia or dilatation of the ventricles, the auricles also proportionably enlarged; it is, however, much more common to find these retaining their natural size even in cases where the ventricles are enormously enlarged. Sometimes also, but more rarely still, the auricles are dilated when the ventricles are of the natural size.

Before we can judge of the extent of this affection we must have precise ideas respecting the natural proportion of the various cavities of the heart. As far as the *cavities* are concerned, we must admit that they are very nearly of equal size; but as the parietes of the auricles are much thinner than those of the ventricles, the former, when simply full and not distended, compose only about one-third of the whole organ,—in other words, the size of the auricles is about one-half that of the ventricles. Both the auricles have the same capacity, although some anatomists have considered the right

---

*Book Third, Chapter 1, Section Fourth. See footnote on page 332.—F. A. W., 1940.

larger, no doubt misled by the greater length of its sinus, and more especially by the distended condition in which it is commonly found after death. A similar distention, though more rarely, takes place also in the left auricle; and this accidental and temporary enlargement is sometimes so considerable, owing to the great extensibility of the auricular structure, as almost to equal the size of the ventricles. In order to distinguish the real from the factitious dilatation, we have only to empty the auricles through the vessels that enter into them, when, in the latter case, these cavities will immediately resume their natural size, and, in the former, they will still nearly retain their acquired volume. There is likewise another mark by which we can at once discriminate the enlargement produced by the accumulation of blood during the few last hours of life, from the permanent increase of capacity of the auricles. In the first case, the parietes of the auricles are greatly distended by the contained blood, and the colour of this appears through the thinnest portions; while, in the latter, the auricles although very voluminous, are still capable of containing more blood, and their parietes remain opaque.

I have never met with decided dilatation of the auricles without some thickening of their walls; and, on the other hand, I have never seen thickening of their walls without an augmentation of their capacity. I may here remark that it requires much experience to judge correctly of hypertrophia of the auricles, as, owing to their great natural thinness, a considerable increase (say double the natural thickness, and the increase is rarely so much) is not obvious to a person little accustomed to such examinations.

The most common cause of dilatation of the left auricle is the contraction of the orifice between it and the ventricle, in consequence of cartilaginous or bony induration of the mitral valve, or of caruncles on its surface. The same causes sometimes occasion the retraction of this valve, and consequently, the permanent patency of the auriculoventricular orifice. In this case dilatation and thickening may arise from the mere action of the ventricle on the auricle. I have never seen any change in the auricles without some alteration in the valves. Dilatation of the right auricle is most commonly the consequence of thickening of the right ventricle. The diseases of the lungs which M. Corvisart reckons among the ordinary causes of this dilatation, seem to me to produce, in general, merely the accidental distention above noticed.

The symptoms of this affection are obscure: M. Corvisart does not distinguish them from those of the corresponding ventricle. I have not myself had yet sufficient experience of the use of the stethoscope in this affection, to speak confidently on the subject. I think, however, there can be little doubt that the signs afforded by it must be confounded with those arising from the disease of the ventricles, or of the valves, of which the auricular affection is the consequence.

Of partial dilatation of the heart, and of the induration of its substance, I have nothing to say in this place.

*PARTIAL DILATATION OF THE HEART**

M. Corvisart found, in the person of a young negro who died from suffocation, a partial dilatation of the left ventricle which was truly aneurismatical. "On the superior and lateral part of this ventricle there was a tumour almost as large as the heart itself.—The interior of this tumour contained several layers of coagulated blood, very dense, and exactly like those found in aneurisms of the limbs. . . . The cavity of this tumour, communicated with the ventricle by a small opening, smooth and polished."† A similar case is cited by M. Corvisart from the *Miscell. Nat. Curios.* I have myself never met with anything of the kind.

There is another rare species of dilatation described by Morand,‡ a second case of which was communicated by me to the Soc. de la Facult. de Med.§ This is a dilatation formed in the middle of one of the lips of the mitral valve, resembling a thimble, or glove-finger projecting into the auricle.

There is still one other variety of partial dilatation of the heart, which I have several times met with, and which is probably, in a great measure, the result of original *malformation.* In the natural conformation of the heart, the right ventricle seems to consist of two distinct parts united together, the one of which descends towards the apex of the heart, while the other, almost at right angles to the former, is directed to the left side, and forwards towards the pulmonary artery. The dilatation to which I now allude, seemed to exist in both these divisions, while the point of union of the two retained its natural dimensions. It is, however, more common to find the anterior or pulmonary division of the ventricle dilated without the other portion; and in every case of dilatation of this ventricle, the former portion is always more dilated than the other. This difference becomes still more evident when the dilatation is conjoined with a certain degree of thickening, as, in this case, the pulmonary portion of the ventricle frequently acquires such a degree of firmness that its parietes do not collapse when laid open, a thing which hardly ever happens to the lower portion of the ventricle.

INDURATION OF THE HEART‖

I have already observed that, in thickening of the heart, the muscular substance possesses an unusual degree of firmness and consistence. Corvisart has seen this so great, that the heart sounded like horn when struck,

*Book Third, Chapter 1, Section Fifth. See footnote on page 332.—F. A. W., 1940.
†Op. Cit. p. 283.
‡Hist. de l'acad. des Sc. 1729.
§Bulletin, No. 14.
‖Book Third, Chapter 1, Section Sixth. See footnote on page 332.—F. A. W., 1940.

and the scalpel experienced great resistance in cutting it. However, the muscular substance of the heart "retained its natural colour, and did not appear to be converted either into the bony or cartilaginous tissue." I have never met with this species of induration, although M. Corvisart has several times. I consider it as the last degree of hypertrophia.

*SOFTENING OF THE HEART**

I have already noticed this condition of the heart. In it the muscular substance is sometimes so soft as to be almost friable, the fingers passing easily through the parietes of the ventricles. Whatever may have been the patient's disease, the heart is rarely filled with blood, and the ventricles equally collapse whatsoever may be their varying thickness. This affection of the heart is almost always attended by some change of colour in the organ. Sometimes this is deeper, and even quite violet; and this is particularly the case in fevers of the kind named *adynamique* by Pinel. More commonly, however, the softening of the heart is attended by a striking loss of colour, so as to resemble the palest dead leaf. This pale or yellowish tint does not always occupy the whole thickness of the heart; sometimes it is strongly marked in the central portions, and very little on the exterior or interior surfaces. Frequently the left ventricle and interventricular septum exhibit this appearance, while the right ventricle retains its natural colour, and even a degree of firmness greater than natural. Again, we sometimes find here and there spots of the natural colour and consistence in hearts which are, everywhere else, much softened and quite yellowish. This variety of yellowish softening is particularly observable in those cases where dilatation is conjoined with a slight degree of thickening. It is also found in simple dilatation, although it is more common to find this state accompanied by that species of softening which is marked by an augmentation of the natural colour of the organ. There is a third variety of softening of the heart, which will be noticed in another place, and which is attended by a pale white colour of the muscular substance. In this, the degree of softening never reaches that of friableness; often it is scarcely perceptible; but the parts are flabby, and the parietes of the ventricles quite fall together on being opened. This condition will be noticed under the head of inflammation of the pericardium, as it is peculiar to that disease.

It would seem that the softening of the heart discovered in subjects whose death has been very gradual, is an acute affection; it is evidently still more so where it exists only partially in the substance of the organ. On the contrare, in cases where the heart is softened and yellowish throughout, it is probable that the affection has existed for a long time. The deep-coloured softness observed in subjects dead of fever, may, I think be compared to that adhesive softness of the other muscles often observed in these cases, and which is also accompanied by a degree of redness greater than

*Book Third, Chapter 1, Section Seventh. See footnote on page 332.—F. A. W., 1940.

natural. This softening of the heart, as well as the analogous *gluey* or *fishy* (gluant ou poisseux) state of the muscles, is particularly observable in putrid fevers, particularly when these exhibit the phenomena formerly considered as marks of putridity—viz: livid intumescence of the face, softening of the lips, gums, and internal membrane of the mouth, black coating on the tongue and gums, earthy aspect of the skin, distended abdomen and very fetid dejections. I cannot assert that this softening of the heart exists in all kinds of continued fevers, but I have met with it constantly in such cases as I have attended to. Could it account for that frequency of pulse which exists, sometimes for several weeks in convalescence from fevers, although the patient continues to regain flesh and vigour?

Cases of total softening of the heart are usually accompanied by a certain degree of cachexy, even when the individuals are otherwise in tolerable health. When such subjects are attacked with dilatation or hypertrophia of the heart, as almost always happens, they do not present the usual swollen and livid state of the face observable in other cases of this sort.

When softening exists along with dilatation of the ventricles, the sound produced by the contraction of these cavities, although loud, is yet dull, and without the clearness which attends common dilatation. When it is complicated with hypertrophia, the sound of the contraction of the ventricles is so obtuse as to be nearly inaudible; and in extreme cases, the impulse of the heart is attended by no noise whatever.

ATROPHY OF THE HEART*

It is an important question whether the heart be susceptible of diminution of size and power like other muscles; and, if so, whether this affords any hope of cure, by debilitating measures, in cases of hypertrophia. This much is certain, that, in cases where there is much emaciation, as in Phthisis and Cancer, the heart is generally found small. From this consideration, I have in many cases of hypertrophia attempted the method of cure proposed by Valsalva in aneurism. Almost all my patients got shortly tired of the extreme severity of the regimen, and alarmed by the frequency of the bleedings. In three cases, however, I have been so far successful that I am led to believe that this disease is not entirely beyond the resources of art and nature. Two of these were young women, the one twelve and the other eighteen years of age, both of whom presented symptoms of hypertrophia in a high degree. The privation of one-half of their ordinary diet, and some occasional general and local bleedings effected the gradual diminution, and, eventually, the complete cessation of all their symptoms. The youngest has now been cured for four years, and has long ago returned to her usual regimen. The other still follows the prescribed regimen, and is

*Book Third, Chapter 1, Section Eighth. See footnote on page 332.—F. A. W., 1940.

now quite reconciled to the diminished quantity of food. Blood-letting has not been found necessary for the last year, and the general symptoms of the disease have disappeared, although the unnatural thickness of the parietes of the heart is still recognizable by stethoscope. The third case is still more conclusive, as I have been enabled to ascertain the state of the heart after death. I shall therefore state it more particularly.

Case 42. A woman, fifty years of age, had been affected for twelve years with all the symptoms of disease of the heart, in a very high degree, viz. strong and frequent palpitations, habitual dyspnoea, breathlessness on using the least exercise, sudden startings from sleep, almost constant edema of the lower extremities, and lividity of the cheeks, nose, and lips. These symptoms had increased during the last year, so that she could scarcely move from her chair without the feeling of suffocation. In this state I recommended the treatment of Valsalva, which she agreed to. I immediaately reduced her aliments to one-fourth of her former allowance, and bled her once a fortnight, either from the arm or by leeches. This mode of treatment gave immediate relief; and in the course of six months all the symptoms had disappeared; and, with the exception of debility (which however was not greater than it had been previously), she enjoyed a better state of health than for many years before. The respiration was now free, and the palpitations, oedema, startings, and lividity of the face had quite disappeared. After this I recommended the bleedings to be decreased in frequency, and I dispensed with them altogether at the end of a year. She also returned gradually to her old regimen, only that now a much smaller quantity of food satisfied her appetite. She lived two years in a state of perfect health, when she was suddenly carried off by an epidemic cholera. Upon examining the body after death I found the heart considerably less than the closed hand of the individual; being only about the usual size of that of a child twelve years old, although this woman was five feet three inches in height. The exterior of the heart resembled, in appearance, a withered apple, the wrinkles running longitudinally. The ventricular parietes were flaccid, but without any notable softening, and of the natural thickness. I am well aware that nothing can be deduced from a single case, but I have thought the above relation might be useful by stimulating others to prosecute this subject more at length.

*FATTY DEGENERATION OF THE HEART**

In medical writings we find many examples of the heart being overloaded with fat in a surprising manner, and to which change of structure various symptoms, and even sudden death of the individuals, were attributed. M. Corvisart thinks that an enormous accumulation of fat around the heart may, in fact, produce such effects, although he has met with no similar, or other permanent derangement, in persons whose hearts were

*Book Third, Chapter 1, Section Ninth. See footnote on page 332.—F. A. W., 1940.

found to be much loaded in this manner. I have also met with a great many cases of hearts, overloaded in this manner, in subjects dead of various diseases. In these the fat was deposited between the muscular substance of the heart and the investing pericardium, and chiefly at the union of the auricles and ventricles, at the origin of the great vessels, and along the tract of the coronary arteries, also along the two edges and at the apex of the heart. Sometimes the posterior face of the right ventricle is covered by this deposition in its whole extent; a circumstance which rarely has place on the surface of the left ventricle.

The fatter the heart is, the thinner, in general, are its parietes. Sometimes these are extremely thin, especially at the apex of the ventricles and the posterior side of the right ventricle. On examining ventricles affected in this manner, they present the usual appearance internally; but on cutting into them from without, the scalpel seems to reach the cavity without encountering almost any muscular substance, the columnae carneae appearing merely as if bound together by the internal lining membrane. In these cases the fat does not appear to be the product of degeneration of the muscular fibres, as these can be separated by dissection. Sometimes, indeed, portions of fat penetrate deeply between the muscular fibres; but, even in this case, the distinction between the two tissues is still very marked, and they are confounded by no mutual gradation of colour or consistence. It would seem probable from this, that, from pressure or some unknown aberration of the powers of nutrition, the muscular substance has wasted in proportion as the investing fat has increased. It would seem reasonable to expect rupture of the heart from an affection of this kind; such an instance, however, has never occurred to me. Very commonly we find, in such subjects, a large quantity of fat in the lower part of the mediastinum, particularly between the pericardium and pleura. This fat, much reddened by its small vessels, and covered by its pleura, assumes the figure of a cock's comb and is firm. The fat surrounding the heart, on the contrary, is almost always of a pale yellow colour. I have not observed, any more than M. Corvisart, any symptoms that could directly denote the existence of an accumulation of this sort. I apprehend it must exist in a very great degree before it gave rise to any serious complaint. This is not, therefore, the condition I wish to denote by the name of *Fatty degeneration of the Heart.* This latter is an actual transformation of the muscular substance into a substance possessing most of the chemical and physical properties of fat. It is precisely similar to the fatty degeneration of the muscles observed by Haller,* and Vicq-d'Azyr.† I have only met with it in a small portion of the heart at one time, and only towards the apex. In these portions the natural red colour is superseded by a pale yellow like that of a dead leaf. This change of structure appears to proceed from without inwards. Near the internal surface of

*Opusc. Pathol.
†Tom. V.

the ventricles, the muscular texture is still very distinguishable; more externally, it is less so; and still nearer the surface it becomes gradually confounded, both in colour and consistence, with the natural fat of the apex of the heart. In such cases, however, even the portions that still retain most of the muscular character, when compressed between two pieces of paper, still grease these very much. This character distinguishes this species of degeneration from simple softening of the viscus. I have never found rupture of the heart attributable to this change, any more than to the morbid accumulation of fat. It is denoted by no symptoms with which I am acquainted.

*CARTILAGINOUS OR BONY INDURATION OF THE MUSCULAR SUBSTANCE OF THE HEART**

I have never met with ossification of the muscular substance of the heart, and only a small number of examples of this are on record. M. Corvisart found, in the case of a man who died of hypertrophia of the left ventricle, the whole apex of the heart, and more partially the columnae carneae, converted into cartilage. (Op. cit.).

Haller (Opusc. Pathol.) found, in a child, whose heart was of the natural size, the inferior part of the right ventricle, the most muscular parts of the left auricle, and the sigmoid valves of the aorta and pulmonary artery, in a state of ossification. M. Renauldin has published, in the Journal de Med. for 1816, a very interesting case of the same kind. The patient was a man thirty-three years of age, much addicted to study, and subject to violent palpitations on the slightest motion. "On applying the hand to the region of the heart a sort of motion of the ribs was felt, and even the slightest pressure produced very acute pain, which lasted long after the pressure was discontinued. On examining the body after death the heart was found extremely hard and heavy. On attempting to cut the left ventricle great resistance was found, owing to the total conversion of the muscular fibre into a sort of *petrifaction,* having in some places a sandy character, in others a resemblance to saline crystallization. The grains of this species of sand were very contiguous to each other, and became larger towards the interior of the ventricle. They were continuous with the columnae carneae, which were themselves converted into a similar substance, but still retained their original form, only much enlarged. Some of these sabulous concretions were of the size of the point of the little finger, and resembled small stalactites shooting in different directions. The ventricle was thickened. The right ventricle and great arterial trunks were sound. The temporal and maxillary arteries, and also a part of both the radial arteries were ossified." We frequently find on the interior surface of the ventricles, especially the left, cartilaginous scales continuous with

*Book Third, Chapter 1, Section Tenth. See footnote on page 332.—F. A. W., 1940.

the lining membrane, and apparently deposited between it and the muscular substance of the heart. These are generally small. I have never found them ossified.

OF CARDITIS*

Inflammation of the heart is a rare affection, and is, consequently very imperfectly known both in a practical and pathological view. There are two varieties of it, the general, or that affecting the whole heart; and the partial, or that confined to a small extent of it. There perhaps does not exist on record a satisfactory case of general inflammation of the heart, either acute or chronic. The greater number of cases so called, and particularly those given by M. Corvisart, are evidently instances of Pericarditis attended by that degree of discoloration of the heart which we shall find frequently to accompany that affection. Nothing proves that the paleness of the heart in such cases is the consequence of inflammation. The affection generally increases both the redness and density of the parts which it occupies;—but the discoloration in the cases alluded to is conjoined, in general, with a perceptible softening of the heart. It is further observable that, in these cases, pericardium was filled with pus while not a particle was found in the substance of the heart itself; now, pus must be considered as the most unequivocal indication of inflammation. The only case which I have met with of general inflammation of the heart possessing this unequivocal mark, is noticed by Meckel in the Mem. de l'Acad. de Berlin. But this case is described with so little precision, as merely to prove the possibility of the fact, and affords no help towards a general description of the disease.

Instances of partial inflammation of the heart, characterized by the presence of an abscess or ulcer in its parietes, are much more common. Bonetus has recorded a good many such cases in his *Sepulchretum*. I have only met with one instance of the kind. In this (in a child twelve years old) the abscess was situated in the parietes of the left ventricle, and might have contained a filbert: it was complicated with pericarditis. In another case, of a man of sixty years old, I found an albuminous exudation, of the consistence of boiled white of egg, and of the colour of pus, deposited among the muscular fibres of the left ventricle. The patient had presented symptoms of an acute inflammation of some of the thoracic viscera, without precisely indicating its site. Orthopnoea, and a feeling of inexpressible anguish, had been the chief symptoms.

Ulcers of the heart have been still more frequently observed than abscess; they have been met with in its external and internal surface.† All the cases, however, recorded under this name are not quite correctly designated. In the *Sepulchretum* we frequently find a case of pericarditis, attended with a rough and uneven pseudo-membranous exudation, mistaken

*Book Third, Chapter 1, Section Eleventh. See footnote on page 332.—F. A. W., 1940.
†Morgagni, Epist. XXV.

for an ulcer of the exterior surface of the heart. This has been noticed by Morgagni (Epist. 20 and 25). That true ulcers of this surface, however, have been observed, is beyond doubt. A case of this kind is described by Olaus-Borrichius in the following words: "Cordis exterior caro, profunde exiesa, in lacinias et villos carneos putrescentes abierat;"* and similar cases are recorded by Peyer† and Graetz.‡ Ulcers on the interior surfaces of the heart are perhaps more common than on the external; or, at least, there are on record a greater number of incontestible examples of the former. Bonetus, Morgagni and Senac have collected a great many of these. I have myself only met with one case of this kind. The ulcer was on the internal surface of the left ventricle, and was an inch long by half an inch wide, and was more than four lines deep in its centre. This patient had laboured under hypertrophia of the left ventricle, which had been recognised before death: this was occasioned by rupture of the ventricle. This terrible and, fortunately, very rare accident, is almost always the result of ulceration of the ventricular parietes. Morand has collected several cases of this kind in the Mem. de l'Acad. des Sciences for the 1732, and Morgagni has described a similar instance—(Epist. 27).

Rupture of the heart from violent exertion, without previous ulceration, is much rarer still; and the number of incontestible examples of this is very small. Several cases, recorded as such, are so imperfectly described, as to leave a doubt whether the alleged rupture might not have been rather the consequence of the incisions of an inexpert dissector. The best authenticated examples of this kind of rupture are those given by Haller (Elem. Physiol.) and Morgagni (Epist. 27).

It is surprising that the great thinness of the parietes of the ventricles, in the cases of accumulation of fat, does not give rise to rupture, more especially towards the apex and posterior part of the right ventricle. This is, however, so far from being the case, that ruptures of the right ventricle are much rarer than those of the left, and that, in this last, the rupture, when it occurs, is very rarely towards the apex.

M. Corvisart has given, for the first time, examples of another species of rupture of the heart, of a less certainly dangerous nature;—that, namely, of the tendons and fleshy pillars of the valves.§

In the three cases related by him the rupture appears to have been the consequence of violent efforts in lifting great weights, etc. A sudden and very intense feeling of suffocation was the immediate result of this accident, which terminated in exhibiting all the usual symptoms of disease of the heart. I shall have occasion to notice in a subsequent section a case of the same kind, only produced, apparently, by ulceration of the tendons.

*Sepulchret., Lib. II., Obs. 86.
†Ibid. Sect. II., Obs. 21.
‡Disput. de Hydr. pericard., Sect. 2.
§Corvisart on the Heart, Obs. 33, 40, and 41.

In the present state of our knowledge it is impossible to ascertain the existence of either an abscess or ulcer of the heart.

OF CARTILAGINOUS AND BONY INDURATION OF THE VALVES OF THE HEART*

The mitral and sigmoid valves of the aorta are subject to become the site of cartilaginous or bony productions, which increase their thickness, alter their shape, and obstruct, sometimes almost totally, the orifices in which they are placed. The tricuspid and sigmoid valves of the pulmonary artery are much less subject to these alterations, although they are not quite exempt from them, as Bichat thought. Morgagni found (Epist. 37), in the case of an old woman, both these partially indurated. He likewise found, in a young woman, the sigmoid valves of the pulmonary artery agglutinated by means of a cartilaginous induration, partly ossified, so as considerably to diminish the diameter of the artery. M. Corvisart has twice met with a cartilaginous induration of the base of the tricuspid valve, and I have myself sometimes observed slight cartilaginous incrustations, both at the base, and on the points of this valve. I am not, however, aware that any one has found these indurated portions completely ossified; nor do I believe that the induration has ever been so considerable as to occasion a serious state of disease. For these reasons I shall confine my remarks to the valves of the left ventricle.

The cartilaginous induration of the mitral valve is sometimes confined to the fibrous bands found in its base. In this case it has the appearance of a very smooth, though unequal roll, lessening the orifice in which it is situated. This sometimes has the consistence of perfect cartilage, sometimes only that of imperfect cartilage. Similar incrustations sometimes are met with in other parts of these valves. The bony indurations present the same characters as to situation and inequality of thickness. Though formed in the interior of the valve, they often project from it quite uncovered. These ossifications are never perfect bone; they are whiter and more opaque, more fragile, evidently contain a greater proportion of phosphat of lime. On this account they have been frequently named *stones* or *calculi*. In fact, they frequently bear a striking resemblance to small pieces of stone, of very irregular surface, recently broken. When they are situated in the floating extremities of the valve, these are sometimes united together, so as to reduce the orifice to a mere slit, which will, sometimes scarcely admit the blade of a knife or a goose-quill. M. Corvisart found the orifice between the auricle and ventricle reduced to a channel three lines wide, and bent like the canalis caroticus, from the thickening of the ossified mitral valves. Sometimes, though rarely, the tendinous cords of the mitral valve are affected in the same manner; and M. Corvisart in one case found the whole of one of its pillars ossified.†

---

*Book Third, Chapter 1, Section Twelfth. See footnote on page 332.—F. A. W., 1940.
†Op. cit., p. 212, 214.

The ossification of the sigmoid valves of the aorta may commence, like that of the mitral, in their base of their loose edges,—and much more frequently in one of these situations than in the intermediate portion. When in the loose extremity, the ossification seems most frequently to originate in the small tubercles known by the name of the *Corpora Sesamoidea.*

When the ossification is confined to the floating edge of the valves, or when the base though ossified is little thickened, the valve may still perform its functions, provided the middle portion of it be still sound. But when the ossification is extensive, the valves grow together, and get incurvated, either towards their concave or convex side, so as to acquire the appearance of certain shells. In this state they are immoveable, being either fixed on the side of the aorta, or in the orifice of the ventricle. Very frequently, of the three valves one is bent in a direction opposite that of the two others. In one case, M. Corvisart found all the three valves ossified in their closed position so as to leave merely an extremely small slit for the passage of the blood. The evil of this was partly obviated by one of the valves, although ossified and very thick, still retaining, at its base, sufficient mobility to allow an increase of one or two lines to the orifice during the action of the heart.

The symptoms of ossification of the mitral valve are somewhat different from those attending the same affection of the sigmoid. According to M. Corvisart the principal sign of the former lesion is "a peculiar rustling sensation, perceived on the application of the hand to the region of the heart." I have often noticed this symptom, which is very readily recognized after being once perceived, although it is difficult to give a description of it. The nearest idea I can give of it is by comparing it to the purring of a cat when pleased. The same sort of quality is said, by M. Corvisart, to exist in the pulse, which, he adds, is weak, but without hardness or fullness. To these symptoms may be added those characteristics of hypertrophia and dilatation of the left auricle and whole right side of the heart, which usually follow the affection of the valve.

I must confess that I have never perceived the peculiar character of the pulse described by M. Corvisart; and that I have frequently found wanting the peculiar vibration in the region of the heart in cases of undoubted disease of the valves. I believe the latter sensation is only perceptible by the hand when the contraction of the orifice is very considerable. In ossification of the sigmoid valves, several signs deduced from the state of the circulation are given by M. Corvisart, but the whole may be reduced to the *purring* sensation above mentioned.

Since I have used the cylinder I have only met with three cases of ossification of the mitral valve accompanied by the purring sensation; and only four cases of the same affection of the sigmoid in a slight degree, and unattended by the purring. In comparing these, however, with the numerous cases I had before studied, I think I can give the following results, if not correct, as, at least, approaching to correctness.

Ossification of the mitral and sigmoid valves does not produce irregularity of the circulation, and cannot therefore be suspected from the state of the pulse, or by the application of the hand to the region of the heart, unless it is so considerable as materially to lessen the orifices of the left ventricle. In ossification of the mitral valve, in a middling degree, the sound which attends the contraction of the auricle becomes much more prolonged, more dull, and with something in its tone which reminds one of the rasping of a file on wood, and sometimes of a bellows smartly compressed. This sound is well-marked when the *purring* is not perceptible to the hand, but it is much more distinct when this is perceptible, and is, indeed, proportional to its intensity.

The ossification of the sigmoid valves of the aorta is shewn by the existence of this sound during the contraction of the ventricle; but this does not exist in slight degrees of the affection, nor in a similar condition of the mitral.

In these cases, as in dilatation and hypertrophia, the alternate examination of the heart under the sternum and between the cartilages of the fifth and seventh ribs, as well as the state of the external jugulars, will always enable us to decide in which side of the heart the disease exists.

*OF ACCIDENTAL OR EXTRANEOUS PRODUCTIONS IN THE HEART**

Of all the organs of the body the heart is perhaps the least liable to these productions, if we except ossifications. Twice only have I found tubercles in its muscular substance, and not once melanosis, medullary sarcoma, or any other species of cancer. M. Recamier, however, informs me that he has found the heart partially converted into a scirrhous matter resembling lard, in a person who also had cancers in the lungs. In the *Sepulchretum* we find several examples of tumours in the heart, which appear to have been cancerous. Columbus found two hard tumours of the size of an egg in the parietes of the left ventricle.† Morgagni relates a case where there were numerous small tubercles on the external surface of the right auricle, in a subject which exhibited similar, but larger, tumours in the mediastinum, lungs, lymphatic glands, and cellular substance of the thorax and abdomen. (Epist. 78.)

Encysted serous tumours are equally rare in this viscus. When they do occur they are most commonly found between the muscular substance and investing pericardium. Examples have been recorded by Baillou, Houlier, Cordaeus, Rolfinckius, Thebesius, Fanton, Dalsalva, Morgagni, and Dupuytren. The latter found cysts of this kind in the parietes of the right auricle, projecting inwardly, and distending it to a size equal to the whole of the

*Book Third, Chapter 1, Section Thirteenth. See footnote on page 332.—F. A. W., 1940.
†De re Anat. lib. XV.

other parts of the heart. Morgagni describes a tumour, which was evidently a hydatid, implanted on the surface of the left ventricle (Epist. 21), and which appears to have been that variety named by Rudolphi *Cysticerous finnus.*

*OF POLYPI OF THE HEART**

It was formerly customary to attribute to the polypous concretions of the heart observed after death, the symptoms which truly depend on the enlargement of that organ. The incorrectness of this opinion is proved by the fact, that these concretions are very frequently found in persons who have never exhibited any symptom of disease of the heart in truth, they are met with in three-fourths of dead bodies. It is equally erroneous to believe, with some modern authors, that polypi never begin to form until the moment of death. Many facts prove that these concretions can be formed during life. The phenomena of aneurisms alone prove this. Haller found the carotid artery and internal jugular vein quite obstructed by very firm concrete fibrine in one case; and the inferior vena cava in another.† Vinckler,‡ Stancari and Banaroli have met with similar cases.§

I have myself observed, in a consumptive subject, an obliteration of the inferior cava for the space of four fingers' breadth. This obstruction was produced by a whitish fibrinous concretion which filled the whole caliber of the vein. The exterior layers of this concretion were like the buffy coat of the blood, only much firmer, and adhered strongly to the inner coat of the vein; the inner portions were, on the contrary, of a yellowish colour, more completely opaque, and of a friable character like certain kinds of cheese. In another case I found a similar obstruction in the carotid artery; and, in a third, I observed the whole of the vessels of the pia mater, in a circumscribed space about the size of the palm of the hand, injected with a similar concretion. None of these individuals had exhibited any symptoms indicative of such an affection; nor did there exist in any of them any obstacles to the course of the blood which might account for them: we must, therefore, attribute them to spontaneous coagulation of the blood, and reasoning, a priori, therefore, nothing is more probable than that the blood may coagulate during life, in the heart also; at least at the very close of life, when the circulation is performed only in an irregular and imperfect manner. M. Corvisart was therefore correct in distinguishing polypi into such as are of a formation posterior to death, and such as have been produced while the individual was still alive. These two kinds are easily distinguished from each other. The former, or those of recent formation, exhibit merely a slight layer of whitish opaque fibrine partially enveloping the coagula of blood contained in the heart and large vessels. This fibrinous or buffy layer never completely surrounds the coagula, and does not adhere

*Book Third, Chapter 1, Section Fourteenth. See footnote on page 332.—F. A. W., 1940.
†Opusc. Pathol. obs. 23, 24.
‡Dissert. de Vasor. lithias.
§Morgagni, Epist. 64.

to the parietes of the heart or vessel in which it is contained. Sometimes this layer is thicker, and, in this case, especially if the subject is dropsical, it is semi-transparent and tremulous like jelly.

On the other hand, the polypi of more ancient formation are of a much firmer consistence, and adhere more or less strongly to the parietes of the heart. In the ventricles and auricular sinuses, this adhesion is partly caused, no doubt, by the intertexture of the concretion with the columnae carneae; but, even here, the principal part of the attachment is independent of any mechanical structure of the parts. These concretions are of a more distinctly fibrinous texture than are the recent formations or the buffy coat of the blood, and they are, further, of a pale flesh or slight violet colour; while the more recent are, as already mentioned, of a white or yellowish colour.

These ancient concretions are found most frequently in the sinus of the right auricle, and in the right ventricle. When in the former, they completely obstruct its cavity, but in the ventricle they only double in thickness its parietes (thereby lessening its cavity) and obstruct the descent of the tricuspid valve. In this case, one may remove all the loose coagulated blood without injuring the concretion; it is even possible that this might be mistaken for the natural boundaries of the cavity.

The columnae carneae to which these concretions are attached, are commonly perceptibly flattened; a circumstance which, of itself, would prove their formation to be anterior to death. M. Corvisart was the first, as far as I know, to observe this flattening of the columnae; in the case noticed by him they were quite *effaced.* I have not met with any case so strongly marked as this; but it is by no means rare to find cases wherein the thing is very perceptible.

There is still a third species of concretion, evidently more ancient than those just described,—of a formation, perhaps, several months anterior to the patient's death. These are found adhering to the parietes of the heart, sometimes so firmly as only to be detached by scraping with the scalpel. Their consistence is less than that of those just noticed; being not at all fibrinous, and resembling rather a dry friable paste or a fat and somewhat soft cheese. They have lost the semitransparency of recently concreted fibrine, and resemble in every respect those layers of decomposed fibrine met with in false aneurisms. I have only met with concretions of this kind in the auricles.

*OF EXCRESCENCES ON THE VALVES AND INTERNAL PARIETES OF THE HEART**

There are two very distinct varieties of this affection. The first has been described by M. Corvisart under the name of *Excrescences of the Valves;* the other, which does not appear to have been hitherto described, I shall

*Book Third, Chapter 1, Section Fifteenth. See footnote on page 332.—F. A. W., 1940.

notice under the name of *globular excrescence.* The first kind might very well be named warty excrescence, inasmuch as they are extremely like warts, especially those of venereal origin on the parts of generation. Like these, the excrescences in the heart sometimes resemble small cherries, in their form and tuberous surface; at other times they are elongated into the form of a small cylinder or cord, and, occasionally, they are so short and so crowded together, as merely to give to the parts on which they are situated a rough or rugged surface; more frequently, however, they are either isolated or ranged in a single line along the loose, or the attached border of the valves. I have never observed any longer than three lines. The colour of these excrescences is sometimes whitish like that of the valves, and hardly so opaque, more commonly they are either wholly or in part tinged with a reddish or light violet colour. Their texture is fleshy, like venereal warts, only of somewhat less firm consistence. They adhere immediately to the subjacent parts; sometimes so strongly as to be only separable by incision; more commonly they are easily removed by scraping. The venereal origin of these excrescences, entertained by M. Corvisart, appears to me very improbable, when we consider their rarity and the frequency of venereal complaints, and when we meet with them, as we do, in individuals who, in all probability, never had this disease. Whatever may be the remote cause of these bodies, the manner of their formation seems to me more explicable. In dissecting the more voluminous excrescences, it has always appeared to me that their texture has borne a strong resemblance to that of the more compact polypous concretions. Frequently we observe in their centre a violet or sanguineous tint; and sometimes I have even found a very small, but distinct, coagulum of blood. From these circumstances I am led to believe, that these excrescences are merely polypi organized by the same process which transforms the false albuminous membranes into true adventitious membranes, or into cellular substance.

In like manner as M. Corvisart, I have only met with these excrescences in the following situations, viz. the mitral, tricuspid, and sigmoid valves, and (much more rarely) the interior of the auricles, especially the left. In general they are more common in the left than the right side of the heart. I may here remark that the view of the formation of these excrescences, given above, proves that they are not likely to occur but in subjects already affected with some serious disease of the heart or large vessels; a circumstance, as we shall find, in another place, which must render their diagnosis very difficult. [In the following notice of a case of this affection, I shall, as in many of the former cases, omit several of the symptoms with the intention of again noticing them in another part of this work.]

Case 43. A man, aged thirty-five, at the period of his coming into hospital, had been affected for five months, with great dyspnoea and violent palpitations on making any considerable exertion, startings from sleep, and occasional spitting of blood. For a few days past he had laboured under a severe diarrhoea. His countenance was tranquil, with some colour, the pulse small, hard, and regular, and the respiration oppressed. The action of the heart was not quite regular, but there was no distention of the jugular veins. This patient died on the third day.

The pericardium contained half a pint of serum. The heart was double the size of the patient's fist. The right ventricle was very large, its parietes being at least four lines thick, and its columnae very large. The tricuspid valves, and the sigmoid of the pulmonary artery, were of a deep violet red colour. The right auricle was sound. The left ventricle was one-third larger than natural, and its walls were six lines thick, and its columnae very thick. One of the tendons affixed to the edge of the mitral valve was ruptured about its middle. This rupture appeared to have been the consequence of progressive wasting of its middle part; and one of the other tendons of the same valve was unequally extenuated, but still whole. The whole floating border of the mitral valve was covered with small excrescences such as I have described, varying in size, form, and consistence. Altogether they gave to the valve a thickened and fringed appearance. The sigmoid valves of the aorta, and the lining membrane of this artery, were extremely red, and exhibited in this respect a striking contrast with the inner membrane of the ventricle. The whole inner surface, and indeed the whole parietes, of the left auricle, were of the same red colour; and, above the opening of the left pulmonary veins, and about two lines from the auriculo-ventricular opening, there was about an inch square coated with a congeries of excrescences similar to those on the mitral valve, and very firmly attached. The muscular substance of the heart was of moderate firmness. The pleura contained about a pint of serum on each side. The lungs were sound.

The *globular excrescences* have a quite different appearance from those just described, resembling little balls or cysts, of a spherical or oval shape, and of a size from that of a pea to a pigeon's egg. The exterior surface of these is equal, smooth, and of a yellowish white colour, and the thickness of their parietes is very uniform, being never more than half a line. The substance composing their parietes is opaque and very similar to that of ancient polypi, its consistence being firmer than boiled white of egg. The inner surface of these parietes (the cyst) is not so smooth as the exterior, and it appears to be composed of a softer substance, which occasionally has the appearance of passing gradually into the matter contained within it. This matter may exist in three different states, all of which may be found in the same subject, but in different cysts. These are, first, a liquid resembling half-coagulated blood, only turbid as if intermixed with some insoluble powder, and sometimes containing a few clots of perfectly coagulated blood; second, a more opaque matter, of a pale violet colour, of a pultaceous consistence, and very like the lees of wine; and third, yellow ish, opaque fluid, like thick pus or thin paste. I have only met with cysts of this kind in the ventricles and auricular sinuses. They are found as frequently in the right as left side of the heart, generally near the apex of the ventricles, and always adherent to the walls of the cavity. They are attached by means of a pedicle, which is often so slightly connected with the columnae carneae as to be detached from them without being ruptured. This pedicle, although forming part of the excrescence, resembles the common polypi more than the other portions, and seems as if it were of more recent formation and less perfectly organized. I have never found these bodies more organized than I have described, and I have considered those containing clots of blood as the newest, those containing a fluid like the lees of wine as next in order, and those containing a puriform matter as the most ancient. I have met with these excrescences in subjects dead of different diseases, but all of whom had remained in a dying state (agonie) for several days or even weeks.

The only case that I have met with in medical writings, which seems to me to agree with the above description, is recorded in the *Miscel. Natur. Curios.* The affection, nevertheless, does not appear to be extremely rare, as I have met with several cases of it.

*OF THE RED COLOUR OF THE INTERNAL MEMBRANE OF THE HEART AND LARGE VESSELS**

In examining dead bodies we frequently find the inside of the aorta and pulmonary artery uniformly reddened, as if stained by the blood they contained. This colouring is of two kinds,—either bordering on scarlet, or violet. The scarlet colour has its seat exclusively in the inner membrane, as, when this is removed, the tunic beneath is found of the natural colour. This colour is quite uniform, as if painted, without any trace of vascularity, only sometimes more intense in one place than another. Sometimes this stain diminishes progressively from the origin of the aorta, but frequently it terminates quite abruptly with irregular edges. Sometimes in the middle of a very red portion we find a circumscribed spot retaining the natural white colour, like the whiteness produced by pressure with the finger on an erysipelatous skin. The origin and arch of the aorta are the situations most commonly reddened, and, with them, the sigmoid and mitral valves. When the pulmonary artery is affected, its valves, as well as the tricuspid, are commonly in the same state. The lining membrane of the ventricles and auricles is frequently colourless when the valves are deeply stained; not infrequently, however, the auricle participates in the affection, but scarcely ever the ventricles. This redness is attended by no sensible thickening of the part, and it entirely disappears after a few hours maceration.

M. Corvisart has slightly noticed this affection; and has avowed his ignorance of its nature and cause. Franck, who has observed it through the

*Book Third, Chapter 1, Section Sixteenth. See footnote on page 332.—F. A. W., 1940.

whole tract of the arteries, considered it as the cause of a particular and uniformly fatal fever. My own observations are far from leading to the same result, although I confess myself ignorant of the nature of this affection. The most natural idea respecting it is, that it is the result of inflammation. But mere redness, without thickening of parts, does not sufficiently characterise this state; while the abrupt termination, and exact circumscription presented by the redness in certain cases, seem not easily to accord with the nature of inflammation. On the other hand, it may, indeed, be said, that in the serous and mucous membranes, this sort of redness by stains is more characteristic of inflammation than the mere sanguineous infarction of the capillaries, which might take place either at, or after, death. The following is an example of this affection.

Case 44. A young woman, fresh-coloured and plump, came into hospital complaining only of intense headache, of three days' duration. At the end of two days the disease assumed the appearance of acute hydrocephalus, the pulse being very slow, very regular and of moderate strength. The cerebral symptoms increasing rapidly, this patient died at the end of ten days from the invasion of the disease, after the application of the usual measures, and particularly the employment of a great number of general and local bleedings indicated by the violence of the headache. For two days before death, the pulse became more frequent, but not stronger, nor more irregular. On examining the body, besides the hydrocephalus, there were found tubercles in the lungs, large tuberculous ulcerations in the intestines, extensive emphysema in several portions of the mucous coat of the intestines, unequivocal marks of confirmed lues, and, finally, a very intense redness of all the valves of the heart, the aorta, and particularly of the pulmonary artery.

One of my pupils informs me that he found in an aorta intensely reddened, some small purulent collections, resembling miliary pustules, situated between the internal and middle coats. This, however, must have been the consequence of disease of the middle coat, itself, as we can hardly suppose that inflammation of the internal coat would terminate in suppuration of its adherent surface. I do not, however, mean to deny the possibility of inflammation of blood-vessels. On the contrary, I think it probable that the affection we have been describing is of this nature; and I would be disposed to consider the various concretions of blood already mentioned, for example, those which produce obliteration of veins, and the warty excrescences, as the result of inflammation.

The second species of redness of the large vessels has a quite different appearance, being, in place of a bright red, of a violet hue. It is also usually extended at the same time to the aorta, pulmonary artery, valves, auricles and ventricles. This variety is not so exactly confined to the lining membrane, as we find the muscular substance of the auricles and ventricles, and even the fibrinous coat of the aorta and pulmonary artery, participating in it, at least partially. I have found this variety of colouring in subjects dead of putrid fevers, emphysema of the lungs, and disease of the heart. All these individuals had remained long in a moribund condition, with suffocation; and I have thought that the violent tint was deep in proportion to the intensity and duration of the latter symptom. From this circumstance I am disposed to consider this condition of the vessels as the effect of deranged circulation and congestion of the blood in the capillaries; being analogous to the livid hue of the cheeks, etc. observable in persons dead of disease of the heart. It is, in fact, an effect of death, or at most produced in articulo mortis.

I would here beg to observe, that it is often difficult to distinguish mere congestion of the capillaries from actual inflammation. The distinction, however, is of great importance, both in morbid anatomy and practical medicine, the more so, as both these affections may exist simultaneously. In proof of this I may refer to the controversy that has for some time existed respecting the condition of the mucous membrane of the intestines in fever.

I am far from denying the influence of irritation, ulceration, aphthae, and consequent inflammation of the intestinal tunics in continued fevers; and, although they have been more or less noticed and appreciated in all ages, M. Broussais has truly benefited his profession by calling the attention of practitioners more particularly to them, and by showing the injurious error of former periods in withholding the employment of general and local bleedings in fevers. But we should fall into as great, although an opposite, error, if we concluded that all continued fevers depended on the intestinal irritation that accompanied them, and that every kind of redness observable in them after death indicates a disorder requiring venesection for its treatment. The mucous membrane of the stomach and bowel is naturally pale only in persons of pale skins; its degree of colour may be judged of by that of the lips, mouth, arms and vulva, in different individuals. No one will set down the livid gums of a dropsical or scorbutic patient, or the swelling and blueness of his hands and feet, to inflammation, or think of treating these affections by blood-letting. Now, in many cases, I conceive, the redness of the mucous coat of the intestines has much more relation to this passive congestion than to inflammation. If, then, such appearances (as is most probable) only took place in such subjects, at the same time as the lividity of the face and of the dependent parts of the body—that is to say, some days or hours before death; it would be absurd to look to such condition of parts for the cause of the fever,—more especially, as we often find, in such cases, traces of as great or greater disorder in almost every texture of the body. For example:—the skin is dry and harsh; the lips, gums, and lining membrane of the mouth are swollen, soft and chopped; the membranes of the brain are gorged with blood and containing serum; the lungs are charged with a sero-sanguinolent fluid; the mucous membrane of the bronchia is swollen and of a violet hue; the heart is flaccid, livid and soft; the blood fluid and imperfectly coagulable; the lining membrane of the arteries or veins livid as if stained by blood; the muscles *fishy* (poisseux); the spleen enlarged; the capillaries of almost every organ, and of the surface, gorged with blood; and lastly, the intestines are in the same state, and their lining membrane livid, ulcerated and thickened in diverse places.—Now, to which of these affections shall we attribute the disease? All are posterior—often many days—to the fever. Is it not, therefore, more rational to consider, that none of these local lesions are the cause, but that, as in smallpox and measles, some unknown cause, acting generally on the system, had produced both the fever and the local affections—whether active or passive—which accompany or follow it?

In the very case where there exists simultaneously aphthae and exulcerations in the intestinal tunics, and redness, lividity, and capillary congestion of the mucous membrane, we ought to conclude, from analogy, that the two former states are the result of inflammation, active or passive,—and the three latter the result of debility of the circulation in the capillaries; that the first may require venesection, but that this very means, carried to too great lengths, may give rise to, or increase the last, by increasing the general debility. The haematemesis and blood fluxes which occur sometimes in continued fevers ought rather, in my opinion, to be attributed to purely passive congestions of the capillaries, than to inflammation. In the instance just mentioned we find the whole of the intestinal tunics in the affected part tinged with blood, and softened, without any notable increase of thickness of the part; while inflammation of every mucous membrane uniformly increases both the thickness and density of the part. We may farther add the fine observation of Bichat, that, of any morbid affection, inflammation has the least tendency to propagate itself by contiguity, especially in membranous parts. Peritonitis and dysentery leave untouched the muscular coat of the intestine, but the lividity consequent on fatal fevers often extends to the whole three tunics.

*OF MALFORMATION OF THE HEART**

There exist two varieties of unnatural communication between the cavities of the heart, viz. the perforation of the septum of the ventricles, and the continued patency of the foramen of Botallus. The first variety is very rare, there being not more than five or six instances of it on record. In all these the unnatural aperture was smooth, evidently very ancient, if not congenital. The continued patency of the foramen of Botallus is much more common. Sometimes this is produced by the imperfect union of the two plates of the foetal valve, so that a probe, or even a female sound, can be passed obliquely from one auricle to the other. This condition of parts is

*Book Third, Chapter 1, Section Seventeenth. See footnote on page 332.—F. A. W., 1940.

not very rare, and does not appear to be productive of any kind of inconvenience. In other cases we find the foramen continue constantly open so as to admit the finger. I have myself seen it sufficiently large to receive the thumb. It is commonly believed that this species of malformation is always congenital; but from some cases which I have met with, I am disposed to believe that such a perforation may be produced by an accident; or, at least, when such a condition of parts exists as above described, that a blow, fall, or violent exertion, may cause the dilatation of the oblique opening, and its progressive enlargement. The history of several cases on record, especially of some of M. Corvisart's, would seem to countenance this opinion, since, in several of these, the individuals had enjoyed good health, without any symptom of diseased heart, until they had experienced some of the accidental causes above mentioned.

I do not know that any of these unnatural communications have existed without consequent thickening and dilatation of either the whole, or part of the heart, especially the right side. The symptoms of the latter affection are, consequently, combined with those of the former. These are principally the four following: 1, a great sensibility to the impression of cold; 2, frequent faintings; 3, the respiration more constantly impeded than in most other diseases of the heart; and 4, a violet or blueish colour of the skin much more extensive than that in any other disease, and, sometimes, even general. This last symptom has been named by several authors *the blue jaundice,* or *the blue disease.* On the other hand, all the above mentioned symptoms have been found to exist in subjects who had no other malformation than the continued patency of the foramen of Botallus; and still more so in those cases where the pulmonary artery was found to originate in the left ventricle, and the aorta in the right, or where the latter has opened at once into both ventricles. In some diseases of the lungs, especially emphysema, the blue colour of the skin is sometimes quite as intense and as extensive as in the case of malformation of the heart. On the other hand, the foramen of Botallus has been found dilated very considerably, without there being present any degree of lividity except on the face and extremities. The case of dilatation noticed by myself, above mentioned, was of this sort.

OF DISPLACEMENT OF THE HEART*

The heart, although retained in its place by the diaphragm, large vessels, and peculiar structure of the mediastinum, and, still more, by the constant state of plenitude of the chest, may, nevertheless, in certain cases, be thrown to the right or left by a solid, liquid, or acriform effusion into either sac of the pleura, by extensive tumours in the lungs, and, as we have already seen, by emphysema of this organ. In like manner, a tumour in the superior mediastinum, or a large aneurism of the arch of the aorta, may press

*Book Third, Chapter 1, Section Eighteenth. See footnote on page 332.—F. A. W., 1940.

it downwards, so that that part of the diaphragm on which it reposes shall project into the abdomen. Sometimes even this depression has taken place without any visible cause, in which case the affection has been named by some authors *prolapsus* of the heart.

These various kinds of displacement produce no perceptible inconvenience when they exist in a slight degree; when more marked, they may produce bad effects; but in this case, they are themselves consequences of lesions much more serious.

CHANGES PRODUCED BY DISEASES OF THE HEART IN THE TEXTURE OF OTHER ORGANS*

On examining the bodies of persons who have fallen victims to organic affections of the heart, besides the organic lesion and the serous effusions which almost always accompany it, we find all the marks of congestion of blood in the internal capillaries. The mucous membranes, especially those of the stomach and intestines, are of a red or violet tint; and the liver, lungs, and capillaries situated beneath the serous, mucous and cutaneous tissues, are gorged with blood. The augmented colour of the mucous membranes varies much in degree and extent. Sometimes it is observed only here and there, under the form of small points or specks, disseminated over the surface of the membrane: at other times it occupies the whole extent of the surface, and has the appearance of being attended by some swelling of the part. These two latter appearances are sometimes so considerable, that, if we looked to them merely, without examining the condition of the heart, and without reference to the history of the patient (who had been found capable of taking into his stomach wine and other stimulant matters without experiencing any pain, even up to the period of his death), we might be tempted to believe that the fatal disease had been a violent inflammation of the stomach and bowels. In fact, the degree of redness of the membranes observed after diseases of the heart, is often much more intense and extensive than is found after true inflammation of these parts, as, for example, in dysentery; a fact, among many others, sufficiently proving the insufficiency of mere redness to characterise inflammation of the mucous membrane of the intestines.

Lancisi and Senac, after Hildanus, consider gangrene of the limbs, as a consequence of disease of the heart and large vessels. The late M. Giraud was of the same opinion, and, since his time, many practitioners have considered the gangrene of old persons as usually caused by ossification of the arteries. M. Corvisart justly doubts whether, in such cases, there is anything else but mere coincidence of independent diseases; and I think that the single circumstance of the rarity of the spontaneous gangrene of the limbs, compared with the frequency of disease of the heart and ossification of the arteries, is sufficient to render the thing quite improbable. This is

*Book Third, Chapter 1, Section Nineteenth. See footnote on page 332.—F. A. W., 1940.

equally the case with the notion of Testa, that ophthalmia, and sometimes the loss of the eye, may be ranged among the consequences of diseases of the heart.*

OF THE CAUSES OF DISEASES OF THE HEART†

The causes of diseases of the heart are, like the diseases themselves, various in their nature. Ossifications are the result of some aberration of the process of assimilation which is not easily understood. I have already stated my opinion respecting the origin of the excrescences on the valves. The dilatation and thickening of the ventricles, diseases of much greater frequency, also may arise from numerous causes; but these are in general more easily traced to their effects, than the former. All diseases which give rise to severe and long-continued dyspnoea produce, almost necessarily, hypertrophia or dilatation of the heart, through the constant efforts the organ is called on to perform, in order to propel the blood into the lungs against the resistance opposed to it by the cause of dyspnoea. It is in this manner that phthisis pulmonalis, empyema, chronic peripneumony, and emphysema of the lungs, act in producing disease of the heart; and that those kinds of exercise which require great exertion, and thereby impede respiration, come to be the most common remote causes of these complaints.

On the other hand, it is found that diseases of the heart, on the same principle of mutual influence, give rise to several diseases of the lungs. They are thus among the most frequent causes of oedema of the lungs and haemoptysis. When, however, diseases of the heart are found to coexist with chronic pleurisy, phthisis, emphysema, and, in general, with chronic disease of the lungs, it will usually be found, on close examination, that the latter are the primary diseases. It follows from these, and other facts noticed under the head of Emphysema and Pulmonary Catarrh, that a *neglected Cold* is frequently the original cause of the most severe diseases of the heart.

To all these causes must be added the congenital disproportion between the size of the heart and the diameter of the aorta. M. Corvisart has, perhaps, gone too far in asserting that there can be no dilatation of the heart without the previous existence of a disproportion of this kind, or of a contraction, or some similar obstruction of the circulation, at a greater or less distance from the heart; it is, however, true, that it is very common to find an aorta of small diameter in cases of hypertrophia or dilatation of the heart. Still, this is not always the case, and however rational such a cause may be, we can readily conceive many others. We know that the energetic and reiterated action of all muscles notably increases their size, as in the case of those of the right arm of the fencer, the shoulder of the porter, and the hands of most artisans. On the same principle we

*Delle Malattie del Cuore. Bologna, 1810.

†Book Third, Chapter 1, Section Twentieth. See footnote on page 332.—F. A. W., 1940.

must admit that even nervous palpitations, or such as originate from moral causes, may, by frequent recurrence, produce a true enlargement of the heart.

There is yet another congenital cause of disease of the heart, which appears to me to be of greater frequency than the small caliber of the aorta, above mentioned,—I allude to a disproportionate thickness of one or both sides of the heart. I am satisfied that in a great many persons the parietes of one or both sides of the heart are either too thick or too thin from birth. In such cases there can be no doubt that the usual exciting causes will be more apt to produce formal disease of the heart than in individuals in whom this disproportion does not exist.

*CHAPTER II. DISEASES OF THE PERICARDIUM**

Of Pericarditis, or Inflammation of the Pericardium

Pericarditis is inflammation of the serous membrane which lines the fibrous sac of the pericardium, the heart, and large vessels. It may be either acute or chronic. This inflammation, like that of all membranes of the same kind, is marked by redness, more or less deep, a concrete albuminous exhalation and a sero-purulent effusion. The redness is almost always but slight in the acute disease. When it exists, it is for the most part only partially. It is most commonly punctuated, and looks as if the surface of the membrane was covered, here and there, with little specks of blood very close to each other. I have never perceived that this redness was accompanied by any thickening of the part. In some cases, wherein, to judge by the thickness of the false membranes, the inflammation appears to have been very great, no redness whatever can be discovered on the serous membrane, on removal of the membranous exudation. This concrete albuminous exudation commonly invests the whole surface of the pericardium, as well on the heart and large vessels, as on the sac. It rarely presents the appearance of an equable membranous layer, like the false membranes of pleurisy; on the contrary, its surface is most frequently marked by a great number of rough and irregular prominences. Sometimes the knobbed appearance of this exudation is very like what would result from the sudden separation of two pieces of slab joined by a pretty thick layer of butter; at other times, it is more like the internal surface of the second stomach of the calf, an observation made, in one case, by M. Corvisart. In certain cases this aspect of the false membrane has given rise to a singular error, having been mistaken for a variolous eruption in subjects dead of the small-pox. The consistence of this exudation is usually greater than that of the false membranes

*Book Third, Chapter 2, Section First. See footnote on page 332.—F. A. W., 1940.

of pleurisy; it is also thicker, and more firmly adherent to the subjacent parts; its colour is, however, the same, being of a pale yellow analogous to that of pus.

The serum effused in inflammation of the pericardium is limpid, of a pale yellow colour, or slightly brownish. It contains few fragments of semi-concrete albumen; at least, it very rarely contains enough of these to give it a milky and turbid character. The quantity of this effusion is usually considerable in the commencement of the disease, often as much as a pound. M. Corvisart found it, in one case, to amount to four pounds. It would seem that the quantity of effused serum diminishes quickly, as soon as the violence of the inflammation begins to subside; as we usually find the proportion of serum and of albuminous exudation nearly equal, while in pleurisy and peritonitis the serum is commonly from twenty to fifty times greater than that of the extravasated lymph. Very commonly even, in very violent cases, we find no effused serum, and only a thick and highly concrete albumen filling the whole cavity of the pericardium, and uniting the heart and large vessels to the exterior or loose portion of this membrane. In this case we may suppose that the effused serum has been quickly absorbed, and the two layers of false membrane cemented together; although it is not impossible that, in some cases, the more solid exudation may be the only one. We have seen that the same thing occasionally takes place in certain partial and sub-acute inflammations of the pleura; and several observations have led me to believe that the cartilaginous patches that sometimes are met with on the exterior of the lungs are produced in the same manner.

When the disease terminates favourably, the pseudo-membranous exudation, after a certain time, is converted into cellular substance, or rather into laminae of the same nature as the serous membranes; that is to say, the laminae are double, the exterior surface being exhalent, and the interior cellular, or adherent, and containing the vessels distributed to the part. Sometimes these laminae are long, sometimes so short that the pericardium seems intimately adherent to the heart.

Before the conversion of false membranes into cellular tissue was well understood, the adhesion of the pericardium to the heart was regarded by divers authors as a cause of various and serious complaints. Lancisi and Vieussens considered it as constantly causing palpitation; Meckel, as rendering the pulse habitually small; and Sénac, as productive of frequent faintings. Even M. Corvisart himself has fallen into some mistakes on this head. He admits three species of adhesions,—all of which I have just described as mere varieties or stages of the same affection. These are, first, a semiconcrete albuminous adhesion, which is the only one recognised by him as the consequence of pericarditis; second, the very intimate or close cellular adhesion, deemed an effect of gouty or rheumatic affections; and third, the extended or long cellular adhesion, the cause of which is not assigned by him.* M. Corvisart is further of opinion that no person can live, and preserve a good state of health, who is affected with a complete and close adhesion of the pericardium to the heart, or of the lungs to the pleura.

I have, however, met with many cases where this condition of parts was found after death, in which no disorder of the respiration or circulation existed during life. A case adduced by M. Corvisart in support of his opinion (Op. cit. p. 34) appears to me rather conclusive against it, inasmuch as the appearances on dissection showed sufficient lesions in other organs to account for the symptoms referred by him to the adhesions between the heart and pericardium.

Sometimes, though rarely, the inflammation is confined to a part only—sometimes a very small part—of the pericardium. These partial inflammations are in proportion to the general, in point of frequency, hardly as one to ten. Their anatomical characters are precisely the same, only that the albuminous exudation is in them confined to the inflamed part. The serous effusion is sometimes as abundant as in the general disease; more commonly, however it is less. The inflammation in this case almost always terminates in being cured, by the transformation of the pseudo-membranous exudation into long serous laminae; scarcely ever are these partial inflammations followed by the intimate adhesion of the parts.

We frequently find on the surface of the heart opaque white patches, sometimes as large as the palm of the hand, more commonly one-half or one-third this size, and often very small. They are nearly of the thickness of the nail, and have a degree of consistence equal to that of the membranes composed of condensed cellular substance, as, for instance, the exterior membrane of the lymphatic glands. They adhere so closely to the parts on which they lie, that it is difficult to ascertain, even by dissection, whether they are situated above or beneath the fine membrane covering the heart and great vessels. M. Corvisart is of opinion that they are beneath it. I have, however, ascertained the incorrectness of this opinion, as I have several times been able to remove the patches, leaving the serous membrane of the pericardium still untouched.

Are these patches the effect of partial pericarditis and the consequent conversion of the effused lymph into a condensed membranous cellular tissue? M. Corvisart considers them as produced without previous inflammation, and seated, as I have already said, beneath the serous surface of the pericardium. Both these notions are, I think, inadmissible, inasmuch as there exists no example of an albuminous exudation on the adherent surface of a serous membrane, and as facts without number prove that pseudo-membranous exudations are always the produce of inflammation.

*See Treatise on the Heart, etc., by M. Corvisart.

I have lately met with a case which appears to me to throw some light on the question of the origin of these spots. In a man dead of peripneumony, I found a thin false membrane, very firm and of a yellowish colour, investing the right auricle and a portion of the ventricle of the same side, all the rest of the pericardium being quite free, only containing in its cavity two or three ounces of a transparent and slightly yellow serum. Some parts of the false membrane, particularly on the auricle, were of a whiter colour and firmer than the rest, and exhibited an appearance, almost the same as the white patches above described.

Chronic pericarditis is always general occupying the whole internal surface of the serous membrane. This is commonly much redder than in the acute disease. The redness is formed by the close approximation of minute points, which look as if applied with a pencil. Rarely the chronic disease is accompanied by a pseudo-membranous exudation; and when this exists, it is thin, soft, friable, and entirely resembling a layer of very thick pus. In every case there exists a more or less copious effusion of a turbid, milky fluid, sometimes having quite a puriform character. I am led to believe that the close adhesion of the pericardium to the heart, is commonly the consequence of the absorption of this fluid, and that the adhesion by the long laminae is the product of the acute disease. In one case I found a close and general adhesion of the pericardium to the heart and large vessels, by means of a false fibro-cartilaginous membrane, in every respect like those of the pleura.

From one case, cited by M. Corvisart, I am led to believe, that there may occasionally arise, subsequently to chronic inflammation of the pericardium, a tuberculous eruption similar to those frequently formed in the false membranes of the pleura and peritoneum. "The portion of the pericardium," he says, "which invests the heart, was of a greyish colour, thickened, unequal, wrinkled, crisp, and containing granulations of which the summit seemed ulcerated." I am the rather led to consider these *granulations* as tubercles, because in the same subject "both lungs, although crepitous, were *granular* throughout."

In many cases of pericarditis, especially in the chronic disease, the muscular substance of the heart has lost its colour and become whitish. This loss of colour is sometimes attended by a notable degree of softening, and, at other times, the consistence is natural. Most writers have regarded this loss of colour as a mark of the inflammation of the heart itself, and most of the examples recorded of Carditis are merely cases of inflammation of the pericardium accompanied by this loss of colour. A great number of those collected by M. Corvisart are of this kind. For my own part I am disposed to doubt the correctness of the opinion that refers this loss of colour to inflammation. We can never be sure of the existence of inflammation in a muscular organ unless we find a deposition of pus among its fibres.

. . . .

1. *Acute Pericarditis.* There are few diseases attended by more variable symptoms, or of more difficult diagnosis, than this. Sometimes it appears with all the symptoms of a very violent disease of the chest; at other times it proves fatal without leading us, in the least, to suspect its existence. Again, we find cases marked by all the symptoms usually attributed by nosologists to this disease, and in the subjects of which, after death we discover no traces of its existence. The same difficulty is acknowledged, or at least encountered, by most practitioners. Corvisart attributes the difficulty to the circumstance of pericarditis being almost "always complicated with pleurisy, peripneumony, or some other disease of the chest, which masks its peculiar symptoms." These complications, which are very common, must, unquestionably, have this effect where they exist; I must, however, confess, that the most completely latent affections of this kind that I have met with, were in subjects whose thoracic viscera were, in every other respect, quite sound, and who had died of disease of the abdomen. These facts seem to prove that inflammation of the pericardium is sometimes a local affection of little violence, and of very inconsiderable influence on the general system or even on the circulation; while, in other cases, it is accompanied by an acute fever, and by such violent disorder of almost all the functions, as to compromise the life of the patient.

M. Corvisart is likewise of opinion that it is when the disease is very acute, that the symptoms are very obscure. "Its invasion," he says, "is sudden, its progress rapid, its termination almost instantaneous." When it exists in a less violent degree, but still acute, he thinks that it can be recognised by the following symptoms: viz. sense of heat in the region of the heart; great difficulty of respiration; greater colour of the left cheek than the right; pulse at first frequent, hard, and rarely irregular,—becoming about the third or fourth day, small, hard, contracted and often irregular; great anxiety, slight palpitations; partial faintings; *peculiar* change of features; and (towards the close of the disease) total or partial cessation of the local pain.

These symptoms are certainly sometimes present in pericarditis; but each, or all of them may be absent, and some of them are very rare. I have never observed the increased colour of the cheek, have rarely heard complaints of local heat or pain, and, in place of the progressive increase of irregularity in the pulse (as described by M. Corvisart), I have uniformly found this irregularly intermitting, wiry, and almost insensible, from the very commencement of the disease.

I must admit that the stethoscope scarcely furnishes us with any more certain signs of this disease. The following appear to me to be the most common symptoms of the inflammation of the pericardium, when not latent; the contraction of the ventricles yields a greater shock, and sometimes a more marked sound, than usual, and, at intervals, feebler and shorter pulsations are perceived, which correspond with intermissions of the pulse, the smallness of which contrasts remarkably with the strength of the heart's pulsation. When these symptoms come on suddenly in a person who had never been affected with disease of the heart, there is great probability of their being the consequence of this disease. In addition, it is further common for the patient to have much dyspnoea and very great anxiety; and to suffer syncope on taking a few steps, or on moving suddenly in his bed.

2. *Chronic Pericarditis.* The signs of this variety are still more uncertain than those of the acute disease. I have attended several cases which I considered, throughout their whole course, as chronic inflammations of the pericardium, but which almost all were cured. In two or three cases only have I been able to verify the correctness of my diagnosis by examination after death; whilst very frequently I have found the pericardium full of pus and in a true state of chronic inflammation, without having been at all led to suspect such an affection. In the cases which have occurred within the last three years, I have found the symptoms to be precisely the same as in the acute disease, only less violent. From one to two years has elapsed before a cure has taken place; and when this has been effected the action of the heart and pulse has become natural and regular.

. . . .

*OF HYDRO-PERICARDIUM, OR WATER IN THE PERICARDIUM**

It is extremely common to find a greater or less quantity of serum in the pericardium; most frequently this does not exceed a few ounces, and can rarely be considered as idiopathic. Most commonly it can only be regarded as taking place in articulo mortis. When there exists a general dropsical diathesis, we occasionally find some water in the pericardium, but, in general, it contains less than the other serous cavities. In the idiopathic hydro-pericardium, on the contrary, the pericardium is commonly the only membrane which contains serous effusion.

The effused serum is sometimes colourless, but more commonly it is yellowish, brownish or reddish, although still perfectly limpid, and without any admixture of flakes of lymph; rarely it is sanguinolent. It is variable in amount. Most frequently it does not exceed one or two pounds, but it has been found in much greater quantity than this. M. Corvisart records an instance wherein eight pounds were found. This effusion is attended by no change in the heart or its coverings. Some authors have, indeed, stated the heart to have been macerated (macéré) in such cases; but I am disposed to consider such statements as the result of imperfect observation and incorrect description. Very frequently before opening a pericardium partially filled with serum, I have distinctly observed an accumulation of air in the cavity. I have seen this occupy a space the size of the

*Book Third, Chapter 2, Section Second. See footnote on page 332.—F. A. W., 1940.

fist, and when as large as this, a distinct hissing sound is perceived in puncturing the pericardium. In place of this continuous mass of air, we more commonly observe a great quantity of small air-bubbles on the surface of the liquid. I am inclined to think that I have found air in the pericardium in cases where there was no serum, but I am not quite assured of the correctness of my observation. At all events, this case of simple *Pneumo-Pericardium* is extremely rare, while the other variety, just described, is by no means so.

Authors vary respecting the symptoms of this affection [hydropericardium]. Lancisi states the principal to be a sensation of an enormous weight in the region of the heart. Reimann and Saxonia assure us that the patient feels his heart swimming in water. Sénac says he has seen the fluctuation of the fluid between the third, fourth, and fifth ribs. M. Corvisart says he has perceived this fluctuation by the touch, and adds the following as marks of the affection:—sense of weight in the region of the heart; inferior resonance on percussion; pulsation of the heart irregular and obscure, and felt over a large space and with variable intensity in the same and different points of this space; pulse small, frequent and irregular; threatened suffocation on lying in the horizontal posture; frequent syncope, but rarely palpitation; oedema. To these symptoms I may apply the same remarks as to those of pericarditis: they may exist, in greater or less number, with or without hydro-pericardium. I am unable to say, from experience, how far, and in what respect, the cylinder will assist the diagnosis of this disease.

OF ACCIDENTAL PRODUCTIONS IN THE PERICARDIUM*

Various species of accidental productions have been found between the pericardium properly so-called, and the pleura; also, between it and the internal and serous membrane; and, lastly, between the serous membrane and the heart. In the Sepulchretum of Bonetus and other collections of cases, we find examples of what appear to be tubercles, cancerous tumours, or cysts, in the different situations just mentioned. But the imperfect knowledge of membranes before the time of Bichat, and the general confusion of all accidental productions under the names of Scirrhus, Carcinoma, Atheroma, etc. renders it impossible to ascertain precisely either the nature or site of such morbid growths. I have already noticed the fatty productions, in the form of a cock's comb, developed occasionally between the pleura and fibrous membrane of the pericardium. Twice or thrice I have found tubercles in the same situation, in subjects which exhibited a great number of these bodies in the lungs and elsewhere. I have also seen a tubercle situated at the point of the origin of the pulmonary artery and beneath the serous membrane of the pericardium.

*Book Third, Chapter 2, Section Third. See footnote on page 332.—F. A. W., 1940.

Once only have I met with an instance of ossification between the layers of the pericardium. As this case was remarkable both for its extent and the effects produced by it, I shall here briefly detail it.

Case 45. A man, aged 65 years, had led an intemperate life, but had, nevertheless, enjoyed good health until his fiftieth year. At this time he appears to have had an attack of pleurisy of short duration, but which was followed by oedema of the lower extremities and subsequently by anasarca of other parts, and by dyspnoea and breathlessness on ascending an elevation, or using any degree of exercise. When he came into hospital, in the end of spring, the dropsical symptoms continued and the lips were swollen and violet. The pulsations of the heart were unequal, irregular, and very distinct, though perceptible over a very small extent of the chest. The pulse was feeble, small, soft, unequal, intermittent and irregular. There was no cough, but copious expectoration. The thorax sounded well superiorly, but badly on the lower parts.

The patient could lie in any posture; slept well, even without having his head raised, and had no sudden startings from sleep.—He died in the course of a few months, the dropsical swellings and dyspnoea having much increased. The brain, lungs, and abdominal viscera were found in a sound state. The heart was enlarged, and adhered throughout to the pericardium, by means of very close cellular attachments. On first touching it, it seemed to be quite inclosed in a bony case, situated beneath the fibrous membrane of the pericardium; but on further examination this incrustation was found to be incomplete. Around the base of the ventricles there was a zone or band, partly bony and partly cartilaginous, of from one to two fingers' breadth, of unequal thickness, flattened, yet somewhat rough on its surface. This band projected into the angle between the ventricles and auricles, and extended along the interventricular septum on both sides, to near the apex of the heart. The whole of this production was contained between the fibrous membrane of the pericardium and the serous membrane which lines it internally. The auricles were enlarged so that each might have contained a large egg. One of the mitral valves contained an ossified point of the size and shape of a French bean.

*OF ANEURISM OF THE AORTA**†

In the following observations I shall adhere to the ancient distinction of *true* and *false* Aneurisms,—the former comprehending dilatation without rupture of any of the arterial coats, the latter with rupture of some of these.

True aneurism of the ascending portion and arch of the aorta is very uncommon. The dilatation usually extends from the origin of the artery to the point were it begins to descend. This dilatation rarely proceeds so

*This chapter is more abridged than the others.—*Trans.* [Forbes].

†Book Third, Chapter 3. See footnote on page 332.—F. A. W., 1940.

far as to produce very serious symptoms, the extreme point of dilatation of the artery not being wider than from two to three fingers' breadth. The convexity of the arch and anterior part of the artery appear to yield more than the other parts of the vessel. When the dilatation exists in the descending aorta, it assumes the form of an ovoid tumour, gradually terminating, at each extremity, in the undilated artery. It is not uncommon to find several dilatations of this kind in the same artery. Sometimes we find the whole tract of the aorta dilated to double its natural size.

Dilatation in the arch of the aorta, in the degree above described, is very common; but this is not usually named *aneurism* unless it arrives at a considerably greater extent. These sometimes are very large. M. Corvisart records one double the size of the heart, and I have seen them of the size of the head of a full-grown foetus. When the *true aneurism* acquires a certain size, the inner coat often is ruptured and a *false* aneurism ensues. The true aneurism is commonly accompanied with a morbid degeneration of the internal tunic of the artery. It exhibits spots of a bright red, slight cracks, and a great number of small ossified points. These latter are usually considered as contained in the substance of the inner coat, but they are, in truth, situated between it and the middle coat.

The false aneurism of the aorta, consequent to the true, is rarer than the simple dilatation of that artery; but it is much more common than that greater degree of simple dilatation which alone usually claims the name of *aneurism*.

The false aneurism is most common in the ascending, and the true in the descending aorta. I have never met with any other species of false aneurism in the ascending aorta, or its arch, but that consequent to the true, or simple dilatation of the part. In the descending aorta, however, false aneurism often takes place without any previous dilatation. The opinion at present current in the Parisian schools, viz. that in aneurism the internal coat remains entire and protrudes, in the form of a hernia, through the ruptured fibrinous tunic, is more untenable, as a general position, than that of Scarpa, who maintains the rupture of the two internal tunics in every case of the disease. Both these opinions are true in certain cases, but not in all.

Aneurisms of the aorta produce various effects on the adjacent organs, according to their volume and position. Simple dilatation, when in a moderate degree, hardly produces any effect, but the most inconsiderable false aneurisms may give rise to very serious disorder. The first and most common of these effects is compression acting on the heart and lungs. When the aneurism is in contact with the lungs, it most commonly merely compresses them; sometimes, however, the substance of these organs gives way, and the aneurism, when it bursts, pours its blood directly into the air-cells. Frequently the aneurism compresses the trachea, or one of the two bronchial trunks, flattens, and eventually destroys a part of them, and death ensues by a species of haemoptysis from the rupture of the tumour. The same thing occasionally happens with the oesophagus, but not so frequently. I have only met with three instances of death from this cause. The ordinary effect of these aneurisms on the heart, is to displace it more or less, downwards or to one side. Sometimes the aneurism bursts into the pericardium (see Morgagni and Scarpa); but I have never met with an example of this. A case is on record of an aneurism of this kind bursting into the pulmonary artery.* The left cavity of the pleura is, by far, the most frequent situation for the rupture of these aneurisms. I have met with one case where the aneurism compressed and destroyed the thoracic duct; and M. Corvisart notices a fatal case of compression of the superior vena cava from the same cause. The most remarkable local effects of aneurisms of the aorta, are those on the vertebral column. They often destroy this to a very great depth. This destruction is entirely the work of interstitial absorption, there never being any mark of caries. On the side next the vertebrae the sac is completely destroyed, and the circulating blood is bounded by naked bone.

Aneurisms of the ascending aorta destroy, in like manner, the sternum by their pressure, so that they are at length covered merely by the skin. I have met with two or three tumours of this sort so large that they could not be completely covered by both hands. The aneurisms of the arch of the aorta, and of the arteria innominata, sometimes project, in like manner, at the top of the sternum or above it, or under the cartilages of the first false ribs of the right side. It is not always the largest aneurisms that most readily make their way externally. Sometimes those of the size of an egg produce this effect, whilst, occasionally, those of the size of the head of a full-grown foetus remain quite covered and are even compressed by the sternum.

. . . .

ANEURISM OF THE AORTA

There are few diseases so insidious as this. It cannot be certainly known till it shows itself externally. It can hardly be suspected, even when it compresses some important organ and greatly deranges its functions. When it produces neither of these effects, the first indication of its existence is often the death of the individual as instantaneously as if by a pistol-bullet. I have known men cut off in this manner, who were believed to be in the most perfect health, and who had not complained of the slightest indisposition. We must, therefore, admit that aneurism of the aorta has no symptoms peculiar to it; all those noticed by authors, and especially by M. Corvisart, being indicative merely of the change or compression of adjoining organs. This will be evident by the enumeration of the principal of these; viz. oppression of the chest,—dissimilarity

*Bulletin de la Faculté de Méd. 1819.—*Trans.*

of the pulse in both arms,—a wheezing or rushing at the top of the sternum, perceptible by the hand,—obscure sound on percussion,—rattling in the throat, and dragging downwards of the larynx, when the tumour compresses the trachea, etc. After what has been said of the symptoms of other diseases of the chest, I need not remark how very equivocal all these are. In the present state of our knowledge there certainly exists no certain means of ascertaining the existence of this disease until it shows itself externally. And hitherto, my experience has been insufficient to enable me to say how far this difficulty is likely to be removed by the use of the stethoscope. Since my employment of this instrument I have met only with a dozen cases of what I conceived to be aneurisms of the aorta. Most of these left the hospital after obtaining relief by blood-letting and proper diet. In two instances of moderate dilatation of the arch, I was enabled to verify by dissection my previous diagnosis afforded by the cylinder; and in a third, which showed itself externally, I was enabled to verify still further the diagnostic indications. In this last case, I found the pulsations of the tumour perfectly isochronous with the pulse at the wrist; they gave, at the same time, a much greater impulse and louder sound than the mere contraction of the ventricles; and the contraction of the auricles was not at all perceptible. This pulsation, which I shall call *simple,* in opposition to that of the heart, which is *double* (including the alternate contraction of auricles and ventricles), was distinctly perceptible between the right scapula and the spine. In some cases, this *simple* pulsation and greater impulse may indicate the disease, but I must confess that I have myself been deceived in three cases notwithstanding these indications. I would, therefore, say that even this *simple* pulsation will not assist us in distinguishing aneurisms of the arch or ascending aorta from dilatation of the ventricles.

Another sign, however, will still remain, though less marked than the *simple* pulsation above mentioned: it is this: If we find under the sternum, or below the right clavicle, the impulse of the circulatory organ isochronous with the pulse, and perceptibly greater than that of the ventricles examined in the region of the heart, we have reason to suspect dilatation of the ascending aorta, or arch,—the more so, as it is extremely rare to feel the impulse of the organ of circulation beyond the region of the heart, even in cases of the most marked hypertrophia.

The whole of my experience on this subject leads me to the following conclusions: first, in several cases aneurisms of the ascending aorta can be ascertained by the cylinder; second, in other cases, it requires the greatest attention to distinguish their pulsation from that of the heart; third, aneurisms of the pectoral aorta can be recognised, more especially when they have produced injury of the vertebral; and fourth, all of them will be often mistaken, because nothing will lead to the examination of the chest, and because there will often be no sign whatever of ill-health.

1825

CALEB HILLIER PARRY

DESCRIPTION OF THE CIRCULATORY PHENOMENA IN EXOPHTHALMIC GOITER

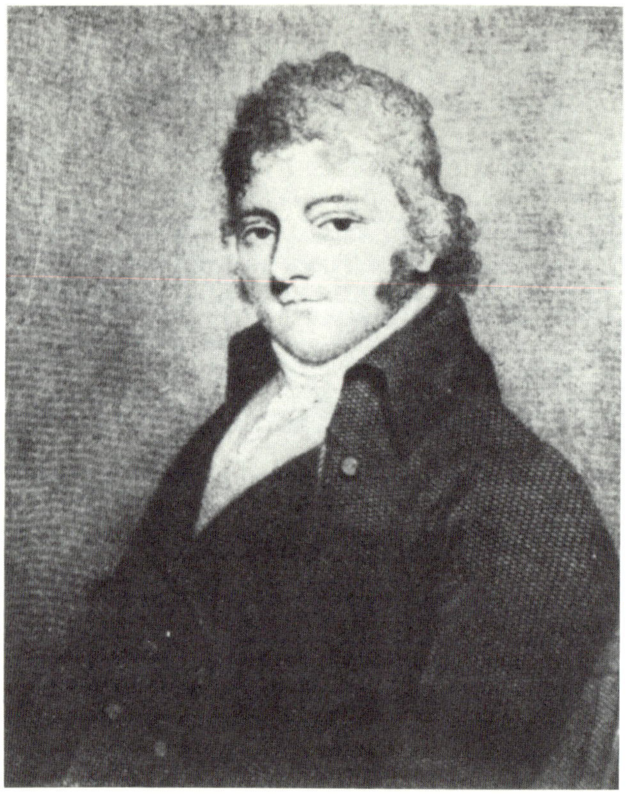

CALEB HILLIER PARRY

Engraving by Philip Audinet from a miniature sketch by John Hay Bell, 1804

(Courtesy Annals of Medical History.)

CALEB HILLIER PARRY

(1755-1822)

CALEB HILLIER PARRY was born on October 21, 1755, in Cirencester in Gloucestershire, the eldest son of a family of ten children. His father, Joshua Parry, was a nonconformist minister.

Young Caleb attended grammar school in Cirencester, where he made the acquaintance of Edward Jenner, a classmate. Jenner and he subsequently became lifelong friends. In 1770, Parry was sent away to school to the Dissenters' Academy at Warrington in Lancashire.

Parry became a student of medicine in 1773, at the University of Edinburgh. At that time the medical department of that institution was dominated by William Cullen, the great teacher.[1] After spending two years at Edinburgh, Parry went to London. In London he lived for a time with Dr. Thomas Denman (1733-1815), obstetrician to the Middlesex Hospital. At London, Parry probably gained some valuable experience. Two years later, 1777, he returned to the University of Edinburgh. He received the degree of Doctor of Medicine in 1778. His thesis was entitled ''De rabie contagiosa vulgo canina.'' Thirty-six years later, in 1814, Parry again wrote on rabies and dedicated the new work to Jenner.

In October, 1778, Parry was married to the daughter of John Rigby of Manchester. Their honeymoon was spent on the Continent, and after the trip they returned to England and settled in Bath in 1779. There Parry spent the rest of his life.

Shortly after choosing Bath for his residence he became physician to the Puerperal Charity Hospital. Later, in 1789, he became physician to the Casualty Hospital.

At Bath, at the beginning of his career, Parry, like many newly graduated physicians of that era, found that the practice of medicine did not demand all his time. He therefore devoted his leisure to the collection of fossils, and in this manner acquired a large collection. In 1781 he published his ''Proposals for a History of Fossils of Gloucestershire.''

In 1788 Parry became a licentiate of the Royal College of Physicians of London. By this time he enjoyed a satisfactory practice. Among his patients were the German astronomer and philosopher, Sir William Herschel, Senior (1738-1822); and Admiral Lord George Rodney (1718-1792). Parry named his third son after the distinguished naval officer. This son died in infancy in 1786. Another son died at the age of twenty-one. His most famous son, William Edward Parry, was destined to become a rear admiral, after having gained renown as a famous Arctic explorer. His eldest son, Charles Henry, became the first physician to the Royal United Hospital in Bath, which was founded in 1826 when the Casualty Hospital merged with the Bath City Infirmary.

Parry, in 1789, presented a paper before the Medical Society of London entitled: ''On the Effects of Compression of the Arteries in Various Diseases, and Particularly Those of the Head, with Hints towards a New Mode of Treating Nervous Disorders.'' This was published in 1792. Therein he observed the beneficial effects,

[1]See page 227, biographic sketch of William Withering.

in the presence of fits, of compressing the carotid artery of the patient and thus causing a diminution of the blood supply to the brain. By applying a tourniquet to the arteries of the limbs, he also observed improvement of patients who had certain diseases of the extremities.

Parry published an important study on angina pectoris in 1799 entitled: ''An Inquiry into the Symptoms and Causes of the Syncope Anginosa, commonly called Angina Pectoris; illustrated by Dissections.''

In 1815 appeared the first volume of Parry's ''Elements of Pathology and Therapeutics.'' He had hoped to publish a second volume but did not live to finish it. His son, Charles Henry Parry, republished this work in 1825, including the unfinished second volume.

In 1816, Parry published the results of some experimental studies he had conducted on animals. It was entitled: ''An Experimental Inquiry into the Nature, Cause, and Varieties of the Arterial Pulse.'' Although some of the observations which he records are inaccurate, his conclusion that the pulse wave is caused by the impulse given to the blood by the systole of the left ventricle is in agreement with present knowledge.

In October, 1816, Parry was stricken with right hemiplegia and aphasia, which prevented him, unfortunately, from producing any more serious works of a medical nature. He devoted his last years to the care of his farm and garden, to reading, and, with his daughter's assistance, to the collecting of miscellaneous items and anecdotes, which were recorded in many volumes.

Parry died on March 9, 1822, at his house in Sion Place, Bath. He was buried in the Abbey Church at Bath, where a memorial was erected to him by his fellow practitioners.

Among Parry's accomplishments of a nonmedical nature was his aid in promoting the wool industry for Great Britain. For his many services he was elected an honorary member of the Farming Society of Ireland. He was also a member of the Royal Society of London and the Society of Natural History of Göttingen in Germany.

In 1825, three years after Parry's death, a collection of his hitherto unpublished medical writings was assembled and published by his son, Charles Henry Parry. Of utmost interest was Parry's description of exophthalmic goiter and the accompanying circulatory phenomena. We are privileged to reprint this classic description. His first case was observed in August, 1786, and thus predated by fourteen years Joseph Flajani's publication in 1800. Of course, Parry's account was made several years before the classic descriptions of Robert Graves and Karl von Basedow.

ENLARGEMENT OF THE THYROID GLAND IN CONNECTION WITH ENLARGEMENT OR PALPITATION OF THE HEART*

By

CALEB HILLIER PARRY

CASE 1.—There is one malady which I have in five cases seen coincident with what appeared to be enlargement of the heart, and which, so far as I know, has not been noticed, in that connection, by medical writers. This malady to which I allude is enlargement of the thyroid gland.

The first case of this coincidence which I witnessed was that of Grace B., a married woman, aged thirty-seven, in the month of August, 1786. Six years before this period she caught cold in lying-in, and for a month suffered under a very acute rheumatic fever; subsequently to which, she became subject to more or less palpitation of the heart, very much augmented by bodily exercise, and gradually increasing in force and frequency till my attendance, when it was so vehement, that each systole of the heart shook the whole thorax. Her pulse was 156 in a minute, very full and hard, alike in both wrists, irregular as to strength, and intermitting at least once in six beats. She had no cough, tendency to fainting, or blueness of the skin, but had twice or thrice been seized in the night with a sense of contriction and difficulty of breathing, which was attended with a spitting of a small quantity of blood. She described herself also as having frequent and violent stitches of pain about the lower part of the sternum.

About three months after lying-in, while she was suckling her child, a lump of about the size of a walnut was perceived on the right side of her neck. This continued to enlarge till the period of my attendance, when it occupied both sides of her neck, so as to have reached an enormous size, projecting forwards before the margin of the lower jaw. The part swelled was the thyroid gland. The carotid arteries on each side were greatly distended; the eyes were protruded from their sockets, and the countenance exhibited an appearance of agitation and distress, especially on any muscular exertion, which I have rarely seen equalled. She suffered no pain in her head, but was frequently affected with giddiness.

For three weeks she had experienced a considerable degree of loss of appetite, and thirst, and for a week had oedematous swelling of her legs

*Parry, C. H.: *Collected Works*, London, 1825, Vol. I, pp. 478-480. We reprint from Major, R. H.: *Classic Descriptions of Disease*, Springfield, Ill., 1932, Charles C Thomas. —F. A. W., 1940.

and thighs, attended with very deficient urine, which was high coloured, and deposited a sediment. Until the commencement of the anasarcous swellings, she had long suffered night sweats, which totally disappeared as the swellings occurred. She was frequently sick in the morning, and often threw up fluid tinged with bile.

Case 2.—August 22, 1803. Elizabeth S., aged twenty-one, was thrown out of a wheel chair in coming fast down hill, 28th of April last, and very much frightened, though not much hurt. From this time she had been subject to palpitation of the heart, and various nervous affections. About a fortnight after this period she began to observe a swelling of the thyroid gland, which has since varied at different times, so as to be once or twice nearly gone. It is now swelled on both sides, but more especially the right, without pain or soreness on pressure. The pulsation of the carotids is very strong and full on both sides; but evidently in the greatest degree on the right. Menses regular; and bowels uniformly open. She voluntarily tells me that she used to be very subject to headaches, which have ceased ever since the commencement of these swellings. Pulse 96, small, hard, and regular.—Mitt^{r} Sanguis è Brachio ad ℥x.

Her head was much relieved by the blood-letting, and the swelling of the thyroid gland was evidently diminished.

On the 25th, she was ordered to take thrice a day a teaspoonful of a mixture of Tincture of Digitalis thirty drops, Syrup of Squills an ounce and a half.

August 31. The medicine made her sick on the second day, but she has continued it ever since without the same effect. Her bowels have been regularly purged once or twice a day, but the palpitation of the heart has been frequent, especially on exercise, which much fatigues her. Swelling of the thyroid, and beating of the carotids, much as before. Pulse 96, Mitt^{r} Sanguis ad ℥x. Pergat in usu Syrupi, 4ter in die.

September 7. Bowels open. No sickness. Palpitation somewhat better. Swellings nearly as before, that on the right being still the largest, and the pulsation of the carotid on that side the greatest.—Pergat.

September 14. All complaints nearly gone. Bowels open without sickness. Pulse about 72, and slightly irregular as to the force of the strokes. Pulsation of the carotids still too strong. Swellings lessened. Menses adsunt.—Pergat in usu Syrupi.

September 24. Yesterday morning she was seized with giddiness and sickness without vomiting. Bowels open yesterday and frequently today. On the 14th ultimo, she was menstruating, and continued to do so for three or four days, during which the swelling of the thyroid almost disappeared; but has since returned, and the beating of the carotid is very strong. She has at this time some catarrh with sore throat.—Pergat in usu Syrupi.

October 1. The symptoms of catarrh are gone; and the swellings are again very much lessened, though the pulsation of the carotids, especially the right, is still too strong. That of the heart, on exercise, is much diminished. Two stools daily, less loose than before.—Pergat in usu Syrupi cum Tincturae Digitalis ʒj. . . .

CASE 3.—Mrs. K., aged about fifty, a very thin woman, had for many years laboured under violent and often irregular action of the heart, accompanied with more or less of shortness and difficulty of respiration. During several aggravations of this disease I attended her, and found her heart violently palpitating, so as to reach 136 beats in a minute; extending its throbbing both downwards and on the right of the thorax, far beyond the due limits, and swelling in a preternatural degree all the arteries which were capable of being felt, and more especially the carotids. The pulse was often unequal both as to frequency and strength. The respiration was greatly hurried, and the head was affected with throbbing pains. The urine was often defective. All muscular exertion aggravated the symptoms, which were occasionally relieved by blood-letting, Squills, Digitalis, and aperients. Still, however, much of the malady continued, and I could never perceive that the pulse was reduced below 120 in the minute.

Mrs. K. was also long affected with an extremely large swelling of the thyroid gland, which began at a period, the relation of which to the commencement of the disorder of the heart, she was unable to recollect.

My last attendance on her was in June, 1813; on the 24th of which, at eight in the morning, I was called to visit her, and found her in bed. Her pulse was 132 in a minute, and very full, hard, and strong, both in the radials and carotids. The beating of the heart extended all over the thorax, and even into the right hypochondrium. The respiration was 24 in a minute, with grunting expiration, and with no elevation of the diaphragm during inspiration. She had occasional cough, with yellowish brown mucous expectoration. The thyroideal swellings projected before the carotids, and involved the sterno-mastoid muscles from their lower insertion to nearly two-thirds of their length upwards. The carotids were driven somewhat forward, and much enlarged; and the external jugulars were swelled and prominent. For about a fortnight she had been affected with an oedematous swelling of her legs, which had gradually increased. The abdomen was also tense, but not fluctuating, and she suffered considerable pain about the navel, where there was soreness on pressure. The bowels had however been open during the night, with griping. The quantity of urine had not exceeded a teacup full in the last forty-eight hours. Some medicines were given, which it is needless to specify, as the patient died at five o'clock the next morning. A dissection was not permitted.

CASE 4.—A woman servant, unmarried, and about thirty years of age, whom during a space of several months, I had at various times seen labouring under a palpitation of the heart, which always more or less existed, and was accompanied with a quick and irregular pulse, great hurry in breathing on an exertion, and an extremely strong beating of the carotid arteries, began at length to have enlargement of the thyroid gland, which had not existed more than a fortnight when I last saw her, and which was much increased from the time when it was first noticed.

CASE 5.—During my attendance on this patient, I was consulted by a married lady, of about forty years of age, from the North of England, who was supposed to be in consumption. She had in fact a very quick pulse, with great shortness and difficulty of breathing, and frequent cough, attended with copious expectoration. She had also an extremely large swelling of the thyroid gland on each side of the neck, with a considerable dilatation of the carotid arteries. The cough having been removed in about a fortnight by blood-letting, Squills, and Citrate of Potash, which were ordered when she first consulted me, I had an opportunity of discovering, at my second visit, that she was afflicted with a most laborious action of the heart, which, from the extent of the pulsation, seemed much enlarged, and suffered a great aggravation of symptoms from any muscular exertion.

This inordinate action of the heart has been of long duration, and considerably preceded the commencement of the thyroideal swelling.

The patient did not remain at Bath long enough for me to know the result of the disease, which, doubtless, would ultimately prove fatal.

My attendance on the three last patients having occurred at the same time, first suggested to me the notion of some connection between the malady of the heart and the bronchocele. I mentioned that opinion to Mr. G. Norman, surgeon, to whom I shewed the lady last mentioned. Shortly afterwards I expressed the same opinion to Mr. Cruttwell, surgeon, to whom it then occurred that he was attending a patient with a similar coincidence, and that in her the bronchocele succeeded to the affection of the heart.

CASE 6.—Anne P., aged about thirty, a married woman, thin, and with a very long neck, who has never had a family, five years ago, at Christmas, when affected with chilblains, for their relief kept her feet in cold water for a quarter of an hour, which made her feet extremely cold. Half an hour afterwards she was seized with a pain about the region of the heart, which was extremely violent; but unaccompanied with cough, fever, or palpitation. Ever since that period she has been subject to attacks of similar pain, which recur frequently. She has also frequent palpitations, which come on more especially after walking or any hurry; though sometimes without any apparent cause whatever. She is often affected also with oppression of breathing, which is sometimes accompanied with globus hystericus, and obliges her to lie high in bed. All pressure about the thorax is uneasy to her; but she lies best on her left side. She is free from cough. At this moment she complains of violent pain on the sternum towards the lower part, which is not sore on pressure. Pulse 112, and weak. Respiration 22. Extremities cold. Skin pale. She is sleepy during the day, but sleeps little at night. Tongue rather furred. Appetite irregular. Urine very various as to appearance. Menses, since the commencement of the malady, defective.

During the palpitation, and indeed at other times, she has long had a violent beating in her head, and a throbbing in her neck. This day fortnight she had an unusual degree of this throbbing, accompanied with a great aggravation of a distracting pain in the head, to which she has been subject ever since she began to be ill, and which is always greatly increased by coming out of the air into a warm room. During the more violent accessions of this affliction of the head, she cannot bear the least conversation, and feels as if she should die. The evening after the last described aggravation, the thyroid gland began to swell at its lower part before, and the swelling has now diffused itself to a considerable degree on each side, without soreness on pressure. The beating of the carotids is very strong.

1827

ROBERT ADAMS

HEART BLOCK

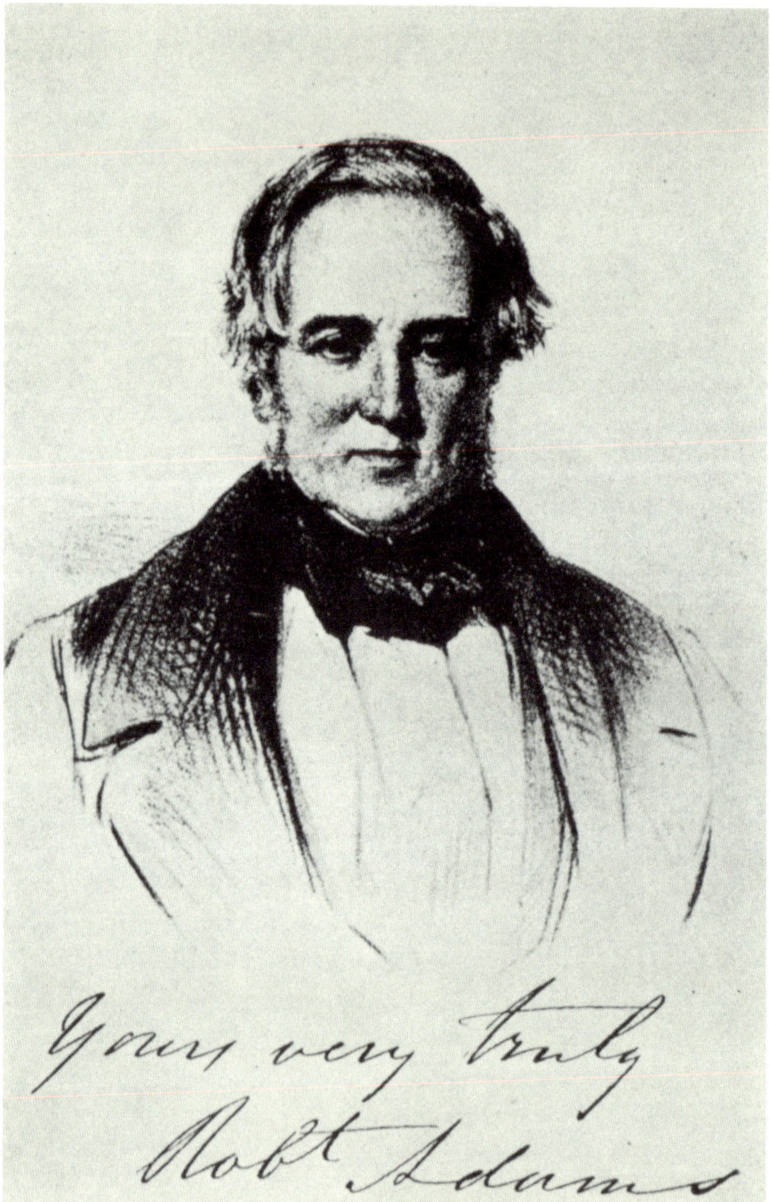

ROBERT ADAMS

(Courtesy Medical Classics.)

ROBERT ADAMS

(1791-1875)

"... that 'Old Guard' of Irish surgery."

—*The Lancet* (London).

ROBERT ADAMS, who was born in Dublin, who spent most of his life there, and who died in the city of his birth at the ripe old age of eighty-four, was, according to the "Lancet," the last of the old guard of illustrious Irish surgeons of the nineteenth century, the roll commencing with the elder Dease and Peile. In the charter granted the Royal College of Surgeons in Ireland by King George IV in 1828, Adams is listed as one of the group to whom the charter was granted. And on the roll of the Supplemental Charter bearing the date of January 24, 1844, his name is the eighteenth that occurs. Immediately preceding his name on this record are the names of Peile, the eminent lithotomist, Crampton, Kirby, Read, Cusack, Jacob, and William Henry Porter.

In 1810 Adams entered the University of Dublin as a student of the liberal arts. He studied intermittently at the University for several years receiving the degree of Bachelor of Arts in 1814, the degree of Master of Arts in 1832, and the degree of Doctor of Medicine in 1842.

The same year that Adams entered college he was apprenticed to William Hartigan, a leading surgeon in Dublin. On Hartigan's death in 1813 Adams apprenticed himself to George Stewart, who at that time was Surgeon-General of the English army in Ireland. In 1815 Adams was licensed by the Royal College of Surgeons in Ireland, and in 1818, at the age of twenty-seven, he was elected a member of that organization. From then on he was very active in the practice of his profession.

At an early date Adams was appointed surgeon to the Jervis Street Hospital in Dublin. When Ephraim McDowell[1] died, Adams was selected to succeed him at Richmond Hospital in the same city. The appointment was contested by John McDonnell and the claims of the two candidates were so evenly balanced that the board experienced great embarrassment as to whom they should select. Richard Carmichael, who was surgeon to the hospital, solved the difficulty by resigning his surgical post to create a second vacancy, declaring that he was unwilling that the institution should be deprived of the services of either candidate, so highly did he estimate the merits of both men.

At some time before his appointment to the Richmond Hospital, Adams, in conjunction with Kirby and Read, had founded the Peter Street School of Medicine. He later broke his connection with the school. But later, at Richmond Hospital, he founded another school, this time with Carmichael and McDowell. This school was later known as the Carmichael School of Medicine and Surgery. There Adams lectured for many years and, while thus occupied, wrote many admirable essays on

---

[1]Possibly a relative of the American, Ephraim McDowell; the ancestors of the American were from North Ireland. *See* Schachner, August: *Ephraim McDowell, "Father of ovariotomy" and founder of abdominal surgery, with an appendix on Jane Todd Crawford,* Philadelphia, 1921, J. B. Lippincott Co., xviii, 331 pp.

abnormal conditions of the joints. These were published in Todd's "Cyclopaedia."[2] He also contributed several important articles on diseases of the heart. These were published in the "Dublin Hospital Reports."

It was in 1826, when he was a surgeon to the Jervis Street Hospital, that Adams noticed the condition now known as "heart block" and frequently called "the Adams-Stokes syndrome." We are reproducing Adams' account, as well as that of Stokes. According to Major,[3] heart block had been described by Marcus Gerbezius in 1719, Morgagni in "De Sedibus" (1761) and Thomas Spens in 1793. Adams' description, however, was the first complete account of this disease entity.

In 1857 he published his classic account of rheumatic gout.[4] In this publication he elaborated his views on chronic rheumatic arthritis, from which he himself suffered for many years previous to his death. In 1861 Adams was appointed surgeon in ordinary to Her Majesty, Queen Victoria, and in the same year he was appointed Regius professor of surgery in Trinity College of Dublin.

Adams was well versed in the writings of Continental surgeons and repeatedly referred to them in his lectures, writings, and even in his consultations. He was much respected by his confrères, who once elected him president of the Dublin Pathological Society, and three times (1840, 1860-1861, 1867-1868) elected him president of the Royal College of Surgeons of Ireland.

Adams died in January, 1875, presumably of cardiac disease. He was buried in Mount Jerome Cemetery in Dublin.

---

[2]Todd, R. B.: *The cyclopaedia of anatomy and physiology,* London, 1835-1859, Longman [and others], 5 volumes in 6.

[3]Major, R. H.: *Classic Descriptions of Diseases,* Springfield, Ill., 1932, Charles C. Thomas, pp. 291-296.

[4]Adams, Robert: *Treatise on rheumatic gout, or chronic rheumatic arthritis of all the joints,* London, 1857, J. Churchill, 362 pp.

CASES OF DISEASES OF THE HEART, ACCOMPANIED WITH PATHOLOGICAL OBSERVATIONS*

By

ROBERT ADAMS, A.B.

Member of the Royal College of Surgeons in Ireland, and one of the Surgeons to Jervis-Street Infirmary, etc.

. . . .

The following case, in many particulars, and in its termination, resembled that above alluded to [the case published by J. Cheyne, in 1818, A case of Apoplexy, in which the Fleshy Part of the Heart Was Converted into Fat]:

An officer in the revenue, aged 68 years, of a full habit of body, had for a long time been incapable of any exertion, as he was subject to oppression of his breathing and continued cough. In May, 1819, in conjunction with his ordinary medical attendant, Mr. Duggan, I saw this gentleman: he was just then recovering from the effects of an apoplectic attack, which had suddenly seized him three days before. He was well enough to be about his house, and even to go out. But he was oppressed by stupor, having a constant disposition to sleep, and still a very troublesome cough. What most attracted my attention was, the irregularity of his breathing, and remarkable slowness of the pulse, which generally ranged at the rate of 30 in a minute. Mr. Duggan informed me that he had been in almost continual attendance on this gentleman for the last seven years; and that during that period he had seen him, he is quite certain, in not less than twenty apoplectic attacks. Before each of them he was observed, for a day or two, heavy and lethargic, with loss of memory. He would then fall down in a state of complete insensibility, and was on several occasions hurt by the fall. When they attacked him, his pulse would become even slower than usual; his breathing loudly stertorous. He was bled without loss of time, and the most active purgative medicines were exhibited. As a preventive measure, a large issue was inserted in the neck, and a spare regimen was directed for him. He recovered from these attacks without any paralysis. Oedema of the feet and ancles came on early in December; his cough became more urgent, and his breathing more oppressed; his faculties too became weaker.

---

*Published in Dublin Hospital Reports 4: 353-453, 1827. We reprint from Medical Classics 3: 633-696, 1939.—F. A. W., 1940.

November 4th, 1819, he was suddenly seized with an apoplectic attack, which in two hours carried him off, before the arrival of his medical attendant.

DISSECTION

56 hours after death

The dura mater presented a natural appearance. The arachnoid membrane was separated from the pia mater by a fluid of gelatinous appearance. The substance of the brain was watery and of a yellowish white colour. There was some water in the ventricles. These cavities did not appear enlarged, but the foramen of communication between them was dilated. The coats of the carotid and middle arteries of the dura mater were quite white and opaque from bony deposition, but were pervious.

The right lung was sound. The left was compressed, and adhered to the side of the thorax; about a pint of serum and quantities of soft fat, of a very deep yellow colour, filled up the space between the anterior mediastinum and the compressed lung, which was impervious to air, and must have been totally useless.

The right auricle of the heart was much dilated. The right ventricle externally presented no appearance whatever of muscular fibres; it seemed composed of fat through almost its whole substance, of the same deep yellow colour as that which occupied the place of the left lung. The reticulated lining of the ventricle, which here and there allowed the fat to appear between its fibres, alone presented any appearance of muscular structure.

The left ventricle was very thin, and its whole surface was covered with a layer of fat. Beneath this, the muscular structure was not a line in thickness; it had degenerated from its natural state; was soft, and easily torn, and a section of it exhibited more the appearance of liver than of a heart. The septum of the ventricles presented the same appearance. In both ventricles, even in the lining fibres, yellow spots, where fat had occupied the place of muscular structure, were to be observed. The whole organ was remarkably light; the valves were all sound, except those of the aorta, which were studded with specks of bone, but elsewhere were cartilaginous and elastic, from which they derived a disposition to remain closed; a fluid gently injected from the ventricle would pass them; still, when the heart was reversed and water poured from the ventricle upon them, their valves retained it; its weight was not sufficient to separate the edges of the thickened valves. There was much fluid blood contained in the heart.

The liver was natural; the vena porta was unusually distended. The spleen was healthy in its structure, although enlarged; the other viscera presented nothing unusual.

In both these cases, No. 1 and No. 2, apoplexy must be considered less a disease in itself than symptomatic of one, the organic seat of which was in the heart; although during life there was much analogy in their symptoms, the examination of the bodies after death disclosed a state of the heart altogether different; in one the ventricle was found nearly an inch in thickness, while in the other, fat had so accumulated at the expense of the muscular structure, that it was scarcely a line in depth. The explanation of the fact how causes so different could have produced effects nearly similar, will, I imagine, be found in the reflection, that anything occasioning an undue distention of the vessels of the brain, may be followed by apoplexy. This over distention may arise from the impulse a tergo being preternaturally strong, or on the contrary, it may be the result of some obstruction in front, as that arising from a contracted arterial opening, or some state of the ventricle incapacitating it from emptying itself with sufficient quickness to relieve the brain. Indeed, upon considering the latter condition of things, where the heart is slow in transmitting the blood it receives, we find, I imagine, even in this a means of accounting for the lethargy, loss of memory, and vertigo, which attends these cases. For the venous blood, which under such circumstances, is supposed to accumulate in the brain, is evidently ill-suited to the functions of this organ. Although the quality of the blood may thus be supposed to have some influence in producing these bad consequences, yet it is probable that the principal causes determining an apoplectic attack where the heart is either actively enlarged, or in a state of atrophy, are mechanical and referable to circumstances in the heart, directly or indirectly producing a state of congestion of the vascular system of the brain.